Recent Results in Cancer Research 161

Springer
Berlin
Heidelberg
New York
Hong Kong
London
Milan
Paris
Tokyo

U. Reinhold W. Tilgen (Eds.)

Chemosensitivity Testing in Oncology

With 75 Figures, Some in Colour, and 45 Tables

Springer

Prof. Dr. Uwe Reinhold
Prof. Dr. Wolfgang Tilgen

Universitätskliniken des Saarlandes
Hautklinik und Poliklinik
66421 Homburg/Saar, Germany

Indexed in Current Contents and Index Medicus

ISBN 3-540-43468-2 Springer-Verlag Berlin Heidelberg New York
ISSN 0080-0015

Library of Congress Cataloging-in-Publication Data
Chemosensitivity testing in oncology / U. Reinhold, W. Tilgen (eds.). p. cm. – (Recent results in cancer research; 161) Includes bibliographical references and index. ISBN 3540434682 (hardcover: alk. paper) 1. Cancer – Chemotherapy – Congresses. 2. Drug resistance in cancer cells – Congresses. 3. Antineoplastic agents – Testing – Congresses. I. Reinhold, Uwe. II. Tilgen, W. (Wolfgang), 1944– III. Series. [DNLM: 1. Drug Resistance, Neoplasm – Congresses. 2. Antineoplastic Agents – therapeutic use – Congresses. 3. Drug Therapy – methods – Congresses. QZ 267C5158 2002]
RC271.C5 C397 2002 616.99'4061–dc21 2002066990

Springer-Verlag Berlin · Heidelberg · New York
a member of BertelsmannSpringer Science-Business Media GmbH

http://www.springer.de

Typesetting: Stürtz AG, 97080 Würzburg, Germany
Cover design: design & production GmbH, 69121 Heidelberg, Germany

Printed on acid-free paper SPIN 10833879 21/3130SM – 5 4 3 2 1 0

Principal Authors

Andreotti, Peter E., PhD, Atlantic Scientific Development Inc., PMB 46, 1511 E. Commercial Blvd., Fort Lauderdale, FL 33334, USA

Bachrach, Uriel, PhD, Department of Molecular Biology Hebrew University-Hadassah, Medical School, P.O. Box 12272, Jerusalem, Israel

Cree, Ian A., MD, Translational Oncology Research Centre, Department of Histopathology, Queen Alexandra Hospital, Portsmouth, PO6 3LY, UK

Fruehauf, John P., MD, PhD, Oncotech Inc., 15501 Redhill Avenue, Tustin, CA 92780, USA

Kaspers, G.J.L., MD, Department of Pediatric Hematology/ Oncology, VU University Medical Center, De Boelelaan 1117, 1081 Amsterdam, The Netherlands

Kobayashi, Hisayuki, MD, Biochemical Laboratory, Nitta Gelatin Inc., 2-22 Futamata, Yao-City, Osaka 5810024, Japan

Kornmann, Marko, MD, Department of General Surgery, University of Ulm, Steinhövelstraße 9, 89075 Ulm, Germany

Kurbacher, Christian M., MD, PhD, Division of Clinical and Experimental Gynecologic Oncology, Department of Gynecology and Obstetrics, University of Cologne Medical Center, Kerpener Straße 34, 50931 Köln, Germany

Kubota, Tetsuro, MD, FACS, Department of Surgery, School of Medicine, Keio University, 35 Shinanomachi, Shinjuku-ku, Tokyo 160-8582, Japan

Mestres-Ventura, Pedro, MD, Institute of Anatomy and Cell Biology, University Hospital, University of Saarland, 66421 Homburg/Saar, Germany

Neuber, Karsten, MD, Department of Dermatology, University Hospital Hamburg, Martinistraße 52, 20246 Hamburg, Germany

Otto, Angela M., MD, Heinz-Nixdorf-Chair for Medical Electronics, Technical University of Munich, Arcisstraße 21, 80290 München, Germany

Sargent, Jean M., MD, Haematology Research, Pembury Hospital, Tonbridge Road, Pembury, Kent, TN2 4QJ, UK

Schadendorf, Dirk, MD, Klinische Kooperationseinheit für Dermatoonkologie (DKFZ) an der Universitäts-Hautklinik Mannheim, Universität Heidelberg, 68135 Mannheim, Germany

Schöndorf, Thomas, PhD, Department of Gynecology and Obstetrics, University of Cologne, Kerpener Straße 34, 50931 Köln, Germany

Ugurel, Selma, MD, Department of Dermatology, The Saarland University Hospital, 66421 Homburg/Saar, Germany

Untch, Michael, MD, Department of Obstetrics and Gynecology, University of München-Großhadern, Marchioninistraße 15, 81377 München, Germany centration of 10 µg/ml and then serially diluted 1:10 for testing. Triplicate cell cultures were tested with antibody dilutions for 4 and 7 days at 37°C in 95% humidity/5% CO_2. Cultures were measured for antibody activity by adding 0.05 ml of liquid extraction reagent (ASD Inc.) to each culture and then transferring 0.05 ml of extracted cell aliquot to counting plates (ASD Inc.) containing dried luciferin-luciferase in each well. Counting plates were measured in a Berthold Detection Systems MPL microplate luminometer and analyzed as described previously for ATP [5, 6].

Luciferase-Transfected Human Tumor Cell Lines

Luciferase (luc) gene-transfected MCF-7 breast and DU-145 prostate tumor cell lines were kindly provided by Dr. Xiao Yun Zhu (Sunol Molecular Corp.) and cultured in IMDM with 10% FBS and 1 mg/ml G418 (Gibco BRL) for selection. For in vitro drug assays performed in triplicate, 2,000 cells/well in 0.2 ml of medium containing serial drug dilutions were cultured in opaque, tissue culture-treated microplates (Dynex Technologies) at 37°C in 95% humidity/5% CO_2. After incubation for 4 days, 0.05 ml of 0.1 M HEPES buffer pH 7.9 containing 0.1% Triton X-100 and 50 µg /ml D-luciferin (Biosynth L-8200) was added to each well. The culture microplate was then incubated at room temperature for 10 min and measured in a Berthold Detection Systems MPL microplate luminometer. Results were calculated as described previously for ATP tumor chemosensitivity assays [5, 6].

In Vivo Imaging Studies

In vivo imaging of luc-transfected tumor cells was performed using 8- to 10-week-old athymic nu/nu female mice injected intravenously with $1–10\times10^6$ MCF-7luc+ or DU-145luc+ tumor cells in 0.1 ml of sterile PBS. For imaging after growth and metastasis of the tumor in vivo, mice were first anesthetized with xylazine (3 mg/ml) and ketamine (7 mg/ml) at 0.12 ml/20 g body weight and then injected i.p. with 4.0 mg of D-luciferin (Molecular Probes L-2912) in 0.1 ml of sterile water. After 2–3 min, mice were then placed in a Berthold Technologies NightOwl Molecular Light Imager and imaged with a two-step process. First, a black-and-white photographic image was acquired with a 15-ms exposure. Next, the luminescent image was acquired with a 5- to 10-min photon integration period. The luminescent image was then processed in software to colorize luminescence intensity and then overlaid onto the black-and-white image for presentation.

Results

Two-Stage TRA

New technologies have been developed for TRA studies with tumor cell lines and clinical specimens including culture microplates with test drugs predried in the wells and counting microplates with ATP extraction reagent and luciferin-luciferase counting reagent predried in the wells (PEA, manuscript in preparation). Dried reagent microplates for both culture and counting procedures have been used for one-stage and two-stage TRA studies. Two-stage studies have been used to evaluate drug sensitivity and resistance of clinical specimens after a standard first-stage TRA. Figure 1 shows results for the first-stage TRA with an ovarian carcinoma specimen tested with both fresh and predried dilutions of paclitaxel, carboplatin, and doxorubicin. Figure 2 shows the second-stage TRA results for the cells that were tested with predried paclitaxel at the 100% TDC concentration in a first-stage TRA. Both TRA assays were analyzed with dried reagent counting plates.

As shown in Fig. 1, in this and other experiments with 12 clinical specimens tested with paclitaxel, carboplatin, and doxorubicin (not shown), no significant difference in drug sensitivity was observed with fresh test drug dilutions compared to drug dilutions that were predried in the culture microplates for 6 months. Using counting microplates with predried ATP extraction and counting reagent for the first-stage TRA makes it possible to perform a two-

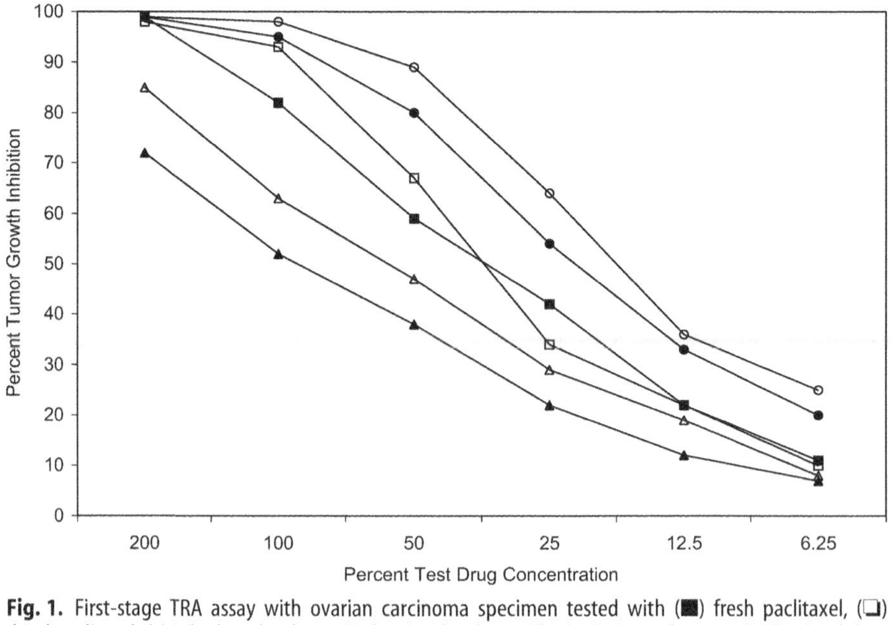

Fig. 1. First-stage TRA assay with ovarian carcinoma specimen tested with (■) fresh paclitaxel, (❑) dried paclitaxel, (▲) fresh carboplatin, (°) dried carboplatin, (●) fresh doxorubicin, and (❍) dried doxorubicin

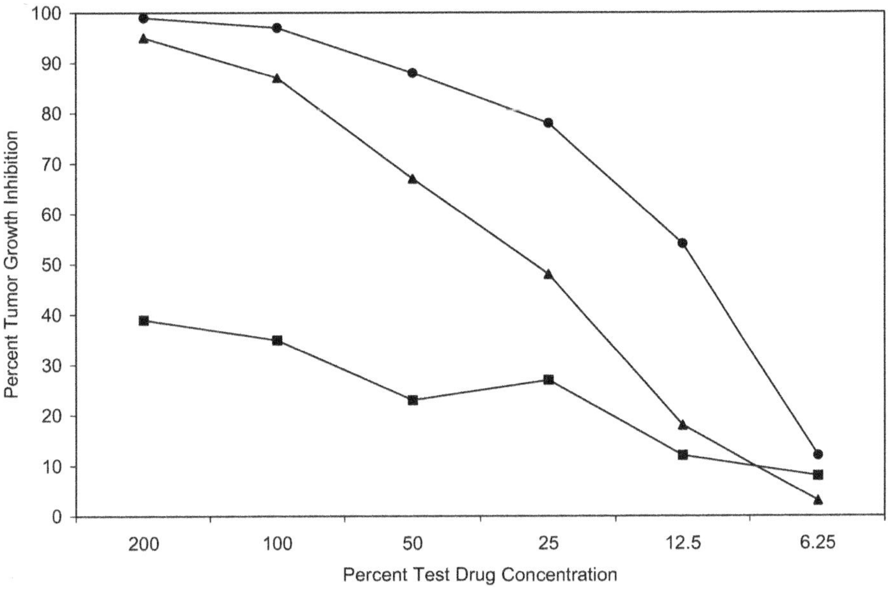

Fig. 2. Second-stage TRA assay with ovarian carcinoma cells cultured with paclitaxel at 100% TDC in first-stage TRA shown in Fig. 1. (●) fresh doxorubicin, (▲) fresh carboplatin, and (■) fresh paclitaxel

stage TRA study to retest cells after initial drug exposure in vitro. As shown in Fig. 2, the ovarian carcinoma cells that survived first-stage exposure to 100% TDC paclitaxel showed the strongest second-stage TRA sensitivity to doxorubicin and, as expected, resistance to paclitaxel.

Monoclonal Antibody TRA

Dried counting reagent microplates have been developed for screening and testing of agents against human tumor cell lines that grow in vitro as adherent monolayers. These counting plates containing dried luciferin-luciferase are used with liquid ATP extraction reagent that is added to adherent cells before the extracted cell samples are transferred to the counting plates. This application for monoclonal antibody testing is illustrated in Fig. 3, which shows results for herceptin monoclonal antibody against MCF-7, MCF-7ADR (doxorubicin resistant), GI-101, and MDA-MB-231 breast tumor cell lines. As shown in Fig. 3, weak herceptin activity at high concentration could be measured against MCF-7 and MCF-7ADR cells but not GI-101 or MDA-MB-231 cells after 7 days of culture. No activity against any of the cell lines could be detected after only 4 days of culture. The observed antibody activity is consistent with a cytostatic effect in vitro manifested after 7 days as a decrease in cell number due to slower cell growth.

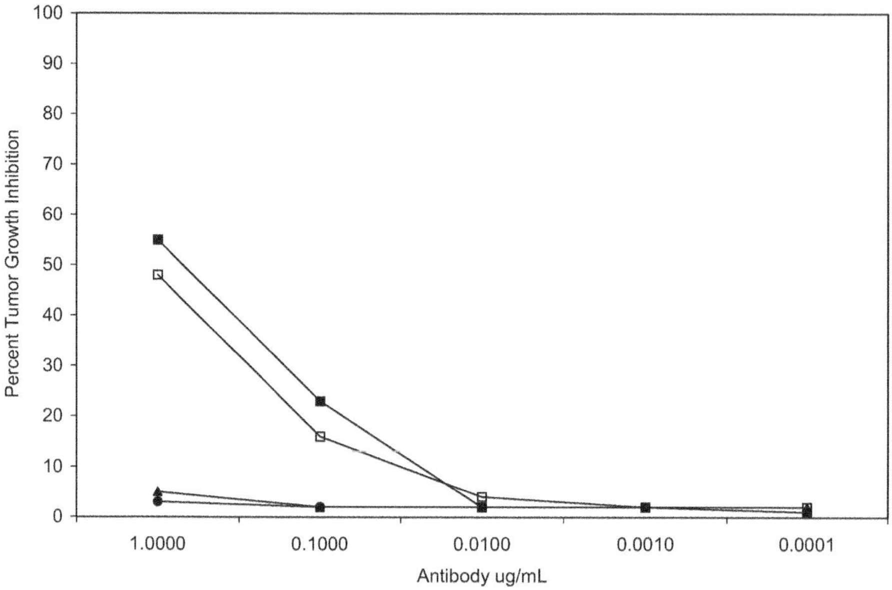

Fig. 3. Herceptin monoclonal antibody tested against human tumor cell lines in 7-day TRA. (■) MCF-7ADR, (□) MCF-7, (▲) GI-101, and (●) MDA 231

Reporter Tumor Cell Lines

An alternative method for screening and testing agents in vitro against human tumor cell lines is to develop reporter cell lines transfected with the *Photinus pyralis* luciferase (luc) gene. The transfected cells, which express the luciferase enzyme and produce endogenous cellular ATP, can be simply measured in TRA studies by adding exogenous D-luciferin in pH 7.9 buffered solution with 0.1% Triton X-100 and counting after 10-min incubation at room temperature. Figure 4 shows results from the use of MCF-7luc+-transfected cells tested with paclitaxel, doxorubicin, an experimental camptothecin analog, and oxaliplatin. As shown in Fig. 4, dose-response activity for all of the test drugs could be measured 4 days after culturing 2,000 cells/well with drug dilutions.

In Vivo Imaging

The in vitro application of reporter tumor cell lines for drug testing, as illustrated with MCF-7luc+ in Fig. 4, can be extended to include in vivo studies using photon imaging to measure growth, metastasis, and drug effects on luc-transfected human tumors in athymic nude mice. Figure 5 shows imaging results acquired 41 days after i.v. injection of 1×10^7 MCF-7luc+ cells into a nude mouse. The image shows metastasis of the tumor cells in lymph nodes and growth in the tail vein at the site of injection. Figure 6 similarly shows imaging

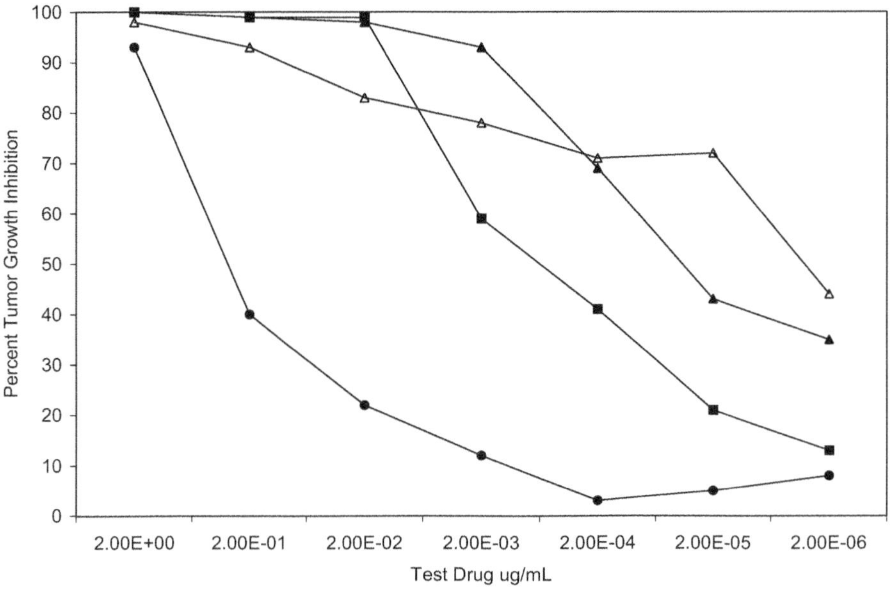

Fig. 4. In vitro assay results for chemotherapeutic drugs tested against luciferase (luc) gene-transfected MCF-7luc+ cells. Results are shown for 4-day assay with (▲) camptothecin, (°) paclitaxel, (■) doxorubicin, and (●) oxaliplatin

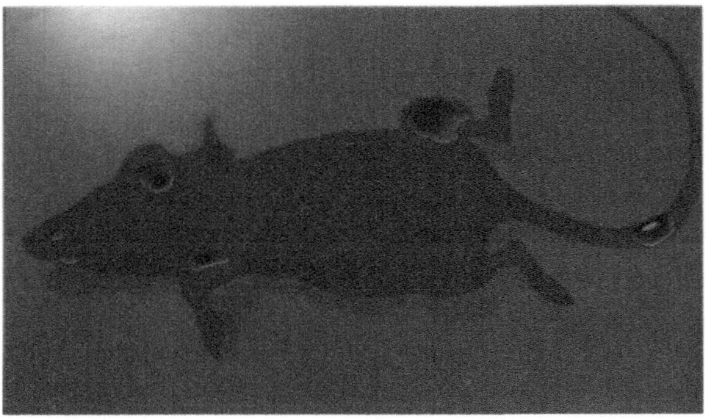

Fig. 5. Photon imaging results showing lymph node metastasis of luc-transfected MCF-7luc+ cells 41 days after i.v. injection of 1×10^7 cells in nude mouse. Tumor growth in the tail at the site of injection can also be observed

results for a subcutaneous tumor 21 days after a mouse was injected s.c. with 1×10^6 MCF-7luc+ cells.

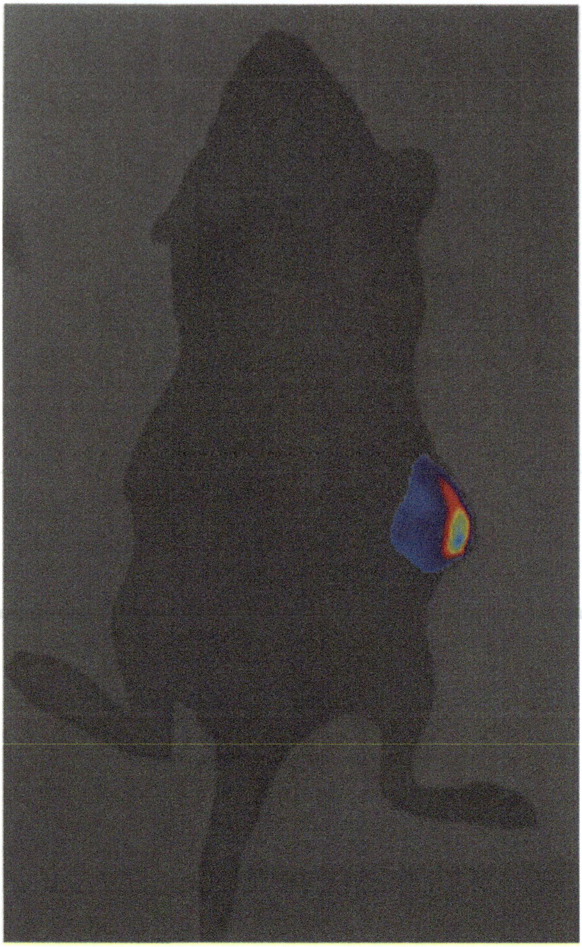

Fig. 6. Photon imaging results showing growth of subcutaneous tumor in nude mouse 21 days after s.c. injection of 1×10^6 MCF-7luc+ cells

Discussion

The ATP bioluminescence assay originally described based on work in different laboratories has proven to be a useful method of new chemotherapeutic drug development concomitant with clinical studies in the United States and Europe showing both good clinical correlation and patient benefit for assay-directed chemotherapy [5, 8, 9–11]. Application of the ATP assay method for high-volume applications has been limited, however, by the relatively high cost of reagents compared with some other methods and the multistep, labor-intensive procedure involving ATP extraction and counting reagent addition required for cell measurement. The TRA studies reported herein describe technical modifications to the ATP assay method that simplify and reduce both labor and materials cost for assays with both cell lines and clinical specimens. These benefits result from the use of culture microplates containing test drug dilutions predried in the culture plate wells and counting microplates containing both extraction and counting reagent, or only counting reagent, predried in the wells. Similarly, culture microplates can be prepared with predried controls and counting plates can be prepared with predried ATP standards (PEA, manuscript in preparation) for quality control.

Development of counting microplates with predried extraction and counting reagent has allowed development of two-stage TRA assay methods to retest cells from clinical specimens that have undergone one cycle of drug exposure in vitro in a standard first-stage TRA. The ability to perform two-stage TRA assays is also a direct benefit of the high sensitivity of the ATP assay method, which requires relatively few cells to measure drug activity. The potential clinical benefit of performing two-stage TRA studies to model first-line drug treatment in vitro and select second-line therapeutic options remains to be determined.

The use of new TRA technologies with human tumor cell lines or clinical specimens combined with the use of luc-transfected reporter cell lines provides an integrated approach for screening and testing new agents for preclinical research and development. Transfected reporter cell lines that grow in continuous culture and can be measured in microplate format with a simple single-reagent procedure are particularly applicable for in vitro screening purposes and are potentially useful for in vivo model studies with nude mice.

References

1. Maehara Y, Miyamoto K, Anai H, et al (1987) The ATP assay is more sensitive than succinate dehydrogenase inhibition test for predicting cell viability. Eur J Cancer Clin Oncol 23:273
2. Kangas L, Gronroos M, Nieminem AL (1984) Bioluminescence of cellular ATP: A new method for evaluating cytotoxic agents in vitro. Med Biol 62:338
3. Sevin B, Peng Z, Perras J, Penalver G, Averette H (1988) Application of ATP bioluminescence assay in human tumor chemosensitivity testing. Gynecol. Oncol 31:191–204
4. Sevin B, Perras JP, Averette H, Donato D, Penalver M (1993) Chemosensitivity testing in ovarian cancer. Cancer 71:1613–1620
5. Andreotti P, Cree I, Kurbacher C, Hartmann D, Linder D, Harel G, Gleiberman I, Caruso P, Ricks S, Untch M, Sartori C, Bruckner H (1995) Chemosensitivity testing of human tumors using a microplate adenosine triphosphate luminescence assay: clinical correlation for cisplatin resistance of ovarian carcinoma. Cancer Research 55:5276–5282
6. Hunter EM, Sutherland LA, Cree IA, Dewar JA, Preece PE, Wood RA, Linder D, Andreotti PE (1993) Heterogeneity of chemosensitivity in human breast carcinoma: use of an adenosine triphosphate (ATP) chemiluminescence assay. Eur J Surg Oncol. 19:242–249
7. Cree IA, Kurbacher CM (1999) ATP-based tumor chemosensitivity testing: assisting new agent development. Anti-Cancer Drugs 10:431–435
8. Cree IA, Kurbacher CM, Untch M, Sutherland LA, Hunter EM, Subedi AMC, James EA, Dewar JA, Preece PE, Andreotti PE, Bruckner HW (1996) Correlation of the clinical response to chemotherapy in breast cancer with ex vivo chemosensitivity. Anti-Cancer Drugs 7:630–635

9. Kurbacher C, Bruckner HW, Cree IA, Andreotti P, Janut MM (1999) A prospective clinical trial on individualized chemotherapy for recurrent ovarian cancer selected by the ex vivo ATP tumor chemosensitivity assay. American Society of Clinical Oncology 1384
10. Kurbacher C, Cree IA, Bruckner H, Brenne U, Kurbacher J, Muller K, Ackermann T, Gilster T, Wilhelm L, Engel H, Mallmann P, Andreotti P (1998) Use of an ex vivo ATP luminescence assay to direct chemotherapy for recurrent ovarian cancer. Anti-Cancer Drugs 9:51–57
11. Kurbacher CM, Cree IA, Bruckner HW, Mallmann P, Andreotti PE (1998) Chemotherapy directed by the ATP tumour chemosensitivity assay improves response rates and survival for patients with recurrent ovarian cancer. Anti-Cancer Drugs 9:51–57
12. Edinger M, Sweeney TJ, Tucker AA, Olomu AB, Negrin RS, Contag CS (1999) Noninvasive assessment of tumor cell proliferation in animal models. Neoplasia 1:303–310
13. Rehemtulla A, Stegman LD, Cardozo SJ, Gupta S, Hall DE, Contag CS, Ross BD (2000) Rapid and quantitative assessment of cancer treatment response using in vivo bioluminescence imaging. Neoplasia 2:491–495

The Use of the MTT Assay to Study Drug Resistance in Fresh Tumour Samples

Jean M. Sargent

Haematology Research, Pembury Hospital, Tonbridge Road, Pembury, Kent, TN2 4QJ, UK
e-mail: jean.sargent@btinternet.com

Abstract

We have found the short-term MTT assay to be a simple, reproducible chemosensitivity technique, suitable for use throughout the time course of disease. We now have 12 years' experience of using this method in a variety of tumour types, both haematological and solid malignancies. Tumour cells are isolated from bone marrow, malignant effusions or solid biopsies and subjected to drug exposure for 48–96 h. Cell survival is measured by re-incubation in MTT for 4 h. We have found a significant correlation of in vitro results with in vivo outcome for acute myeloid leukaemia (AML) and for ovarian cancer (both $p<0.0001$) with an assay sensitivity of 98% for AML and 81% for ovarian cancer. Furthermore, the 5-year survival of ovarian cancer patients treated with a drug found sensitive in vitro is significantly higher than that for patients treated with a drug found resistant in vitro ($p=0.033$). We have correlated assay results with drug resistance markers. For example, expression of the newly described half transporter BCRP is related to daunorubicin resistance ($p<0.05$). The MTT assay is also suitable for screening for modulation of drug resistance. We have found that the DNA polymerase inhibitor aphidicolin markedly increases in vitro sensitivity to the platinum drugs in ovarian cancer and cytosine arabinoside in AML in the majority of patients. The greatest effect was seen for patients deemed resistant in vitro to these agents. We have identified novel drug combinations which demonstrate significant synergism using this methodology and have also used it to study the emergence of drug resistance in cell line models with a view to its prevention. In conclusion, we have found the MTT assay to be a simple, repeatable, adaptable technique which produces accurate information to help the clinician select suitable treatment for individual cases.

Recent Results in Cancer Research, Vol. 161

Drug Resistance

Despite substantial advances in the biological and molecular characterisation of cancer, drug resistance remains a major problem of cancer chemotherapy whether it is intrinsic or, as is more common, acquired after previous exposure to chemotherapeutic agents. Ever since chemotherapy first entered the clinic, attempts have been made to address this problem, and clearly further development of alternative strategies is still essential.

One such alternative is the use of chemosensitivity testing to identify drug resistance in tumour samples taken directly from patients. This offers the chance to spare patients toxicity associated with agents which turn out to be clinically ineffective, and so allows customisation of therapy for individuals.

Clinical drug resistance is multifactorial, consisting of host or pharmacological factors alongside cellular factors. Host factors can include inadequate tumour cell exposure, lack of bioactivation or dose-limiting normal tissue toxicity. We are particularly interested in the cellular factors which can be categorised broadly into alterations in drug transport, altered drug activation or inactivation and enhanced repair or tolerance to DNA damaging agents. Table 1 contains a list of some of the drugs with which we have most experience, along with their putative resistance mechanisms.

MTT Assay

We have been working in the field of drug resistance for over 12 years, and we always commence our investigations by using the short-term MTT assay to identify drug resistance in clinical samples before the patient receives chemotherapy. We have studied a wide variety of tumour types, both haematological and solid malignancies. The MTT assay was first used for chemosensitivity

Table 1. Cytotoxic drugs with their putative cellular resistance mechanisms

Drug	Mechanism
Topoisomerase inhibitors	
Daunorubicin	
Doxorubicin	
Idarubicin	Altered target enzyme
Mitoxantrone	(*topoisomerase inhibitors only*)
Etoposide	Altered drug transport
Topotecan	Altered detoxification
Platinums	DNA repair
Cisplatin	
Carboplatin	
Antimetabolites	
ara-C	Altered drug activation
Fludarabine	DNA repair
6TG	

testing in 1953 with thin tissue sections [1], but it was not until the advent of microtitre technology that this technique became widely used [2]. This semi-automated assay was then adapted for pre-clinical drug development, enabling screening of large numbers of compounds against a series of human tumour cell lines [3]. The dogma at the time suggested that this technique was not applicable to clinical samples; however, this was proved wrong by a number of groups who first used it for clinical studies [4–6]. We have found the MTT assay to be simple, rapid (producing results within a clinical time scale), repeatable throughout the course of the disease and relatively inexpensive. The success rate is high, with results being obtained in around 80% of cases [5, 7, 8] and most importantly of all, it provides a good correlation with the clinical outcome after therapy [9, 10]. We have noticed one disadvantage of this technique compared with others, and that is the relatively high number of cells that are required per well to give an adequate signal. As these cells from clinical samples are mainly quiescent (G_0/G_1), their metabolic activity is not as high as is seen in established cell lines. Therefore, more cells are required to give a reading. Other more sensitive techniques such as the ATP assay, which measures the end point of cell metabolism, are preferred for small samples such as fine needle aspirates or superficial tumours such as TCC of the bladder [11] or squamous cell tumours.

The methodology for the MTT assay consists of sample preparation and drug exposure followed by the measurement of cell survival. Briefly, cells are isolated from biopsies of solid tumour by mechanical disaggregation, and this is followed by density gradient centrifugation, which is also used for bone marrow samples and malignant effusions to remove red blood cells and necrotic cells. Continuous drug exposure for 48 or 96 h against a range of concentrations at pharmacologically achievable levels is followed by removal of drug by inversion and re-incubation of cells in MTT for approximately 4 h. The MTT assay is based on the fact that there is a linear relationship between the number of live cells per well and the amount of formazan produced by intracellular dehydrogenase enzymes. We use acidified isopropanol as a solvent for any formazan crystals formed, and the plate is read at 570 nm (reference 690 nm). A dose-response curve is drawn for every test, and sensitivity or resistance is assessed by using previously defined criteria which we have found give us the best predictive accuracy [5, 8]. We have repeatedly reported a marked variation in drug effect between cells from patients with the same disease [5, 7, 8, 12]. We now have a large database of information on tumour cells taken from approximately 3,500 patients, concentrating mainly on the haematological tumour acute myeloid leukaemia (AML) and ovarian cancer as an example of a solid tumour.

Correlation with Clinical Outcome

Acute Myeloid Leukaemia

These results, however, would be meaningless if they did not predict clinical outcome after therapy. When we first started using this technique we compared the in vitro cell kill of blast cells from patients with AML with the clearance of blast cells from the peripheral blood of the same patients over the same period of time. We were very encouraged to find that the two were strongly related ($p<0.0001$; [5]). We then proceeded to look at the relationship between in vitro MTT assay results and the induction of remission in this disease. In 1997, we published a highly significant correlation between in vitro results and in vivo response to treatment in almost 80 patients with AML, showing an overall predictive accuracy of almost 90% [9]. We found that sensitivity to the anthracyclines appeared to predict remission induction. Since then, we have found that initial sensitivity to cytosine arabinoside (ara-C) is more important in the long term. Patients whose blast cells were found resistant to ara-C in vitro tended to relapse early with a median disease-free survival of 28 weeks compared with 63 weeks for the ara-C-sensitive group ($p=0.022$). These results are in agreement with those found by Klumper et al. when studying the use of the MTT assay for chemosensitivity testing in AML [13].

Ovarian Cancer

Most of our experience in solid tumours has been derived from ovarian cancer. We have studied cells isolated both from biopsies of solid material and malignant effusions. The clinical relevance of the data produced from 120 patients has been demonstrated in a recent report [10]. Again, we found a highly significant correlation of in vitro MTT assay results with clinical outcome ($p<0.0001$), predicting resistance with an 83% degree of accuracy. This was not as high as we had achieved for AML patients, perhaps because host factors, such as adequate tumour cell drug exposure, are probably more important in solid tumours.

Despite all of these patients having advanced disease, FIGO stage III–IV, we found that patients treated on presentation with a drug which was found sensitive in vitro lived twice as long as patients treated with drugs found resistant in vitro, with a 5-year survival of 24% compared with 12% ($p=0.033$; [10]). This suggests that chemosensitivity testing can provide a significant improvement in the existing management of this devastating disease.

Drug Resistance Mechanisms

Once we had identified drug resistance in these clinical samples, a natural extension of our studies was to attempt to identify the mechanism involved with a view to overcoming this resistance in vivo.

Over the past few years we have studied a plethora of resistance markers using a variety of techniques (Table 2). Mainly we have looked at protein expression using immunocytochemistry or immunofluorescence. We have also carried out some functional studies including intracellular drug accumulation. Unlike reports using tumour cell models, generally, we have been unable to find a strong correlation between resistance markers and in vitro sensitivity in these clinical samples. For example, we were not able to establish an overall, statistically significant correlation between expression or function of and in vitro sensitivity to daunorubicin or doxorubicin in AML [14] P-glycoprotein (P-gp). We concluded that this lack of correlation might be due to the wide variation in these parameters found between patients, but this also clearly demonstrates the multifactorial nature of drug resistance at this cellular level. We did find, however, that blast cells from certain patients behaved in the expected fashion, with overexpression of Pgp teamed with resistance to the anthracyclines which was modulated in vitro by inhibitors of multidrug resistance (MDR), but, as stated before, this was not always the case.

One of our more recent studies involved a newly described member of the ABC transmembrane transporter superfamily, breast cancer resistance protein (BCRP). BCRP is so called because it was first found in an MCF-7 human breast cancer cell line which had been selected in doxorubicin + verapamil [15]. Transfection and enforced expression of BCRP has been shown to confer resistance to mitoxantrone and topotecan, often with cross-resistance to doxorubicin and daunorubicin. Interestingly, these cells remain sensitive to the

Table 2. Markers of drug resistance and resistance modulators studied in clinical samples

Resistance mechanism	Resistance markers	Resistance modulators
Altered drug transport	Intracellular drug accumulation [14, 25]	Cyclosporin A [14, 23, 25, 36]
	P-glycoprotein (MRK 16, UIC2) [14, 23, 25, 35, 36]	PSC 833 [14, 23, 25, 36]
	BCRP (BXP-34) [19]	GF120918 [14]
	LRP (LRP 56) [36]	Verapamil [9, 23]
		Tamoxifen [9, 23]
Altered detoxification	Intracellular GSH levels [26]	BSO [9, 24, 26]
	MRP1 (MRPm6) [26, 36, 37]	Ethacrynic acid [9, 37]
	GST α, μ and π [37]	Probenecid
		Indomethecin
Altered drug activation	ara-CTP accumulation and retention [38]	Bryostatin 1 [38]
Altered DNA repair	NT	Aphidicolin [12, 30]
Altered apoptosis	BCL2/Bax ratios [39, 40]	NT
	HSP 70 [40]	

NT, not tested.

vinca alkaloids and the taxanes, distinguishing them from cells demonstrating the protein product of other members of the ABC transporter superfamily such as P-gp (see [16] for review). We used immunocytochemistry with the BXP-34 monoclonal antibody (kind gift from Prof Rik Scheper, Amsterdam) on cytospin preparations of the final cell preparation from ovarian cancer and from AML. Only 2 of 32 (6%) samples from ovarian cancer stained positively agreeing with Scheffer et al. [17], who found that BCRP expression was low or undetectable in a panel of human tumour samples mainly from solid malignancies. However, when we turned our attention to blast cells from patients with AML we found that 6 of 22 (27%) samples were positive with up to 95% of cells showing a strong intensity of staining. This result agrees with the findings of Ross et al., who studied BCRP gene expression in AML blast cells with RT-PCR and found that 33% expressed high levels of BCRP mRNA [18]. Whilst we were unable to demonstrate any significant correlation between BCRP positivity and resistance to mitoxantrone, topotecan or doxorubicin in this small data set, we did find a striking relationship between BCRP and resistance to daunorubicin with five of the six positive samples showing high daunorubicin LC_{50} values. Indeed, the median LC_{50} was over fourfold higher at 0.89 μM compared with 0.21 μM for the BCRP negative samples ($p<0.05$; [19]).

These results, therefore, suggest that BCRP may be involved in drug resistance in AML and could account for some of the anomalies associated with studies of the expression and function of other members of the ABC superfamily such as P-gp and MRP1. Further studies are justified to confirm these findings and establish the clinical implications of this transporter in drug resistance. As daunorubicin is considered an extremely effective agent in AML, these results have important clinical significance particularly because we were previously unable to establish a strong relationship between P-gp and this agent [14]. The fact that statistical significance was found in this present, relatively small study suggests to us that BCRP may have even more importance as a xenobiotic transporter in AML than P-gp. Several compounds have been shown to inhibit BCRP in vitro, for example, the acridone carboximide GF120918 [20], and this is an area we intend to investigate further.

Drug Resistance Modulation

The MTT assay provides the ideal environment for the study of drug resistance modulation. Whilst some clinical MDR modulation regimens have shown promise, generally early results have been disappointing [21]. This is particularly true for solid tumours [22], possibly because most patients do not have the benefit of in vitro screening before treatment. As modulators can have a variety of biological effects, screening with the MTT assay provides an insight into cellular resistance with all relevant mechanisms in play together. We have studied a variety of compounds in our system and have found a marked variation in their effect among patients [23–26]. Sometimes we even

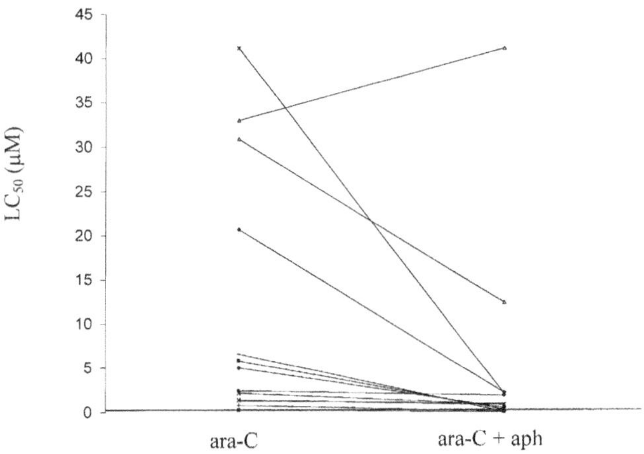

Fig. 1. The effect of aphidicolin on ara-C resistance. Lines represent the change in ara-C LC_{50} on co-incubation with aphidicolin for individual patients (n=13)

see significant increases in sensitivity in the absence of the expected resistance markers and vice versa, emphasising yet again the importance of in vitro screening before therapy. Table 2 itemises some resistance modulators, grouped according to mechanism, that we have studied in the past.

One of these modulators stands out as the most effective agent we have come across in recent years. Aphidicolin is a reversible inhibitor of DNA polymerases α, δ and ε [27,28]. As the glycinate ester, it underwent phase I trial as an anticancer agent but showed little antitumour activity in its own right [29]. As is often the case with such agents, further clinical development ceased. Yet, with the recent upsurge in interest in DNA repair we decided to study its effect as a resistance modulator in fresh tumour samples. To study resistance modulation with the MTT assay, cells are co-incubated for 48 h in the drug under test with and without the putative modulator at a fixed non-toxic dose. Cell survival is then measured by the MTT assay in the usual way but using cells incubated in the modulator alone as control. A sensitisation ratio of the drug LC_{50} over that for drug + modulator gives a measure of modulation effect. After demonstrating a marked increase in sensitivity to the platinum drugs in cells derived from patients with ovarian cancer for this agent [30], we turned our attention to the agents routinely used to treat AML especially as alteration in DNA repair appears to be a common mechanism responsible for resistance to these drugs (Table 1). Whilst aphidicolin did not appear to have a significant effect on the majority of these agents, we were very encouraged to find striking increases in sensitivity to ara-C on co-incubation with aphidicolin, anything up to 80-fold with a median increase of 4.75-fold overall (Fig. 1). Furthermore, this effect was seen for the majority of samples tested (70% showing more than twofold increases in sensitivity) suggesting that increased DNA repair may be a major player in ara-C resistance [12]. When samples were grouped according to ara-C sensitivity, it became apparent that aphidicolin had greater effect in those found resistant (median 8.9-fold increase in sensitivity compared to 2.12-fold for the sensitive group; $p<0.01$). This suggests that aphidicolin targets the population most requiring rescue. It is possible that increased effect in vitro could lead to increased toxicity in vivo. To test this possibility we used the MTT assay to calculate the therapeutic index for ara-C and compare it with that for ara-C + aphidicolin. To do this we compared the sensitivity of both blast cells and normal cord blood cells to ara-C with or without aphidicolin and we found that the combination was slightly less toxic than the drug itself, providing a good therapeutic index [12]. We have since progressed to a joint, collaborative, in vitro study of cells from childhood leukaemias, both AML and ALL, with Gertjan Kaspers' group in Amsterdam.

We firmly believe that this in vitro evidence is more than enough to support the renewed clinical application of aphidicolin, albeit as a resistance modulator. Furthermore, aphidicolin glycinate showed limited toxicity in phase I trial, reinforcing its suitability [29].

Drug Combination

Our techniques lend themselves to screening for the best combination chemotherapy for individuals. Previously, we have found that combining drugs in vitro leads to an additive effect rather than synergism [31]. Additivity can be very important, but the search for synergism continues, allowing scaling down of drug dosage and thereby decreasing toxicity. We have undertaken a pilot study of the promising combination of daunorubicin with the topoisomerase I inhibitor topotecan. Blast cells from patients with AML were incubated with a range of concentrations of the two drugs both singly and together at a constant ratio. The effect of combining the drugs was assessed using CalcuSyn software (Biosoft, Cambridge, UK). So far, we have tested samples from 12 patients and found true synergism in the blast cells from 8 (66%) of these patients using this combination. Again, this could represent a very effective drug regimen for certain patients [32].

Prevention of Drug Resistance

All the studies I have mentioned above hinge on the use of the MTT assay to identify drug resistance in fresh tumour samples from patients. The MTT assay is also widely used for in vitro chemosensitivity testing in human tumour cell lines as cancer cell models. It provides the ideal environment to study the development of drug resistance in these cell lines when they are selected in increasing concentrations of cytotoxic agents. Most studies of drug resistance have concentrated on overcoming resistance once it has become apparent. There are very few studies addressing the issue of drug resistance prevention.

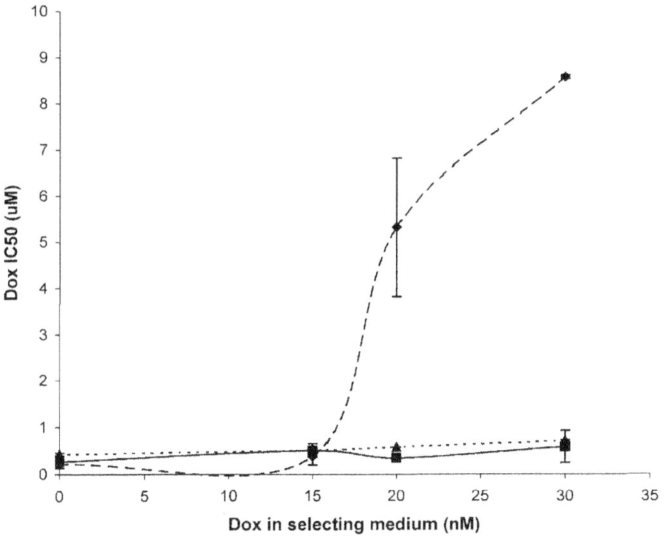

Fig. 2. Dexrazoxane affects the emergence of resistance to doxorubicin. K562 cells were selected in stepwise increasing concentrations of doxorubicin in the presence (solid line) and absence (dashed line) of dexrazoxane. The MTT assay was used to measure drug sensitivity (IC_{50} values) in the resultant sublines. The dotted line represents the addition of the MDR inhibitor, PSC 833 to the chemosensitivity test showing modulation of doxorubicin resistance in the cells selected in doxorubicin alone

The idea that emerging resistance could be delayed or indeed prevented is a novel concept that we have been investigating recently.

There is some clinical evidence to suggest that the bisdioxopiperazine dexrazoxane may affect the development of resistance. Dexrazoxane is now given routinely alongside anthracycline-containing regimens in advanced breast cancer in the United States. It has proven to be a very effective cardioprotectant in this setting [33]. In the course of their statistical analysis, Swain et al. [33] were intrigued to find that patients initially sensitive to doxorubicin who were also given dexrazoxane lived twice as long as those given doxorubicin + placebo and furthermore, this increase in survival was independent of cardiac events. They were unable to explain this finding. As drug resistance is a major cause of treatment failure in this disease, it is possible that dexrazoxane was preventing the development of resistance. As classical MDR is a major mechanism of resistance to doxorubicin, we decided to induce resistance using stepwise increasing concentrations of doxorubicin in the presence and absence of dexrazoxane in a cancer cell model, the human myeloid leukaemia cell line K562. We used the MTT assay to measure any developing resistance in the resultant sublines. In the absence of dexrazoxane, we found the expected increase in doxorubicin IC_{50}, which was related to the dose of doxorubicin in the selecting medium [34] (Fig. 2). When the MDR modulator PSC 833 (kind gift from Novartis) was added into the chemosensitivity test, this completely overcame the increase in resistance to doxorubicin, suggesting an

MDR-based mechanism. However, cells which were selected in doxorubicin + dexrazoxane remained sensitive to doxorubicin, providing evidence to suggest that dexrazoxane can prevent the emergence of drug resistance in K562 cells. Measurement of MDR1 mRNA by RT-PCR, P-gp expression (MRK 16 and flow cytometry) and function in terms of intracellular drug accumulation confirmed that cells selected in doxorubicin showed an MDR1 phenotype whereas those selected in doxorubicin + dexrazoxane remained MDR1 negative. On continuous culture of these sublines in the appropriate media, cells selected in doxorubicin + dexrazoxane remained MDR1 negative for a period of 5 months. Then weak expression of MDR1 mRNA was followed by a rise in P-gp expression with an attendant fall in intracellular drug accumulation which, after a further 3 months, led to a steep rise in doxorubicin IC_{50} [34]. So it appears that dexrazoxane does not totally prevent the emergence of resistance but certainly delays it. As these cells have been continuously exposed to drugs, this could translate into a considerable length of time given the pulsed therapy normally employed for patients.

Conclusions

After working in the field of chemosensitivity testing over the past decade, we have found the MTT assay to be simple, very adaptable and repeatable throughout the course of the disease to identify developing resistance. It clearly demonstrates a marked variation in drug effect among patients comparable to that seen in the clinic. Most importantly of all, there is a good correlation with the clinical outcome after therapy. It also provides the ideal tool for screening drugs both singly and in combination. All these factors strongly suggest that chemosensitivity testing using fresh tumour samples should be considered for inclusion into pre-clinical drug development.

The multifactorial nature of drug resistance is strongly evident to anyone undertaking chemosensitivity testing routinely. Perhaps, further significant advances in cancer chemotherapy will not occur until the topic of customisation of therapy is properly addressed. For example, we sometimes find a cohort of patients whose tumour cells appear resistant in vitro and express a particular resistance marker which is susceptible to modulation with known inhibitors of that specific mechanism. However, more often than not this is not the case. The MTT assay, or indeed any cell survival assay, measures the total effect of all resistance mechanisms in play at any particular time, providing a snap-shot of each tumour. It is quite possible that when one resistance mechanism is inhibited the cell switches to the use of another pathway. These, after all, are the same mechanisms which have evolved over millions of years to protect our cells from a variety of chemical and other toxic insults. Therefore, paradoxically, it is these same protection mechanisms that must first be overcome if drug resistance is to be circumvented.

Chemosensitivity assays can be technically demanding, requiring a certain expertise. However, with the correct training, suitable procedures for sample collection and determination to see it through, it is possible to set up these techniques in any diagnostic laboratory. The wealth of evidence suggests that the clinical implications of chemosensitivity testing are huge and that the use of these techniques could lead to a significant improvement in the management of cancer.

Acknowledgements. These studies were made possible by the dedication and determination of my colleagues, particularly Alena Elgie and Christine Williamson. I would also like to thank Colin Taylor and Kurt Hellmann for their discussions on the clinical implications of our findings and Helen Coley, Grazyna Lewandowicz and the numerous clinicians who sent us samples from their patients.

References

1. Black MM, Speer FD (1953) Effects of cancer chemotherapeutic agents on dehydrogenase activity of human cancer tissue in vitro. Am J Clin Pathol 23:218–227
2. Mosmann T (1983) Rapid colorimetric assay for cellular growth and survival: application to proliferation and cytotoxic assays. J Immunol Methods 65:55–63
3. Carmichael J, De Graff WG, Gazdar AF, Minna JD, Mitchell JB (1987) Evaluation of a tetrazolium-based semi-automatic colorimetric assay. Cancer Res 47:936–942
4. Pieters R, Huismans DR, Leyva A, Veerman AJP (1988) Adaption of the rapid tetrazolium dye based (MTT) assay for chemosensitivity testing in childhood leukaemia. Cancer Lett 41:323-332
5. Sargent JM, Taylor CG (1989) Appraisal of the MTT assay as a rapid test of chemosensitivity in acute myeloid leukaemia. Br J Cancer 60:206–210
6. Twentyman PR, Fox NE, Rees JKH (1989) Chemosensitivity testing of fresh leukaemia cells using the MTT colorimetric assay. Br J Haematol 71:19–24
7. Wilson JK, Sargent JM, Elgie AW, Hill JG, Taylor CG (1990) A feasibility study of the MTT assay for chemosensitivity testing in ovarian malignancy. Br J Cancer 62:189–194
8. Taylor CG, Sargent JM, Elgie AW, Reid FDA, Alton PA, Hill JG (1998) The clinical relevance of chemosensitivity testing in ovarian cancer. Cancer Detect Prev 22:305-312
9. Sargent J, Elgie A, Williamson C, Taylor C (1997) The use of the MTT assay to study drug resistance in acute myeloid leukaemia - an update. Adv Blood Dis 3:33–41
10. Taylor CG, Sargent JM, Elgie AW, Williamson CJ, Lewandowicz GM, Chappatte O, Hill JG (2001) Chemosensitivity testing predicts survival in ovarian cancer. Eur J Gynaecol Oncol 22:278–282
11. Gontero P, Sargent JM, Hopster DJ, Lewandowicz GM, Taylor CG, Elgie AW, Williamson CJ, Sriprasad SI, Muir GH In vitro chemosensitivity to mitomycin C in transitional cell carcinoma of the bladder and its relationship with P-glycoprotein and apoptotic factors. (submitted)
12. Sargent JM, Elgie AW, Williamson CJ, Lewandowicz GM, Taylor CG (2001) Circumvention of resistance to ara-C by aphidicolin in blast cells from patients with AML. Br J Cancer 84:680–685
13. Klumper E, Ossenkoppele GJ, Pieters R, Huismans DR, Loonen AH, Rottier A, Westra G, Veerman AJP (1996) In vitro resistance to cytosine arabinoside, not to daunorubicin, is associated with the risk of relapse in de novo acute myeloid leukaemia. Br J Haematol 93:903–910
14. Elgie AW, Sargent JM, Williamson CJ, Lewandowicz GM, Taylor CG (1999) Comparison of P-glycoprotein expression and function with in vitro sensitivity to anthracyclines in AML. Adv Exp Med Biol 457:29–33
15. Doyle LA, Yang W, Abruzzo LV, Krogmann T, Gao Y, Rishi AK, Ross DD (1998) A multidrug transporter from human MCF-7 breast cancer cells. Proc Natl Acad Sci USA 22:15665–15670

16. Ross DD (2000) Novel mechanisms of drug resistance in leukemia. Leukemia 14:467–473
17. Scheffer GL, Maliepaard M, Pijnenborg ACLM, van Gastelen MA, de Jong MC, Schroeijers AB, van der Kolk DM, Allen JD, Ross DD, van der Valk P, Dalton WD, Schellens JHM, Scheper RJ (2000) Breast cancer resistance protein is localised at the plasma cell membrane in mitoxantrone- and topotecan-resistant cell lines. Cancer Res 60:2589–2593
18. Ross DD, Karp JE, Chen TT, Doyle LA (2000) Expression of breast cancer resistance protein in blast cells from patients with acute leukemia. Blood 96:365–368
19. Sargent JM, Williamson CJ, Maliepaard M, Elgie AW, Scheper RJ, Taylor CG (2001) Breast cancer resistance protein and resistance to daunorubicin in blast cells from patients with AML. Br J Haematol 115:257–262
20. Maliepaard M, van Gastelen MA, Tohgo A, Hausheer FH, van Waardenburg RCAM, de Jong LA, Pluim D, Beijnen JH, Schellens JHM (2001) Circumvention of breast cancer resistance protein (BCRP)-mediated resistance to camptothecins in vitro using non-substrate drugs or the BCRP inhibitor GF120918. Clin Cancer Res 7:935–941
21. Covelli A (1999) Modulation of multidrug resistance (MDR) in hematological malignancies. Ann Oncol 10 (Supp 6): 53–59
22. Kaye SB (1999) New drug development: its role in reversing drug resistance. Br J Cancer 80:116–121
23. Sargent J, Elgie A, Alton P, Taylor C (1995) Identification of drug resistance in fresh blast cells from acute myeloid leukaemia and its modification in vitro. Contrib Oncol 49:109–116
24. Sargent J, Elgie A, Taylor C, Wilson J, Alton P, Hill JG (1994) The identification of drug resistance in ovarian cancer and breast cancer: application of the MTT assay. Contrib Gynecol Obstet 19:64–75
25. Coley HC, Sargent JM, Williamson CJ, Titley J, Scheper R, Gregson SE, Elgie AW, Lewandowicz GM, Taylor CG (2002) Assessment of the classical MDR phenotype in epithelial ovarian carcinoma using primary cultures: a feasibility study. Anticancer Res 22:69–74
26. Lewandowicz GM, Britt P, Elgie AW, Williamson CJ, Coley HM, Hall AG, Sargent JM (2002) Cellular glutathione content and the effect of BSO modulation in tumour biopsies derived from patients with advanced ovarian cancer. Gynecol Oncol 85:298–304
27. Ikegami S, Taguchi T, Ohashi M, Oguro M, Nagano H, Mano Y (1978) Aphidicolin prevents mitotic cell division by interfering with the activity of DNA polymerase-alpha. Nature 275:458–460
28. Yamade K, Itoh R (1994) Involvement of DNA polymerase δ and/or ε in joining UV-induced DNA single strand breaks in human fibroblasts (comparison of effects of butylphenyldeoxyguanosine with aphidicolin). Biochim Biophys Acta 1219:302–306
29. Sessa C, Zucchetti M, Davoli E, Califano R, Cavalli F, Fristaci S, Gumbrell L, Sulkes A, Winograd B, D'Incalci M (1991) Phase I and clinical evaluation of aphidicolin glycinate. J Natl Cancer Inst 83:1160–1164
30. Sargent JM, Elgie AW, Williamson CJ, Taylor CG (1996) Aphidicolin markedly increases the platinum sensitivity of cells from primary ovarian tumours. Br J Cancer 74:1730–1733
31. Sargent JM, Taylor CG, Elgie AW (1993) Study of drug combinations in acute myeloid leukaemia (AML) using the MTT assay. In: Kaspers GJL et al (eds) Drug resistance in leukaemia and lymphoma – the clinical value of laboratory studies. Harwood Academic, London, pp 293–297
32. Taylor CG, Elgie AW, Williamson CJ, Sargent JM (2001) The combination of topotecan and daunorubicin shows striking synergism in vitro in AML. Leukemia 15:492 (abst O44)
33. Swain SM, Whaley FS, Gerber MC, Ewer MS, Bianchine JR, Gams RA (1997) Delayed administration of dexrazoxane provides cardioprotection for patients with advanced breast cancer treated with doxorubicin-containing therapy. J Clin Oncol 15:1333–1340
34. Sargent JM, Williamson CJ, Taylor CG, Hellmann K (2001) Dexrazoxane significantly impairs the induction of doxorubicin resistance in the human leukaemia line, K562. Br J Cancer 84:959–964

35. Faulkner Pulsford J, Sargent J, Elgie A, Taylor C (1995) Comparison of P-glycoprotein expression with in vitro drug sensitivity in fresh blast cells from acute myeloid leukaemia. Br J Biomed Sci 52:188–194
36. Sargent JM, Coley HM, Williamson C, Taylor CG (1998) Evidence of ABC transporters in fresh tumor cells from patients with ovarian cancer. Int J Pharmacol Therapeut 36:64–66
37. Sargent JM, Williamson C, Hall AG, Elgie AW, Taylor CG (1999) Evidence for the involvement of the glutathione pathway in drug resistance in AML. Adv Expl Med Biol 457:205–209
38. Elgie AW, Sargent JM, Alton P, Peters GJ, Noordhuis P, Williamson CJ, Taylor CG (1998) Modulation of resistance to ara-C by bryostatin in fresh blast cells from patients with AML. Leuk Res 22:373–378
39. Balkham SE, Sargent JM, Elgie AW, Williamson CJ, Taylor CG (1999) Comparison of BCL-2 and BAX protein expression with in vitro sensitivity to ara-C and 6TG in AML Adv Expl Med Biol 457:335–340
40. Elgie AW, Sargent JM, Williamson CJ, Taylor CG (2001) Bcl-2, bax, hsp 70 expression and drug sensitivity in patients with AML. Leukemia 15:489 abst P17

Chemosensitivity Testing of Human Tumors Using Si-sensor Chips

Pedro Mestres-Ventura

Institute of Anatomy and Cell Biology, University Hospital,
University of Saarland, 66421 Homburg/Saar, Germany
e-mail: anpmes@uniklinik-saarland.de

Abstract

Chemotherapy is, on its own or in combination with other treatments, a very effective anticancer therapy. Introduced in the middle of the last century, chemotherapy today still faces the problem of determining which specific agent or agents are able to yield the desired clinical therapeutical effect for a particular tumor and patient.

Numerous tests in vitro have been developed to detect chemosensitivity and chemoresistance and also for screening new drugs.

Three groups of tests can be defined: 1, cell viability tests; 2, measurements of cell metabolism; and 3, clonogenic assays.

Test time, tissue preparation, complexity of test performance, and correlation with the clinical progress of the disease are criteria used to judge how successful the tests are. The introduction of Si-sensor chips, which are able to detect metabolic changes in living cells, has opened up new possibilities in this field.

Basically two sensor principles or types can be considered: (a) the light-addressed potentiometric sensor (LAPS) and (b) the multisensor array (MSA). Whereas LAPS measures one, MSA registers online many parameters (for instance, impedance, pH, O_2, temperature). The aim of this chapter is to review this technology and to present recent applications using cells, tissue slices, and biopsies.

Introduction

Chemotherapy is today a highly effective type of cancer therapy, together with surgery and radiotherapy. The chemotherapy of tumors began in the last century with the introduction of nitrogen mustards. In comparison with bacterial diseases, the chemotherapy of tumors shows a number of basic differences. In

Recent Results in Cancer Research, Vol. 161

Table 1. Chemosensitivity tests/drug-screening assays

1. Human tumor stem cell assay
2. Kern assay
3. MTT assay
4. ATP bioluminescence assay
5. Fluorescence cytoprint assay (Analytical Biosystems, Inc.)
6. Sulforhodamine blue assay
7. Extreme drug resistance assay (Oncothec, Inc.)
8. Flow cytometric analysis (FACS)
9. Cytotoxicity tests (trypan blue exclusion, LDH colorimetric test)
10. Fluorometric microculture cytotoxicity assays
11. Nuclear damage assay
12. Screening assay using nude mice and isotopic evaluation
13. In vitro chemosensitivity test based on immunohistochemical detection of certain enzymes [for instance, ODC (ornithine decarboxylase) as proliferation marker] in individual cells
14. In vitro chemosensitivity test using a three-dimensional culture matrix (collagen gel-embedded cells; sponge gel-supported histoculture drug-response assay, see also *cytoprint assay*)
15. Evaluation of chemosensitivity in terms of apoptosis (cell counts)

the case of infectious diseases the therapy was oriented to the sensitivity of bacteria to the chemical agents available. In the case of tumors the histological structure was considered one of the more important criteria. However, tumors with the same or similar histological structure may react differently to chemotherapy. The possibility of making predictions of the chemical sensitivity of a tumor is a fundamental aid to individually defining the corresponding tumor therapy. Comparing the antibiogram with the in vitro chemosensitivity assays for tumors, it cannot be ignored that there are a number of parallelisms in their rationales. The introduction some time ago of the term anti-oncogram for these assays reflects these similarities, but as far as efficacy is concerned the divergencies are considerable (Bellamy 1992).

In Table 1 the more important tests are summarized. The list does not claim to be exhaustive but indicates trends in the development of such methods. Although the usefulness of such tests has not yet been convincingly demonstrated, clinicians still consider such assays necessary. In the opinion of physicians and clinicians, research focusing on the development of new test strategies and/or the improvement of others already existing is indispensable, because of the requirement for an appropriate therapy that is singular and specific in relation to both tumor and patient.

The main criticisms against numerous assays could be expressed in four points:

1. All known tests are "end point tests."
2. The basic parameters only deal with cell processes such as cell death and cell proliferation.
3. The preparation of cell or tissue cultures is very laborious and requires a lot of manpower and time.

4. The adaptation of the tumor cells to the in vitro conditions is accompanied by changes in the phenotype, and consequently the sensitivity to the drugs could change, differing in the tumor cells from that of the originals in vivo. The extrapolation of results to the patient might therefore become difficult.

In view of these considerations, and although some groups have published very promising results (Bachrach et al. 1994; Kurbacher et al. 1998; Kobayashi et al. 2001; Manni et al. 2001), it seems to be necessary to continue the search for new techniques to achieve a high grade of efficiency in the prediction of chemosensitivity in the field of tumor diseases. Such an advance might be possible with the aid of sensor chip technologies (Owicki et al. 1994; Wolf et al. 1998). Under laboratory conditions these types of systems have already yielded promising results; however it is not yet clear whether they are able to cope with the day-to-day problems of medical care (chemosensitivity prediction).

Biosensors

In general, biosensors are defined as devices composed of both a biological and a physical element. They are designed to measure the activity of biomolecules, cells, and cell tissues. The physical element acts as a transducer of the signals received from the biomolecules, cells, and cell tissues, allowing such signals to be quantified. In fact,biosensors might be considered as chemoreceptors, because the quality of the signals has a chemical character, but the inclusion of biological elements into the system justifies the use of the prefix "bio." In numerous situations the biological element detects changes of the environment that can then be analyzed and measured. One example is the combination of nerve cells and a sensor chip for the detection of toxic gases (Gross et al. 1995; Morefield et al. 2000; Frommherz 2001). In other cases, the biological element is also the unknown variable while the sensor chip detects functional changes that can be expressed in electrochemical terms (Wolf et al. 1998; Stenger et al. 2001).

The material currently used to manufacture the sensors is silicon. It is used in plates on which metallic structures – of palladium, for instance – can be installed and allows a relatively high number of parameters to be measured (Table 2).

In Table 3 the main families of sensors that seem relevant to our topic are classified.

The Impedance

Some years ago Giaever and Keese (1984) used a sensor technology to establish the basis of a method of measuring changes in cell shape associated with adhesion to substrate and consequently those related to cell locomotion. Cells

Table 2. Parameters that can be measured with a Si-sensor chip

Electric current, electric potential, intensity and phase of electromagnetic radiation (usually visible light), mass, electric conductance, electric impedance, temperature, viscosity
Of all these parameters, those primarily relevant in the context of chemosensitivity testing are: 1. Impedance (cell-chip contact, i.e., cell adhesion and cell shape) 2. pH (cell metabolism) 3. Oxygen concentration and consumption (cell metabolism) 4. Temperature (culture conditions) Ionic or chemical composition of fluids in the sensor chamber (special chip membranes are necessary)

Table 3. Families of relevant sensors

The family of electrochemical biosensors:
1. Amperometric "enzyme electrode" (detection of products such as glucose) 2. FET (field effect transistor). These are semiconductors with ion-sensitive surfaces 3. ISFET (ion-sensitive field effect transistor). The chip is covered by a polymer selectively permeable to the analyte ion 4. ESFET (enzyme field effect transistor) The family of optical biosensors: 1. LAPS: light-addressed potentiometric semiconductors 2. MLAPS (multi-LAPS)

in suspension are applied to dishes fitted with gold electrodes. Cells become adherent and spread out on the gold surface, developing contacts of differing extent. Modifications of the size of the area of contact, originating through locomotion or other circumstances reducing the grade of adherence, cause variations in the electric flow between the medium and the gold electrodes. When the adherence is high the impedance is also high and vice versa. With regard to time, this parameter can give information not only about the grade of adhesion but also on dynamic cell processes in response to changes of the medium (Ehret et al. 1998). Coating the surfaces with certain biomolecules (for instance, fibronectin, laminin, bovine serum albumin, vitronectin) can strongly influence the cellular adhesion, because it is possible to quantify impedance and to express these cell behavioral changes in terms of this electrical parameter. When adherent cells round up and become detached, this could be a sign of a toxic effect. In such cases the impedance will reveal the intensity and also the chronological progression of this phenomenon. In relation with chemosensitivity the impedance can be used as an indicator to determine the response of the cells to chemical substances or antimetabolites. However, it is important in such experiments to know the cytological composition (tumor vs. nontumor cells) of the specimen as well as whether the substance or substances tested target one or many cell types. The necessity of including very well established standards and controls should be stressed here.

Investigations using small pieces of tumor tissue from biopsies or tumor slices have shown that interactions with the electrodes are quite different from those known for cell suspensions. In general only single cells spreading out from a tissue block seem to be able to directly create firm contacts with the substrate (electrode), whereas the block of tissue does not.

The recent development of multisensor arrays as a new generation of sensor chips is an attempt to overcome such handicaps (Henning et al. 2001). In these chips the electrodes are made of palladium and give satisfactory results (Lehmann et al. 2001). Current investigations with scanning electron microscopy (SEM) reveal aspects of contacting cells that are relevant for the interpretation of very fine variations in the impedance. Investigations with interferential reflexion microscopy have shown that cells anchor with the substrate by means of thin processes called filopodia, which terminate in small feet. Between the membrane of the feet and the substrate there is a thin gap of a few nanometers in width that is passed by the electric current. Light microscopy is generally unable to discriminate these very fine surface profiles and contact sites. In contrast, SEM and, nowadays, environmental SEM (ESEM) yield very precise images, allowing the study of the architecture of the cell surface. Cell reactions to anticancer drugs or simply a certain substrate material in vitro are accompanied by changes in the cell surface and adhesion morphology (Figs. 1, 2). Using quantitative approaches, the impedance measurements can be correlated with these ultrastructural data.

The Pericellular Acidification

The acidification of the immediate environment of cells express, under standard conditions, an increment in cell metabolism. Increases in glycolysis and respiratory activity result in a release of protons through the cell membrane that causes a diminution of pH outside the cell (Fig. 3).

Of the numerous sensors available (see Table 3), the type developed by Owicki et al. (1994), a light-addressed potentiometric sensor (LAPS), seems so far to be a very successful one. On the basis of such sensor principles Molecular devices, Inc. have developed a device in which the cells can be incubated under supravital conditions for a relatively long period of time and exposed to the action of drugs and the changes in pH can be detected. This system is called a microphysiometer and is commercially available under the trade name Cytosensor. Basically the device is composed of an incubation chamber for the cells or tissue, a setup providing nutrient fluids for the cells, and a control unit with a computer regulating the regime of the different system parameters and storing the data (Fig. 4).

In a recent publication Hafner (2000) revises the scientific background of this technique and discusses numerous applications in cell biology, pharmacology, etc. A central question in this review is the global character of microphysiometric measurements. In fact, the data collected refer not to a single cell but to many cells placed in the chamber. A potential difficulty of pH global measurements could be the interpretation of the results in terms of signal pathways and metabolic processes. Hafner (2000) describes a number of stra-

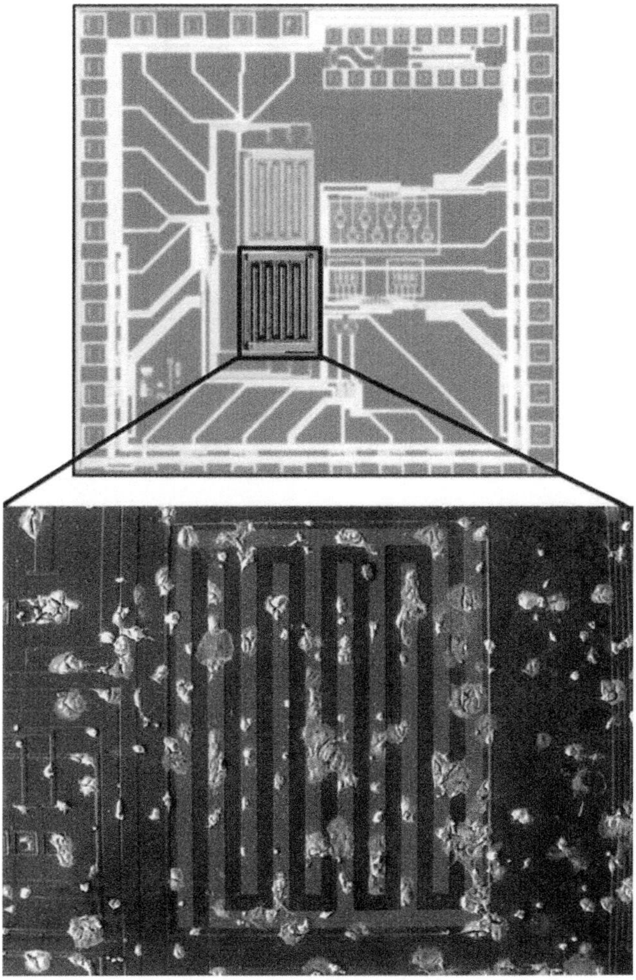

Fig. 1. Scanning electron microscopy of a sensor chip with MCF-7 cells. The insert in the upper part shows the area with the specific sensor for impedance. In the lower part the cells appear adhered to the palladium gates

tegies in which pharmacological approaches help considerably to focus the problem and to distinguish less relevant variables.

Studies performed in our laboratory with the aim of demonstrating the validity of the "microphysiometric" principle have shown interesting results at least in two situations: (1) ligand-receptor interactions in genetically modified cells and (2) cellular reactions of cell monolayers and "slices" to the medium and to pharmacological agents.

The stimulation of CHO cells that have been genetically transformed and that overexpress muscarinic acetylcholine receptors (ATCC, Teddington, UK) shows a dose-response correlation with the possibility of repeating the experi-

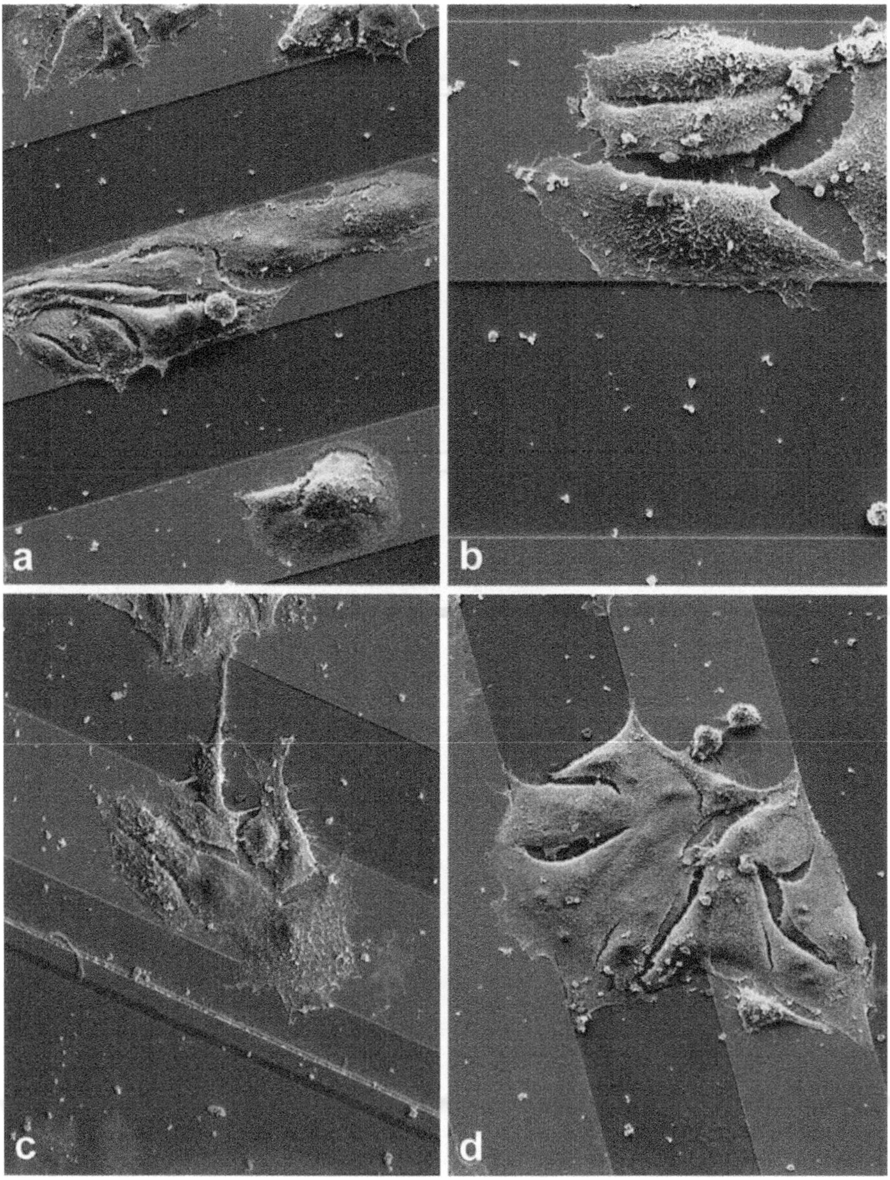

Fig. 2a–d. Scanning electron microscopy of MCF-7 cells cultivated on a sensor chip. The cells display numerous surface profiles varying between robust processes and fine filopodia. The contact area of cell with substrate is defined by the summation of all contact sites, large (cell body) and very small (each single filopodium). a, b At this cell concentration (early culture stage) the cells show a certain preference for palladium surfaces. c, d Some cells aggregate and try to cross the Si-surface located between two palladium gates. These pictures correspond to a cultivation of 24 h. With longer cultivation time they become more dense, occupying the Si-surfaces, too. This phenomenon probably depends in part on the surface conditioning through the medium proteins

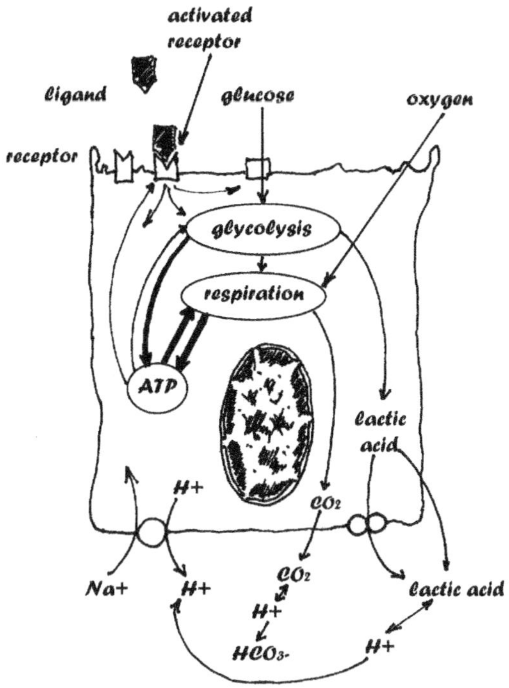

Fig. 3. Diagram with essentials about the metabolic background of the pericellular acidification. (Slightly modified from Molecular Devices, Inc.)

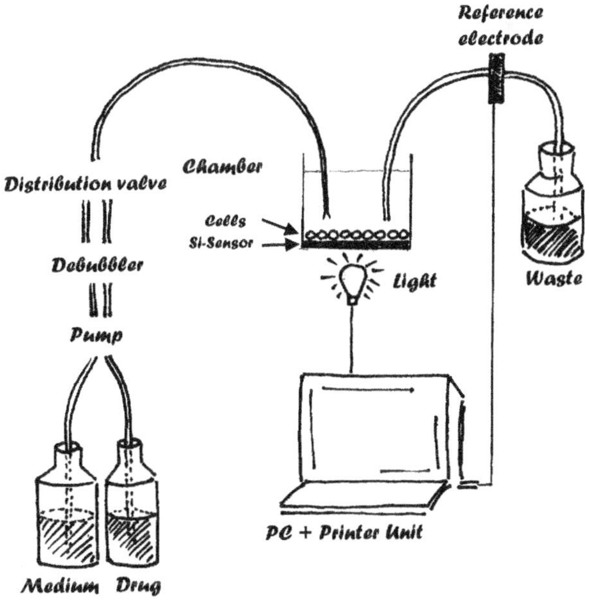

Fig. 4. Diagram showing the basic structure of a microphysiometer. (Inspired by a drawing of Ekelund et al. 1998)

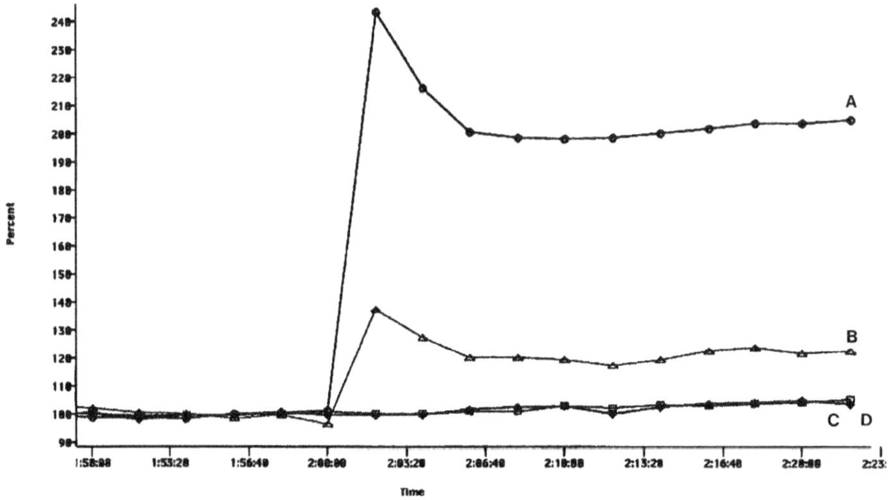

Fig. 5. Stimulation of cell metabolism in CHO-M1 cells. This is a cell line that was transfected with muscarinic acetylcholine receptor M1. In A, 30 µM carbachol was applied as agonist. In B, carbachol was used at a concentration of 3 µM. The controls (without carbachol) are represented in C and D. The increase of acidification is represented in % on the Y-axis, whereas the real time is indicated on the X-axis

ment many times (Fig. 5). This type of cell represents a very useful tool as a control object for studies on chemosensitivity and as a standard for the performance of the sensor chip.

The comparison between monolayers and tissue fragments is relevant in the case of tumors because the preparation of monolayers, i.e., the dissociation of the original tissue, might cause considerable changes in both cell types present in the specimen and a loss in the three-dimensional cell arrangements, considerably modifying the cell interaction frame. For these reasons we try to prepare the tissue maintaining the three-dimensional structure in a minimal volume. A proper approach seems to be the production of slices with a thickness that permits an adequate diffusion of nutrients and agents from the medium into the inner part of the tissue sample. Experiments with rat livers have demonstrated the suitability of this approach. Cell monolayers, or slices, of the rat liver were incubated in a Cytosensor and exposed to an agonist and antagonist on the adrenergic receptor (Fig. 6). Although the course of the experiment was very satisfactory, one point, however, remained unclear and that was whether the response observed referred to the cells located at the surface of slices or whether it means that cells located in deeper parts of the slices were likewise involved. These and similar questions are currently the subject of studies in our laboratory, serving as a foundation for further more specific investigations into the tumor tissue of patients. In this connection the assessment of vitality and structural/functional preservation of the specimen during

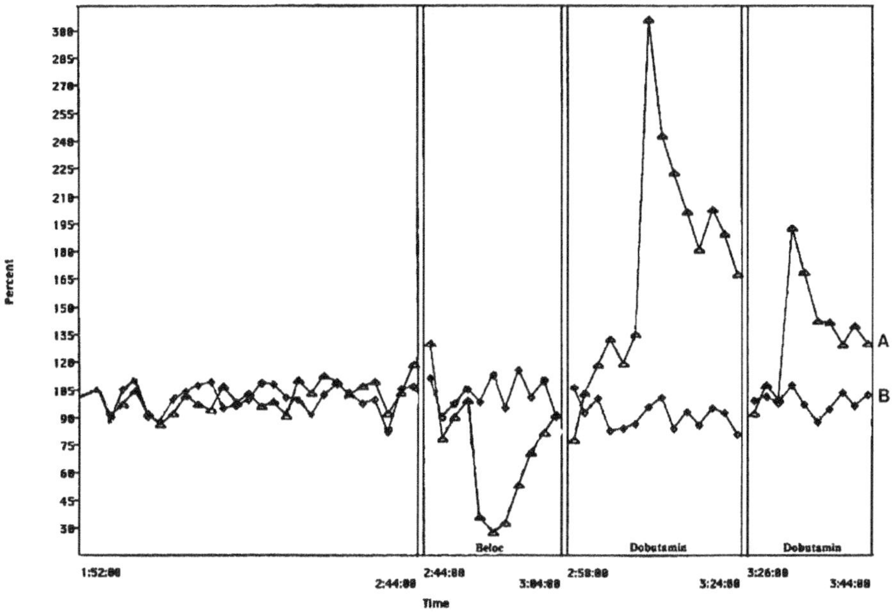

Fig. 6. Treatment of liver slices with dobutamine, an agonist of beta-1 adrenoreceptors with no vasoconstrictor effect, and with an antagonist called Beloc, a beta-blocker. The liver tissue was maintained at a temperature of approximately 8°C and slices of 300 µm were prepared. Pieces of 3- to 4-mm diameter were cut and transferred into the microphysiometer. After 1 h of adaptation time, the drugs were applied. Dobutamine increases the cell metabolism (curve A), whereas Beloc decreases it (curve B)

and at the end of an investigation with a sensor chip device seems to be essential.

Studies with Prospective Clinical Relevance

The application of sensor chip technologies to determine the chemosensitivity of tumors has until now received only scant attention in the literature. The study of Ekelund et al. (1998) and more recently the investigations of Metzger et al. (2001) using the system of Molecular Devices are remarkable exceptions and represent the first attempt to bridge over the gap between laboratory and medical routine, showing the practice-oriented application of a novel technique. The advantage of obtaining data on chemosensitivity in only a few hours and with almost minimal manipulation of the specimen was recognized in these studies. Both groups have shown that the dynamic profile of reactions between cells and drugs can be highly specific for tumors and also for the drugs tested. Both groups work with a Cytosensor from Molecular Devices.

Ekelund et al. (1998) have stressed the basic necessity not only of determining the mechanism of action of the drugs but also of improving the technical resources for predicting drug sensitivity to combat the tumor of a patient. In their publication the authors describe very precisely adequate tissue preparation methods for a microphysiometer. The objects of these studies were cell lines and primary tissue from clinical probes. The more relevant message of the microphysiometer is probably the description and quantification of metabolic activity patterns. Comparisons with data obtained by using methods for determining the cell viability of the tumor in vitro (for instance, fluorometric microculture cytotoxicity assay) serve validation purposes. According to these authors the possibility of following online the metabolic state of the cells exposed to a drug seems to be one of the fundamental advantages of the method. The online character of the measurements allows critical moments in the dynamic process of the test to be noted, such as the detection of changes in cell viability and the moment in which the irreversibility (point of no return) of these phenomena is reached. Knowledge of the critical moments makes it possible to stop the drug exposure and insert a recovery phase as well as to try a new test with the same cells and, for instance, with another drug. The number of clinical cases evaluated in this study is not yet sufficient for a validation of the test in clinical terms. However, it is a very promising reference.

The investigation of Metzger et al. (2001) largely confirms the statements of Ekelund et al. (1998) and in addition greatly extends the clinical correlations. Of particular interest is the fact that these authors have pointed out the capacity of a microphysiometric approach to determine not only the chemosensitivity but also the chemoresistance. These authors have developed a test method called "Chemo-Select" in which a light-addressed potentiometric sensor is used. The resolution of this test seems to be very high, detecting changes of pH on the order of 1/1000 of pH units and with less than 500 cells. The results of the testing now in progress of "Chemo-Select" within the frame of a clinical study involving at least 18 hospitals will be of great importance for research following this paper.

Horizons

Despite the evident importance of continuing with the development of tissue preparation and tumor analysis for test purposes it is no less significant to improve the physical side of these technologies, i.e., to enhance the skills and capacities of the sensor chips.

Along this line of thinking, one should emphasize the developments of Wolf and coworkers (Ehret et al. 1998; Henning et al. 2001; Lehmann et al. 2001) around the creation of multisensor arrays in which different sensor types dealing with different parameters can be integrated in a single Si-chip. This represents another, very new attempt to progress in this field. The increased number of parameters permits a more detailed analysis of tumor cell dynamic patterns, being at the same time a challenge in data management and in handling of tumor probes. These objectives are being pursued in a national project led by Prof. Wolf (TU Munich) in which university hospitals in Munich and Homburg are involved.

Acknowledgements. The author is indebted to Prof. Dr. W. Schmidt and coworkers (Department of Gynecology and Obstetrics, University of Saarland) for supplying tumor material and for advice on clinical questions and to Norbert Pütz, Gabi Kiefer, Anette Schofer, and Tinka Reichmann for excellent aid in many technical matters. These investigations were generously supported by SPV-Saar (Me 2000–2001), Molecular Devices, Inc. (Munich, Germany) and Micronas (Freiburg, Germany).

References

Bachrach, Shayovitz U et al (1994) Ornithine decarboxylase – a predictor for tumor chemosensitivity. Cell Mol Biol 40(7):957–964

Bellamy WT (1992) Prediction of response to drug therapy of cancer. A review of in vitro assays. Drugs 44(5):690–708

Ehret R, Baumann W et al (1998) On-line control of cellular adhesion with impedance measurements using interdigitated electrode structures. Med Biol Eng Comput 36(3):365–370

Ekelund S, Nygren P et al (1998) Microphysiometry: new technology for evaluation of anticancer drug activity in human tumor cells in vitro. Anticancer Drugs 9(6):531–538

Frommherz P (2001) Interfacing von Nervenzellen und Halbleiterchips. Physikalische Blätter 57(2):43–48

Giaever I, Keese CR (1986) Use of electric fields to monitor the dynamical aspect of cell behavior in tissue culture. IEEE Trans Biomed Eng 33(2):242

Gross GW, Rhoades BK et al (1995) The use of neuronal networks on multielectrode arrays as biosensors. Biosens Bioelectron 10(6–7):553–567

Hafner F (2000) Cytosensor microphysiometer: technology and recent applications. Biosens Bioelectron 15(3–4):149–158

Henning, Brischwein T et al (2001) Approach to a multiparametric sensor – chipbased tumor chemosensitivity assay. Anticancer Drugs 12(1):21–32

Kobayashi H, Higashiyama M et al (2001) Examination of in vitro chemosensitivity test using collagen gel droplet culture method with colorimetric endpoint quantification. Jpn Q J Cancer Res 92(2):203–210

Kurbacher CM, Cree IA et al (1998) Use of an ex vivo ATP luminescence assay to direct chemotherapy for recurrent ovarian cancer. Anticancer Drugs 9(1):51–57

Lehmann M, Baumann W et al (2001) Simultaneous measurement of cellular respiration and acidification with a single CMOS ISFET. Biosens Bioelectron 16(3):195–203

Manni, Astrow A et al (2001) Immunohistochemical detection of ornithinedecarboxylase in primary and metastatic human breast cancer specimens. Breast Cancer Res Treat 67(2):147–156

Metzger, Deglmann R et al (2001) Towards in-vitro prediction of an in-vivo cytostatic response of human tumor cells with a fast chemosensitivity assay. Toxicology 166(1–2):97–108

Miller, Olson DL et al (1993) Cholinergic stimulation of the Na^+/K^+ adenosine triphosphatase as revealed by microphysiometry. Biophys J 64(3):813–823

Morefield SI, Keefer EW et al (2000) Drug evaluations using neuronal networks cultured on microelectrode arrays. Biosens Bioelectron 15(7–8):383–396

Owicki JC, Bousse LJ et al (1994) The light-addressable potentiometric sensor: principles and biological applications. Annu Rev Biophys Biomol Struct 23:87–113

Stenger DA, Gross GW et al (2001) Detection of physiologically active compounds using cell-based biosensors. Trends Biotechnol 19(8):304–309

Wolf B, Brischwein M et al (1998) Monitoring of cellular signalling and metabolism with modular sensor-technique: the PhysioControl-Microsystem (PCM). Biosens Bioelectron 15;13(5):501–509

Multiparametric Sensor Chips for Chemosensitivity Testing of Sensitive and Resistant Tumor Cells

Angela M. Otto, Martin Brischwein, Helmut Grothe, Elena Motrescu, Bernhard Wolf

A.M. Otto (✉)
Heinz-Nixdorf-Chair for Medical Electronics, Technical University of Munich, Arcisstraße 21, 80290 München, Germany
e-mail: angela.otto@ei.tum.de

Abstract

Many different assays have been developed for testing the chemosensitivity of tumor cells in vitro, usually based on a single biochemical or cellular parameter. A multiparametric test system has been developed that accommodates on a single chip numerous sensors for metabolic parameters, ΔpH and ΔpO_2, as well as for morphological changes. The cells grow directly on the chips and can be continuously monitored online up to several days. The effects of various chemotherapeutic drugs on the metabolic profile of several tumor cell lines have been investigated. In colon carcinoma-derived LS174T cells, cytochalasin B markedly increased oxygen consumption while decreasing the rate of extracellular acidification. These effects, which reflect the biochemical action of cytochalasin B, were reversible on drug removal. In contrast, chloroacetaldehyde markedly reduced respiration, which recovered when the drug was removed. Primary breast cancer cells also responded to chloroacetaldehyde with a marked reduction in ΔpO_2, followed by a reduced rate of acidification. Comparing the metabolism of doxorubicin-sensitive and -resistant mouse sarcoma S180 cells, the rates of acidification and respiration were inhibited by doxorubicin only in the sensitive cells, whereas in the resistant cells oxygen consumption even increased. These examples demonstrate that this chip-based test system provides rapid and important information for assessing chemosensitivity of tumor cells.

Introduction

The dilemma of choosing the "right" chemotherapeutic agents for treating a patient with a particular tumor is "knowing" whether the specific tumor of this patient will respond and regress. Although statistics may favor the prediction of a positive outcome, the diversity of seemingly similar tumors and the

Recent Results in Cancer Research, Vol. 161

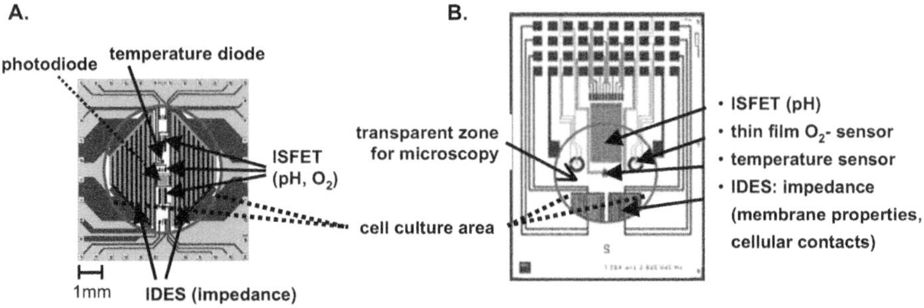

Fig. 1. Schematic view of (A) a silicon chip and (B) a glass chip

systemic individuality of each organism cast great uncertainty on such predictions. Unnecessary chemotherapeutic treatment, which means distress and valuable time lost for pursuing other promising treatments, could be avoided if at least the resistance of the patient's tumor for a drug or drug combination could be tested before deciding on the treatment.

Obviously, achieving this goal has been the motivation for developing numerous assays thought suitable for predictive testing. The test parameters include:

- Cell counting
- DNA synthesis
- Cell viability
- Clonogenic potency
- Energy metabolism, e.g., the activity of mitochondrial enzymes, ATP production, and extracellular acidification

The biochemical methodologies often require procedures leading to irreversible damage of the cells and cell death. As a rule, all these assays require multiple replicates of samples if different time points are to be included in the protocol.

The multitude of different biochemical assays that can be employed to detect changes in cellular metabolism, growth behavior, and cell death calls for a multiparametric test system that would:

- Accommodate several such parameters
- Be applicable to even a single tissue sample
- Collect data without damaging (or otherwise affecting) the cells

A test system answering to these demands has been developed during the last years. It is based on growing cells or tissues on multiparametric sensor chips. At the heart of this system is a chip made of silicon or glass decorated with various sensors (Fig. 1). The size of the culture area on the chip ranges from a few square millimeters to 100 mm^2, thus requiring only small cell or tissue samples. The main difference between these two chip materials is that glass chips can be used for microscopy, whereas silicon chips are easier to produce. The sensors on both chips can include, for example:

- FET: field effect transistors or
- Electrode structures for detecting changes in O_2
- ISFET: ion sensitive field effect transistors, which are used to measure changes in extracellular pH
- IDES: interdigital electrode structures, which can detect changes in the electric current depending on the cells' membrane properties and morphology

Because the tissue or cells grow directly on the sensor, the measurements document changes in the immediate environment of the cells.

Basic Experimental Setup

A prerequisite for the biological and medical application of the glass hybrid or silicon chips is that cells will retain their functional and growth properties when in contact with the sensor material. Numerous experiments have demonstrated that carcinoma cells of various origins will adhere and grow under appropriate culture medium conditions (Ehret et al. 1997; Lehmann et al. 2001). The chips, associated growth chambers, and tubing can be sterilized with sodium hypochlorite. An important feature of the test system is that the cells are perfused with culture medium, thereby ensuring a continuous supply of nutrients while metabolic waste products are removed.

Adherent tumor cell lines LS174T as well as S180 and its doxorubicin-resistant counterpart were used. Cells were trypsinized, seeded on to the chips at $2\text{–}4\times10^3$ cells/mm^2, and precultured under standard conditions in medium (RPMI) with 10% FCS. The chips were set into the apparatus immediately before beginning the measurements. To increase the sensitivity of the measurements, the culture medium used for the perfusion (at 37°C) was modified (Henning at al. 2001), mainly omitting bicarbonate and HEPES buffers; the volume on the chip was about 50 µl. Sensor signals were monitored during time intervals when the fluid flow was interrupted, and online data was collected on a PC with appropriate software. At the end of the experiment, the cells were lysed with 0.1% Triton X-100 to give baseline sensor signals.

Breast cancer explants from surgery were minced and enzymatically disintegrated to obtain a collection of single cells. These were seeded on to the chips and preincubated before beginning the measurements within 24 h after explantation. Further details have been published by Henning et al. (2001).

Application of Sensor Chips for Chemosensitivity Testing

Tumor Cell Lines

To establish the applicability of the sensor chips for biomedical testing, cancer cell lines were tested for their growth behavior. The human colon carcinoma cell line LS174T has been used for studying the effect of various drugs on metabolic parameters, namely changes in pH and O_2 consumption. The metabolic profile of these cells shows a steady increase in the rate of oxygen consumption during a 24-h incubation period, whereas the rate of acidification remains fairly constant.

The epithelial-like properties of these cells are manifested in a basolateral orientation to the growth substrate and by the formation of a monolayer. This allows morphological changes to be monitored by following changes in the electrical capacity of the cell population.

The addition of cytochalasin B to these cells, which not only results in disruption of the actin filaments but also inhibits glucose uptake, has profound and rapid effects on cellular morphology and metabolism (Fig. 2) (Ehret et al. 2001). Within minutes, cellular metabolism was suppressed as indicated by a diminished rate of acidification, which reflects a reduction in glucose utilization, i.e., glycolysis. At the same time, there is an increased consumption of oxygen , which is indicative of a compensatory oxidative utilization of amino acids. The increased capacitance values of the impedance sensors in the cell

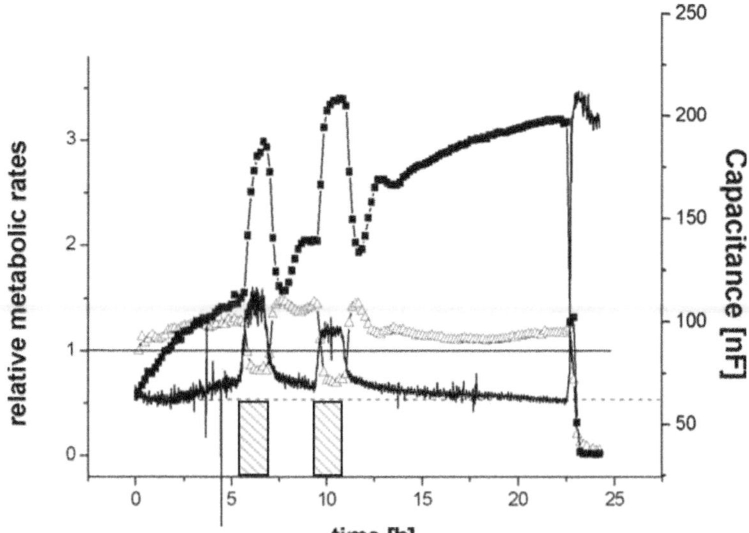

Fig. 2. Effect of cytochalasin B on metabolic and morphological parameters of LS174T cells as detected by a multiparametric glass sensor chip. Bars indicate the time interval at which cytochalasin B (1 μg/ml) was present in the culture medium. ■, changes in pO_2; °, changes in pH; –, capacitance

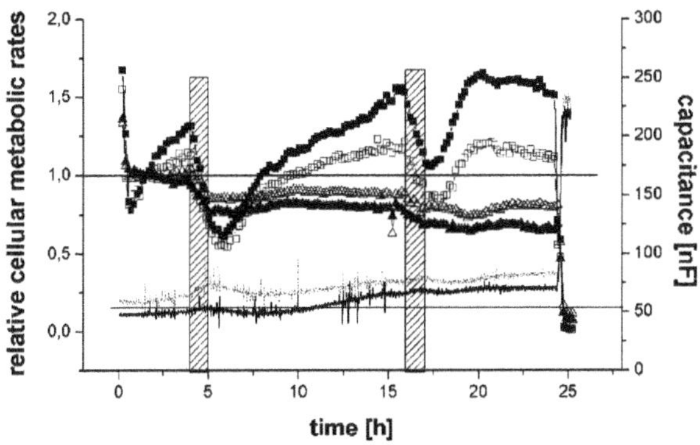

Fig. 3. Growth of colon carcinoma cell line LS 174T on silicon chips: Effects of transient exposure to chloroacetaldehyde (50 μM) at the times indicated by the bars. Each condition was done in two parallel setups. Depicted are rate of changes in pO_2 (❑, ■) and in pH (°, ▲), and capacitance (–, –)

culture reflects retraction of cell–cell contacts and less substrate adhesion, which was confirmed by microscopic observations. On removal of cytochalasin B, the cells quickly returned to their normal metabolic and morphological state. Thus this experiment demonstrates that anaerobic and aerobic metabolic functions, along with morphological changes, can be monitored rapidly and simultaneously in the same cell culture.

Another experiment with LS174T cells growing on silicon chips demonstrates the transient effects of chloroacetaldehyde, an alkylating metabolite from the cytostatic drug ifosfamide (Fig. 3). This type of drug has been shown to act on nucleic acids, proteins, and membrane phospholipids (Skipper et al. 1951), and it also had marked, albeit different, effects on the cellular metabolism: Within minutes the rate of respiration (i.e. O_2 consumption) was reduced, with little change in the acidification rate. On removal of the drug, cellular respiration recovered, with biphasic kinetics in the first instance and a more rapid and uniform recovery in the second instance. At the same time, little change was observed in the impedance measurements, suggesting that, at least for the monitored incubation time of 25 h, the drug had apparently no prolonged effect on cellular morphology or membrane properties.

To demonstrate the reproducibility of the measurements, two parallel cultures were used each for control and for the treatments: Fig. 3 shows that the results of the parallel cultures were virtually identical.

Monitoring Sensitive and Resistant Tumor Cells

For predictive chemotherapeutic testing with the multiparametric sensor chip, a central question is by which criteria sensitive and resistant cells can be distinguished. To compare the metabolic and morphological changes on drug treatment, the mouse sarcoma cell line S180 and doxorubicin-resistant S180dox cells were used. The latter cell line is characterized by overexpressing

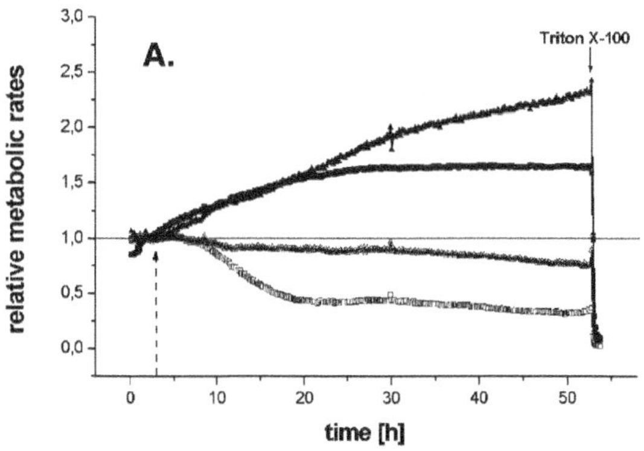

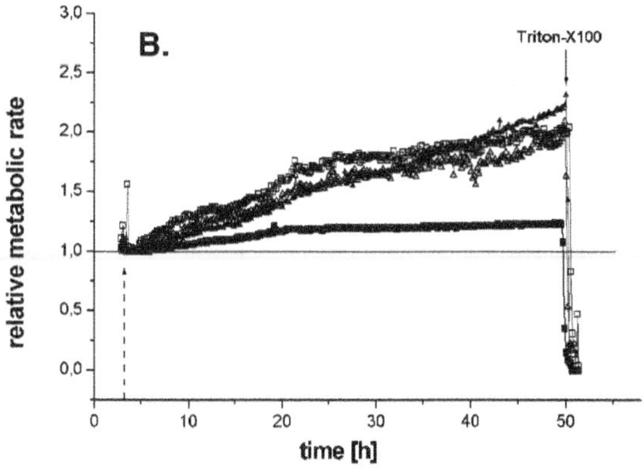

Fig. 4. Effect of doxorubicin on the metabolism of (**A**) sensitive S-180 cells and (**B**) resistant S-180dox cell cultures grown on glass sensor chips. Depicted are the rate of changes in pO_2 (■) and pH (▲) in control cultures, and the rate of changes in pO_2 (❑) and pH (°) upon perfusion with doxorubicin (10 µg/ml) beginning at the time indicated by the dashed line

glutathione *S*-transferase-π and shows a 340-fold resistance toward doxorubicin (Volm et al. 1992). This drug intercalates into DNA and produces semichinon radicals, which cause DNA strand breaks. As shown in Fig. 4A, the drug-sensitive S180 cells plated on glass chips grow well over an incubation period covering 52 h, as indicated by the continuous increase in the rate of extracellular acidification and in the rate of oxygen consumption for at least up to 20 h. Treating these cells with doxorubicin resulted in the expected growth inhibition, which is seen in a reduction in the rate of extracellular acidification and, more markedly, in a reduced rate of oxygen consumption (Fig. 4A).

Cultures of the drug-resistant S180dox cells growing without doxorubicin show changes in the metabolic parameters similar to those of their untreated "normal" counterparts. However, addition of doxorubicin had no inhibitory effects on S180dox cells and, on the contrary, even led to a increased rate of oxygen consumption (Fig. 4B). The metabolic profiles of these cells, therefore, reflect their differences in drug sensitivity.

The differences between S180 and S180dox cells were also manifested when impedance was monitored after repeated additions of doxorubicin (not shown). Growth of untreated S180 and S180dox cells gradually increased impedance. Addition of doxorubicin suppressed this increase in the sensitive S180 cells, whereas doxorubicin had no effect on the impedance of the resistant S180dox cells, which is consistent with the unaffected metabolic parameters (Fig. 4B).

Tumor Specimens

With these results, the next step was to use the multiparametric sensor chips for monitoring tumor tissue. Figure 5 shows the growth of primary tumor cells from a breast cancer explant on multiparametric glass sensor chips. There is more heterogeneity in the signals than with cell lines, probably because of the heterogeneous properties of the cell population. In general, in untreated cultures little overall change was observed in O_2 consumption, whereas the acidification rate increased, indicative of cell proliferation. In contrast, the parallel culture, which had received chloroacetaldehyde, showed a very rapid decline in the respiration rate to a basal signal level within about 2.5 h, whereas the acidification rate of the culture declined more gradually up to about 22 h. Thus, as also observed in the previous experiments, changes in pH and pO_2 did not follow the same kinetics, indicating that different regulatory mechanisms underlie these processes. Most importantly, this experiment shows that the sensitivity of a tumor explant to drug treatment can be monitored on sensor chips.

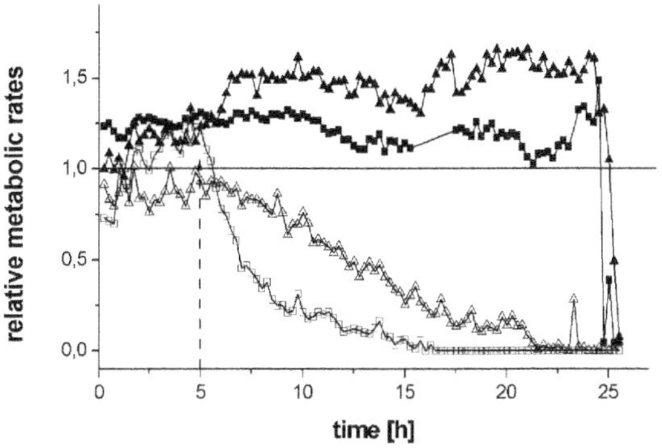

Fig. 5. Growth of breast cancer explants on glass sensor chips, one culture without and the other culture with addition of chloroacetaldehyde at the time indicated by the dashed line. Control cultures: rate of changes in pO_2 (■) and pH (▲); perfusion with chloroacetaldehyde (50 μM): rate of changes in pO_2 (❑) and pH (°)

Discussion

Multiparametric sensor chips were developed for monitoring in a cell culture or on a tissue probe metabolic activities and rapid changes in membrane properties continuously and virtually simultaneously. The experimental results demonstrate that this sensor technology can indeed serve chemotherapeutic testing by virtue of fulfilling criteria expected of a reliable chemosensitivity assay, the first and foremost being the monitoring of living cells, the rapid and continuous acquisition of data (up to at least 50 h), the low amount of cellular sample required, and reproducibility. The cardinal feature of the sensor system combined with a perfusion fluidic system, however, is the possibility of multiparametric monitoring of both metabolic and morphological signals.

The metabolic monitoring of tumor cells or cell lines may by itself already give important information on the state of the cells. Although the colon carcinoma-derived cell line LS174T is characterized by an increase in the rate of respiration (Figs. 3, 4), the oxygen consumption levels off in sarcoma cell line S180. On the other hand, S180 continuously increase their rate of acidification, whereas there is little change in the pH in LS174T cultures. Thus these two cell types differ in their basic metabolism: The LS174T appear to have a high rate of oxidative metabolism, whereas glycolysis has a greater part in the S180 cells.

Differences in the metabolic profile also occur depending on the drug treatment and may thereby provide information on a possible mechanism of action: Whereas cytochalasin B increases oxygen consumption but inhibits acidification, i.e., glycolysis (Fig. 3), chloroacetaldehyde decreases the oxidative metabolism dramatically and acidification lags behind with a gradual and moderate decrease (Figs. 4A, 5). Whether a prolonged increase in oxygen consumption is a characteristic of drug resistance, as might be concluded from the response of the S180dox cells to doxorubicin (Fig. 4B), remains to be established with further drugs and tumor cells.

In the future, the metabolic profile of tumor cells and of drug-treated cells will be expected to provide valuable information, which could help to distinguish between resistant and sensitive tumors and to decide on the most promising treatment. Moreover, monitoring morphological changes, reflecting cell-cell and cell-substrate contacts, will complement our judgment on the integrity and social behavior of tumor tissue.

References

Ehret R, Baumann W, Brischwein M, Schwinde A, Stegbauer K, Wolf B (1997) Monitoring of cellular behaviour by impedance measurements on interdigitated electrode structures. Biosens Bioelectron 12:29–41

Ehret R, Baumann W, Brischwein M, Lehmann M, Henning T, Freund I, Drechsler S, Friedrich U, Hubert M.-L, Motrescu E, Kob A, Palzer H, Grothe H, Wolf B (2001) Multiparametric microsensor chips for screening applications. Fresenius J Anal Chem 369:30–35

Henning T, Brischwein M, Baumann W, Ehret R, Freund I, Kammerer R, Lehmann M, Schwinde A, Wolf B (2001) Approach to a multiparametric sensor-chip-based tumor chemosensitivity assay. Anti-Cancer Drugs 12:21–32

Lehmann M, Baumann W, Brischwein M, Gahle H-J, Freund I, Ehret R, Drechsler S, Palzer H, Kleintges M, Sieben U, Wolf B (2001) Simultaneous measurement of cellular respiration and acidification with a single CMOS ISFET. Biosens Bioelectron 16:195–203

Skipper HE, Bennet HL, Langham WH (1951) Overall tracer studies with C14-labeled nitrogen mustard in normal and leukemic mice. Cancer 4:1025

Volm M, Efferth T, Mattern J, Pommerenke EW (1992) Resistance mechanisms in murine tumors with acquired multidrug resistance. Arzneim Forsch 42:1163–1168

Development of a New In Vitro Chemosensitivity Test Using Collagen Gel Droplet Embedded Culture and Image Analysis for Clinical Usefulness

Hisayuki Kobayashi

Biochemical Laboratory, Nitta Gelatin Inc., 2-22 Futamata, Yao-City, Osaka 5810024, Japan
e-mail: hi-kobayashi@nitta-gelatin.co.jp

Abstract

The results of chemotherapy are not fully satisfactory in many cases, particularly solid cancers. Therefore, it seems useful if the effective anticancer drugs can be selected for each patient using the screening methods. In such a background, we developed a new anticancer-drug sensitivity testing method that overcame several defects in the existing method, which is the collagen gel droplet embedded culture drug sensitivity test (CD-DST) and satisfies the following requirements: a high success rate, ability to assay biopsy specimens, and quantification of the anticancer effects without contamination with fibroblasts. Under the biological exposure condition, the sensitivities of the cancers were similar to their clinical response rate and there was a statistically significant correlation between clinically reported response rates and the response rates obtained by CD-DST ($P<0.01$). Furthermore, the true positive rate was 79.8%, and the true negative rate was 88.8%. Sensitivity and specificity were 88.2% and 80.6%, respectively, resulting in an overall predictive accuracy of 84.1% (154/183). The CD-DST not only shows high predictive accuracy for humans, but because of the high correlation between the results of in vitro and nude mice assays, if it also is practical as a pre-clinical screening, it can easily provide these predictions.

Introduction

The prediction of chemosensitivity of a patient to the use of an anticancer drug not only contributes to the improvement of a cancer chemotherapy as regards the medical treatment results, but can also avoid medication with an invalid anticancer drug. For effective cancer chemotherapy, chemosensitivity testing of anticancer drugs should be performed with fresh surgical specimens and biopsy obtained from the cancer. The results of chemotherapy are not fully satisfactory in many cases, particularly in solid cancers. Therefore, it seems useful if effective anticancer drugs can be selected for each patient by the screening methods. In the 1990s, a number of new drugs (paclitaxel, docetaxel, vinorelbine, gemcitabine, etc.) became available to treat solid cancers in Japan. Although we now have many choices, there is no single drug that shows high clinical response. Therefore, it has been more important to select the most effective drug for each patient with chemosensitivity screening methods. The development and clinical introduction of the chemosensitivity test for realizing the effective and proper use of an anticancer drug have been desired strongly in the clinical setting. Various chemosensitivity tests have been studied and developed. The nude mouse method [1–3] proposed by Rygaard [4] in 1969 was expected to be an ideal model for predicting the antitumor effects in humans. However, it has not been used as a routine method for clinical use because of its low efficiency and high cost and the long time required for evaluation. For similar reasons, the subrenal capsule assay (SRC) proposed by Bogden [5, 6] has not been used widely. As evaluation systems, the human tumor clonogenic assay (HTCA) [7–9] thymidine incorporation assay (TIA) [10–12], succinic dehydrogenase inhibition assay (SDI) [13] and MTT assay [14, 15] have been developed, but no methods that have yet been applied practically to clinical cases. In such a background, we developed a new anticancer drug sensitivity testing method that overcame several defects in the existing method, which is the collagen gel droplet embedded culture drug sensitivity test (CD-DST), and its clinical practicality has been reported [16–18]. In this review, we introduce recent results and describe the clinical usefulness of CD-DST method.

The Characteristics of CD-DST

At first, we would like to describe the collagen gel droplet embedded culture method itself. A human solid cancer consists of cancer cells, normal cells, blood cells, and extracellular matrix (ECM). We tried to reproduce a minimum environment that mimicked the in vivo situation by using type I collagen gel as shown in Fig. 1. As advantages of this culture method, high colony

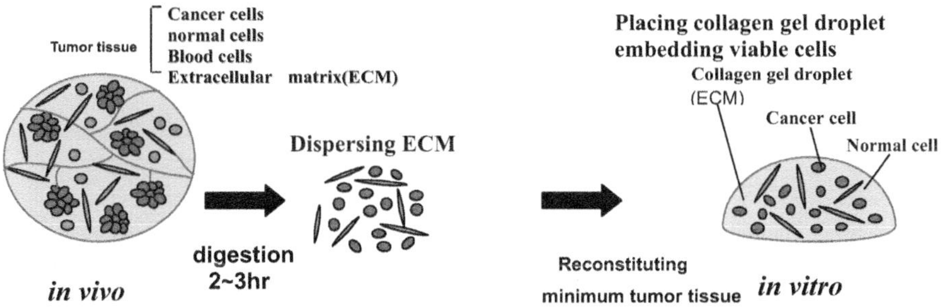

Fig. 1. The concept of the collagen gel droplet embedded culture

Table 1. The exposure conditions in CD-DST

Drug	Concentration (μg/ml)	Exposure time (h)	Clinical dose	AUC (in vitro/human)[a]
MMC	0.03	24	20 mg/body	1.05
CDDP	0.2	24	100 mg/m^2	1.67
DXR	0.02	24	60 mg/m^2	0.98
VDS	0.01	24	2 mg/m^2	0.8
VP-16	1.0	24	300 $mg/m^2 \times 3$	1.94
5-FU	1.0	24	600 mg/m^2 (bolus)	0.92
CBDCA	2.0	24	450 mg/m^2	0.72
DOC	0.1	24	60 mg/m^2	0.83
NVB	0.05	24	25 mg/m^2	1.05
PAC	1.0	24	210 mg/m^2	1.03
EPI	0.1	24	40 mg/m^2	1.2

[a]1.0=same as clinical AUC.

efficiency in primary cancer cell culture, behavior of cells similar to that in vivo, and a possible reproduction of in vivo phenomena have been reported, and its usefulness was indicated [19–23]. The cell number was reduced to 3×10^3 per droplet in the present CD-DST. This has an advantage over HTCA or TIA, both of which require 5×10^5 cells/well. Moreover, when this method was applied to the anticancer drug sensitivity test, anticancer activity was evaluated at drug concentrations similar to those secured in vivo (Table 1). Sensitivity matching closely with clinical efficacy and a high prediction rate of clinical efficacy has been obtained [17]. Particularly, in the case of the area under the drug concentration-time curve (AUC)-dependent anticancer drugs, a high correlation with anticancer activity was obtained [24] when in vivo pharmacokinetics was reproduced in CD-DST. And we introduced the new method of colorimetric quantitative determination on images for evaluation of anticancer effect in simple live cancer cells alone, which was based on the difference in the proliferating morphology and stainability with neutral red of cells within collagen gel drops, using video-micro scope and the NIH Image macro-program. The CD-DST satisfies the following requirements:

- A high success rate for primary culture
- A small number of cells being required for the test
- Easy quantification of the anticancer effects without contamination with fibroblasts
- Good correlation of anticancer effects with clinical response
- A rapid and simple method

In Vitro Drug Sensitivity Test

Collagen Gel Droplet Embedded Culture

Figure 2 shows the process of the CD-DST method. Briefly, primary human solid cancers were prepared from fresh specimens collected at the time of surgery or biopsy. Each sample was treated with Dispersion Enzyme Cocktail EZ (Nitta Gelatin Inc., Osaka, Japan). The cell suspension obtained was inoculated into collagen-coated flasks (CG-flask, Nitta Gelatin Inc.) and cultured in preculture medium PCM-1 [containing 10% fetal bovine serum (FBS)] at 37°C in 5% CO_2 overnight. Next, collagen gel was digested with 0.05% collagenase (type I, Sigma-Aldrich Japan, Tokyo, Japan) and viable cancer cells were obtained. Type I collagen (Cellmatrix Type CD, Nitta Gelatin Inc.), 10x F-12 medium, and reconstitution buffer were mixed together in ice water in a ratio of 8:1:1. The prepared cancer cell suspension was added to the collagen solution with the final density being 1×10^5 cells/ml. Three drops of the collagen-cell mixture (30 μl/droplet) were placed in each well of a six-well multiple plate on ice and allowed to gel at 37°C in a CO_2 incubator; the final concentration was about 3×10^3 cells per collagen gel droplet. DF medium containing 10% FBS was overlaid on each well 1 h later and incubated in a CO_2 incubator at 37°C overnight.

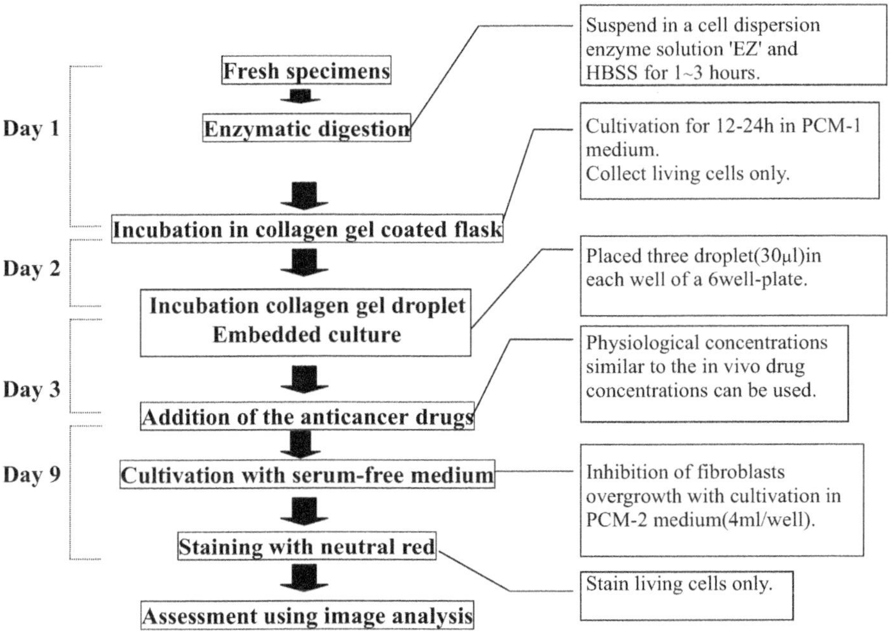

Fig. 2. The process of the CD-DST method

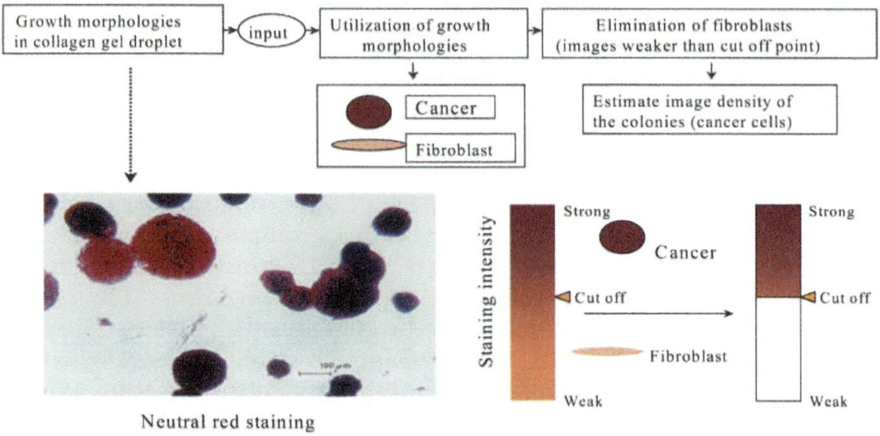

Fig. 3. Principle of measurement by imaging colorimetric quantification method. Step 1: Acquire image of cancer cells (deeply stained) and fibroblasts (lightly stained) in collagen gel stained with neutral red. Step 2: Eliminate fibroblasts on the image by critical value procedure. Step 3: Convert image density of the remaining cancer cells on the image to optical density. (From [18])

In Vitro Chemosensitivity Test

The anticancer drugs were added at the final concentrations shown in Table 1 and incubated for 24 h. After removal of the medium containing the anticancer drugs, each well was rinsed twice with 3 ml of Hanks' balanced salt solution (HBSS) each time, overlaid with 4 ml of PCM-2 medium (serum-free medium, Nitta Gelatin Inc.), and incubated for a further 7 days. At the end of the incubation, neutral red was added to each well at a final concentration of 50 μg/ml and colonies in the collagen gel droplets were stained for 2 h. Each collagen droplet was fixed with 10% neutral-buffered formalin, washed in water, air dried, and quantified by image analysis (Fig. 3). The growth rates of control incubations were calculated as the image density on day 7/image density on day 1. Cases with more than 0.8 growth rates were regarded as evaluable cases.

Growth of Human Cancer Cells in Collagen Gel Droplet

Figure 4 shows the growth of cancer cells in collagen gel and soft agar. In collagen gel droplet embedded culture, the colonies are much larger in size and more colonies are formed than in soft agar culture. The cloning efficiency of lung, breast, colon, and gastric cells cultured in collagen gel droplet is overwhelmingly higher than that for the soft agar culture (Fig. 5) [25]. The morphology of human lung cancer cells grown in the collagen gel droplets is shown in Fig. 6. As we reported previously [17], lung cancer cells in collagen gels grew with a three-dimensional spherical morphology, mimicking their in

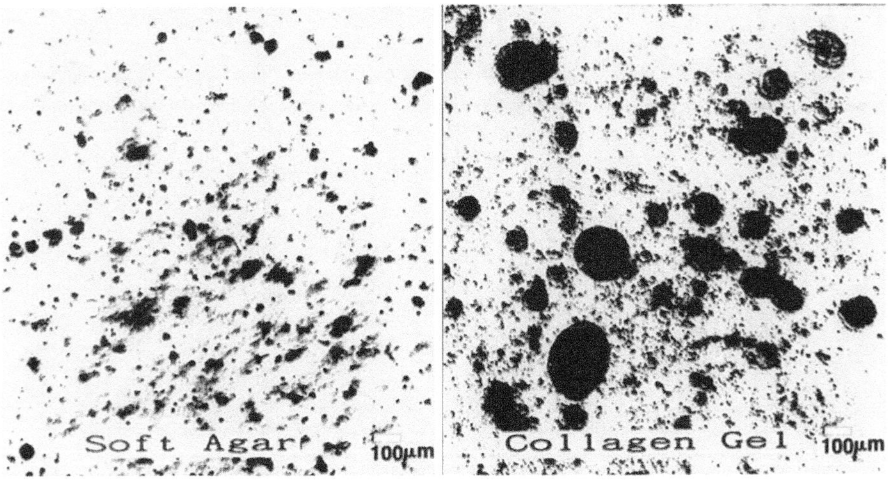

Fig. 4. Growth of colon cancer cells in soft agar and in collagen gel droplet (10-day culture) In collagen gel droplet culture, the colonies were much larger in size and a much larger number of colonies were formed than in soft agar culture. (From [25])

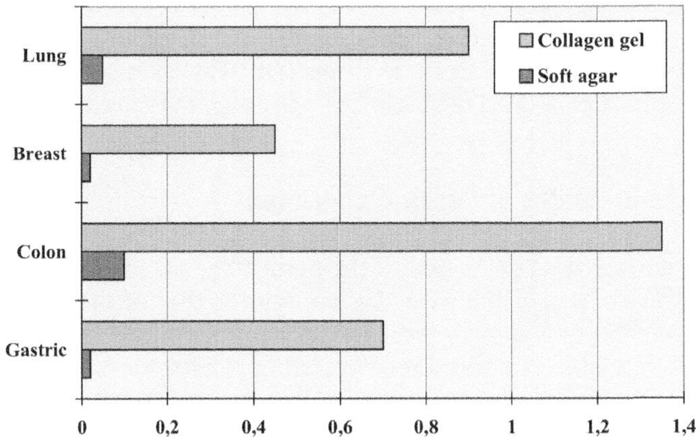

Fig. 5. Comparison of cloning efficiency between collagen gel (CG) and soft agar culture

vivo characteristics, whereas fibroblasts showed a bipolar extension (Fig. 6A). Furthermore, lung cancer cells were densely stained with neutral red, whereas staining was light for fibroblast cells, as shown in Fig. 6B.

Establishing the In Vitro Exposure Conditions of Anticancer Drugs

The in vitro exposure conditions of MMC, CDDP, VDS, VP-16, 5-FU, and DOX were established by means of correlation between the results of the clinically equivalent dose (CED) nude mice assay and those of CD-DST [16]. It was re-

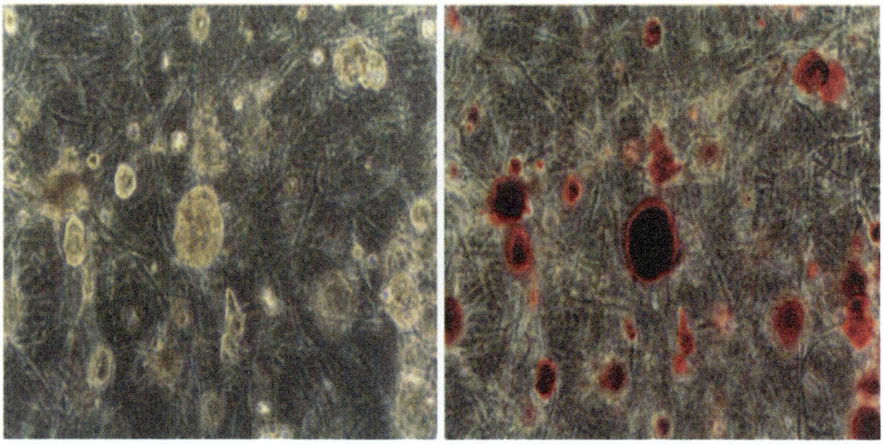

A B

Fig. 6. Morphologies of human primary cancer cell and fibroblast cell in collagen gel droplet (7-day culture). **A** Stained with 10% neutral buffered formalin. **B** Stained with neutral red. Bar, 100 µm

ported that the results of the CED nude mice assay showed a good correlation to the clinical response rate [26, 27]. As each in vitro AUC of the six drugs investigated closely resembled the clinical AUC, we tried to establish the exposure conditions of other anticancer drugs (CBDCA, DOC, PAC, EPI, CPA and VNR) by reproducing those AUCs of the administered clinical dose (Table 1).

Assay-Evaluable Rates of Surgical Specimens

In vitro sensitivity was expressed as the percentage T/C ratio, where T was the image optical density of the treated group and C that of the control group; a T/C ratio of 50% or less was regarded as demonstrating in vitro sensitivity. The overall evaluable rate was 83%, consisting of 82% for 659 lung cancer cases, 81% for 163 breast cancer cases, 85% for 92 gastric cancer cases, 83% for 107 colon cancer cases, 85% for 13 esophagus cancer cases, 100% for 17 pancreas cancer cases, 100% for 8 biliary tract cancer cases, and 88% for 32 metastatic brain tumor cases (Table 2). The reasons for why some of the cases were not evaluable included an insufficient number of tumor cells (less than 1×10^5 in the initial assay) and incomplete growth of control cells during the culture period. There were no statistically significant differences in the evaluable rates of the different carcinomas by χ^2-test.

Drug Sensitivity Studies

In vitro sensitivity and clinical response rate are shown in Table 3. We used a χ^2-test for statistical analysis. There were no statistically significant differ-

Table 2. Evaluable rates of surgical specimens in the CD-DST

	Lung (NSCLC)	Breast	Gast.	Colon	Eso.	Panc.	Bil.	Metast. brain	Total
No. of cancers treated	659	163	92	107	13	17	8	32	1,091
Evaluable cases	543	132	78	89	11	17	8	28	906
Evaluable rate(%)	82	81	85	83	85	100	100	88	83

Table 3. In vitro sensitivity (IVS) and clinical response rates (CRR) of several cancers to individual drugs

Cancer type		MMC%	CDDP%	5-FU%	DXR%	VDS%	VP-16%
Lung[a]	IVS	23.9	23.4***	ND	ND	30.1	30.4
	CRR	19	25	ND	13	22	18
Breast	IVS	14.8**	13.8*,**b	27.9*,**	36.1*,***	ND	ND
	CRR	20	8	26	37	15	6
Gastric	IVS	26.8	14.3*	35.3*	19.5*	ND	ND
	CRR	31	25	23	34	0	8
Colon	IVS	17.9	6.0***	16.1	7.1***	ND	ND
	CRR	18	0	17	5	8	ND

In vitro drug sensitivity was defined as positive when T/C ratio was 50% or less.

*$P<0.05$; **$P<0.01$; ***$P<0.001$ by χ^2-test.

[a]Non-small cell lung cancer.

ND, not done. Complete response (CR) and partial response (PR) were regarded as effective.

*Range of response rate (%); **No. of response/No. of evaluated patients.

ences in the sensitivity of non-small lung cancer to MMC, CDDP, VDS, and VP-16. The sensitivity of breast cancer to 5-FU was significantly higher than to MMC and CDDP ($P<0.01$), and the sensitivity to DXR was significantly higher than to MMC ($P<0.05$). The sensitivity of gastric cancer to 5-FU was higher than to CDDP and DXR ($P<0.05$). The sensitivity of colon cancer to CDDP and DXR was significantly lower than that of lung and breast cancer, respectively ($P<0.001$). The sensitivities of all cancers were similar to their clinical response rate (CRR), and there was a statistically significant correlation between clinically reported response rates [28–31] and the response rates obtained by CD-DST ($P<0.01$, $r=0.702$) [17].

Assay-Evaluable Rates of Biopsy Specimens

The biopsy specimens of 5–10 pieces were collected from various internal organ cancers, and enforcement of CD-DST was tried. The samples tested included 136 specimens of lung cancer, 58 specimens of breast cancer, 25 specimens of gastric cancer, and 13 specimens of esophagus cancer. The evaluable

Table 4. Evaluable rates of biopsy specimens in the CD-DST

	Breast	Lung			
	Incisional or VCNB	Bronchoscopy	Pleural fluid	Gastric endoscopy	Esophageal endoscopy
No. of cancers treated	58	129	7	25	13
Evaluable cases	49	45	5	18	9
Evaluable rate(%)	85	35	71	72	69

Major factors limiting culture included insufficient cell yield (<10^4cells).
VCNB; vacuum-assisted core needle biopsy.

rates of breast (incisional or vacuum-assisted core needle biopsy), lung (bronchoscopy and pleural fluid), gastric (endoscopy), and esophageal (endoscopy) cancer were 85%, 35%, 71%, 72%, and 69%, respectively (Table 4). The major limiting factor of culture was insufficient cell yield (less than 10^4 cells). The evaluable rates of all specimens except those resulting from bronchoscopy were generally more than 70%, so these results showed the possibility of clinical usefulness of CD-DST. In contrast, about 74% of the bronchoscopical specimens in lung cancer could not be set up because of poor viability cells (less than 10^4 cells). This suggested that a new resection method was required.

Predictive Accuracy

One hundred eighty-three patients with measurable lesions who received chemotherapy tested by CD-DST had their in vitro sensitivities compared with the clinical response. All patients received chemotherapy with a single agent or a combination regimen using the anticancer drugs listed in Table 1. Clinical response was assessed according to WHO criteria, with complete response (CR) and partial response (PR) being regarded as clinical responders. Seventy-five patients were evaluated as being true positives, 79 patients were assessed as true negatives, and 19 patients were regarded as being false positives. There were 10 false negative cases; the true positive rate was 79.8%, and the true negative rate was 88.8%. Sensitivity and specificity were 88.2% and 80.6%, respectively, resulting in an overall predictive accuracy of 84.1% (154/183) (Table 5).

The Possibilities of CD-DST

Some results of the clinical research that adopted the CD-DST are introduced in the following section.

Table 5. Predictive accuracy in the CD-DST

CD-DST/Clinical response	S/S	S/R	R/S	R/R	Total
Lung (NSCLC)	44	13	5	46	108
Breast	24	3	4	26	57
Gastric	4	3	0	3	10
Esophagus	2	0	1	1	4
Brain	1	0	0	3	4
Total	75	19	10	79	183

True positive rate: 79.8% (75/94); true negative rate: 88.8% (79/89); predictive accuracy: 84.1% (154/183).

S; sensitive; R; resistant. Sensitivity: 88.2% (75/85); specificity: 80.6% (79/98).

Non-Small Cell Lung Cancer

In Japan, the rate of lung cancer is increasing every year, and 80% of cases are the so-called non-small cell lung cancer. Among these, the ratio of operation adaptation will remain about 30%, and about 70% of cases will depend on radiotherapy and chemotherapy by anticancer drugs. When stage I cancer cases are removed from the cases of operation adaptation, the prognosis is very poor and the medical treatment strategy at the time of a recurrence is a big issue. In such a situation, we are examining whether chemosensitivity determination by CD-DST is useful for the chemotherapy of non-small cell lung cancer. To clarify the usefulness of CD-DST, it is important to prove that survival period is extended by treatment based on a chemosensitivity examination. In our investigation, it is becoming clear that chemosensitivity and prognosis are independent factors. The MST of a resistant group treated with the effective drug obtains a result significantly better than that of the resistant group receiving standard medical treatment, radiotherapy, and the best supportive care [32]. Moreover, the results of CD-DST with the surgically resected specimens of primary non-small cell lung cancer correlated significantly with chemotherapeutic response in patients with postoperative recurrence. This result significantly exceeded the results of experiential chemotherapy by clinicians [33].

Breast Cancer

The CD-DST result with biopsy specimens performed before operation for recurrence or advanced breast cancer and the results of a neoadjuvant chemotherapy are compared. The CE (cyclophosphamide+epirubicin) treatment or the DOC (docetaxel) treatment was enforced as a neoadjuvant chemotherapy. The evaluation of good efficiency of CD-DST with biopsy specimens was over 80%, and its practicality was strongly suggested. Moreover, the predictive accuracy of biological markers, such as P-gp, bcl-2, p53, erbB-2, MIB1, and ER, was also examined simultaneously. The results accumulated so far suggest that the highest predictive accuracy resulted from CD-DST. And the time to progression of the sensitive group treated with the effective drug is obtaining a result significantly better than that of the resistant group which received one of chemotherapies [34]. Future research on non-small cell lung cancer and breast cancer must collect and evaluate more data.

Future of CD-DST

CD-DST made it possible to test with fewer cells than the conventional in vitro examining method (MTT assay, HTCA). I think that a chemosensitivity testing method must be a growth assay for us to predict the clinical effect. In fact, CD-DST is a growth assay method and its evaluable rate is high [17]. In recent years, development of the cell viability assay (ATP-CVA) [35] and tumor chemosensitivity assay (ATP-TCA) [36–38], with sensitivity higher than that of the MTT assay and the possibility of using a low few number of cells, has been reported. In particular, ATP-TCA is a growth assay, and the high evaluable rates of this method in a breast cancer or an ovarian cancer have been reported [39]. Moreover, reports have mentioned that because the fibroblast cells of the tumor tissue affect sensitivity, chemosensitivity testing in conditions with coexisting fibroblast cells is important [40, 41]. However, fibroblast cells will not increase but will die from the floating cultivation by agar or culture medium, without the opportunity for performing functional discovery, because the fibroblast cell is an anchorage-dependent cell. Therefore, the cultivating method using ECM, which can carry out functional discovery of the fibroblast cell for reproducing the sensitivity of the in vivo situation, is suitable. For this reason, CD-DST included three-dimensional culture using a collagen gel with ECM. Moreover, because CD-DST with serum-free medium includes minimum essential growth factors, function of the fibroblast cell is promoted rather than proliferation. Consequently, we think that this method might lead to high predictive accuracy for clinical response. In future, we think the in vitro chemosensitivity test will have to meet the following requirements: (1) a quick adaptation in a new anticancer drug, (2) a prediction of clinical response by the improved combination of chemotherapy and prescribing method for the individual patient (for example, 5-FU civ injection, Taxol weekly injection, etc.), and (3) a relation with molecular biological factors. These requirements must be met for the global spread of in vitro chemosensitivity testing. Regarding the possibility of quick adaptation in a new anticancer drug and improved predictability of clinical response to treatment by the prescribed method, this seems to be easy because the anticancer drug exposure conditions of CD-DST can be set up by reproducing pharmacokinetics in the living body. The CD-DST can actually reproduce some methods of prescribing 5-FU for the patient by changing exposure time and concentration. And the result approximates the clinical effect in colon cancer and gastric cancer (Table 6).

Table 6. Effect of 5-FU by exposure condition

Material	10 µg/ml 3 h	1.0 µg/ml 24 h	0.2 µg/ml 120 h	0.4 µg/ml 120 h
Gastric	30.8%[a]	35.3%	18.5%	–
Colorectal	0%	16.1%	10.5%	–
Meta-liver (colorectal)	–	–	–	40.9% (9/22)

[a]In vitro sensitivity rate.

Conclusion

To improve a cancer patient's chemotherapy results and QOL, after the so-called research of chemosensitivity can begin, a considerable time has passed. Various methods have been developed and verified in the period. In Japan, CD-DST, the MTT assay, and HDRA have been adopted by many researchers and clinicians. Moreover, in the U.S., the extreme drug resistant assay (EDRA) [42, 43] and the DiSC-assay [44, 45] have been adopted. In Europe, ATP-TCA, the DiSC assay, and the MTT assay have been adopted by many researchers. To reach worldwide acceptance of these methods, it cannot be overemphasized that it is necessary to carry out RCT (randomized control trial). We think it is necessary to convince a clinician or physician logically. With the possibility of meeting their requirement for more closely reproducing the environment in the living body, we think that the CD-DST method can be equivalent to various anticancer drugs or the most standard prescribing method. CD-DST not only shows high predictive accuracy for humans, but because of the high correlation between the results of in vitro and nude mice assays [24], if it also is practical as a pre-clinical screening, it can easily provide these predictions. This required that many researchers evaluate the clinical usefulness of CD-DST by itself.

Acknowledgements. I greatly appreciate all those who were very helpful to me in the writing of this review: Prof. S. Noguchi, Dr. Y. Takamura, Prof. K. Kobayashi, Dr. M. Kawamura, Dr. K. Kodama, Dr. M. Higashiyama, Dr. Koezuka, Prof. S. Kodaira, Dr. Y. Hanatani, Dr. T. Mori, Dr. T. Yamaguchi, Dr. M. Morishita, Dr. K. Aiba, Prof. M. Kitajima, and Dr. T. Kubota. Moreover, I express my thanks to those who provided technical support: Mr. K. Minamigawa, Ms. N. Yoneda, and Mr. T. Takano.

References

1. Osieka R et al (1977) Chemotherapy of human colon cancer xenografts in athymic nude mice. Cancer 40:2640–2650
2. Countenay VD, Mills J (1978) An in vitro colony assay for human tumours grown in immune-suppressed mice and treated in vivo with cytotoxic agents. Br J Cancer 37:261–268
3. Fujita M et al (1984) Chemosensitivity of human gastrointestinal and breast cancer xenografts in nude mice and predictability to clinical response of anti-cancer agents. In: Immune-Deficient Animals. 4th Int workshop on immune-deficient animals in exp res. Karger, Basel, pp 311–315

4. Rygaard J, Povlsen CO (1969) Heterotransplantation of a human malignant tumour to "Nude" mice. Acta Pathol Microbiol Scand 77:758–760
5. Bogden AE (1978) A rapid screening method for testing chemotherapeutic agents against human tumor xenografts. In: Symposium on the use of athymic (nude) mice cancer research. Gustav, New York, pp 231–250
6. Bogden AE (1984) Predictive testing with the subrenal capsule assay. Cancer Treat Rev 11:113–124
7. Salmon SE (1978) Quantitation of differential sensitivity of human-tumor stem cells to anticancer drugs. N Engl J Med 298:1321–1327
8. Von Hoff DD et al (1981) Human tumor cloning: feasibility and clinical correlations. Cancer Chemother Pharmacol 6:265–271
9. Rozencweig M et al (1984) In vitro growth of human malignancies in a cloning assay. Recent Results in Cancer Res 94:1–7
10. Tanigawa N et al (1982) Rapid assay for evaluating the chemosensitivity of human tumors in soft agar culture. Cancer Res 42:2159–2164
11. Kern DH et al (1985) Development of miniaturized, improved nucleic acid precursor incorporation assay for chemosensitivity testing of human solid tumors. Cancer Res 45:5436–5441
12. Tanigawa N et al (1992) In vitro growth ability and chemosensitivity of gastric and colorectal cancer cells assessed with the human tumor clonogenic assay and thymidine incorporation assay. Eur J Cancer 28:31–34
13. Kondo T et al (1966) In vitro test for sensitivity of tumor to carcinostatic agents. Jpn J Cancer Res 57:I13–121
14. Mosmann T (1983) Rapid calorimetric assay for cellular growth and survival, application to proliferation and cytotoxicity assays. J Immunol Methods 65:55–63
15. Carmichael J et al (1987) Evaluation of a tetrazolium-based semiautomated colorimetric assay: Assessment of chemosensitivity testing. Cancer Res 47:936–942
16. Kobayashi H et al (1995) Development of new in vitro chemosensitivity test using collagen gel droplet embedded culture and its clinical usefulness. Jpn J Cancer Chemother 22 (13):1933–1939 (in Japanese)
17. Kobayashi H et al (1997) An in vitro chemosensitivity test for solid human tumors using collagen gel droplet embedded cultures. Int J Oncol 11:449–455
18. Kobayashi H et al (2001) Examination of in vitro chemosensitivity test using collagen gel droplet culture method with colorimetric endpoint quantification. Jpn J Cancer Res 92 Feb:203–210
19. Jason Y et al (1979) Sustained growth and three-dimensional organization of primary mammary tumor epithelial cells embedded in collagen gels. Proc Natl Acad Sci USA 76:3401–3405
20. Lawler EM et al (1983) Significance of three-dimensional growth patterns of mammary tissues in collagen gels. In Vitro 19:600–610
21. Enami J et al (1987) Growth of normal and neoplastic mammary epithelial cells of the mouse by mammary fibroblast conditioned medium factor. In: Enami J, Ham RG (eds) Growth and differentiation of mammary epithelial cells in culture. Scientific Societies Press, Tokyo, pp 125–153
22. Miller BE et al (1985) H. Factors affecting growth and drug sensitivity of mouse mammary tumor lines in collagen gel cultures. Cancer Res 45:4200–4205
23. Sinha DK, White CJ (1988) Collagen gel culture of rat mammary tumor cells as an assay system for determination of therapeutic efficacy of chemotherapeutic agents. In Vitro Cell Develop Biol 24:525–529
24. Inaba M et al (1996) In vitro-in vivo correlation in anticancer drug sensitivity test using AUC-based concentrations and collagen gel droplet embedded culture. Oncology 53:250–257
25. Koezuka M et al (1993) Drug sensitivity test for primary culture of human cancer cells using collagen gel embedded culture and image analysis. Int J Oncol 2:953–959
26. Inaba M et al (1986) Evaluation of response rates to various antitumor agents of human gastric tumors implanted in nude mouse. Jpn J Cancer Res 77:190–196

27. Tashiro T et al (1989) Responsiveness of human lung cancer / nude mouse to anticancer agents in a model using clinically equivalent doses. Cancer Chemother Pharmacol 24:187–192
28. Bakowski MT (1983) Chemotherapy of non-small cell lung cancer: a reappraisal and look to the future. Cancer Treat Rev 10:159–172
29. Haskell CM et al (1985) Breast cancer. In: Haskell CM (ed) Cancer treatment, 2nd edn. pp137–180
30. Ramming KP, Haskell CM (1983) Stomach cancer. In: Haskell M (ed) Cancer treatment, 2nd edn. pp 257–271
31. Tominaga T (1986) Chemotherapy for advanced and recurrent colorectal cancer. Jpn Cancer Chemother 13 (7):2298–2306 (In Japanese)
32. Kawamuta M et al (2001) Order-made therapy for early lung cancer patients. Kyobu Geka 54:962–967 (in Japanese)
33. Higashiyama M (2001) Cisplatin-based chemotherapy for postoperative recurrence in non-small lung cancer patients: Relation of the in vitro chemosensitive test to clinical response. Oncol. Reports 8:279–283
34. Takamura Y et al (2002) Prediction of chemotherapeutic response by collagen gel droplet embedded culture drug sensitivity test in human breast cancers. Int J Cancer 98:450–455
35. Koechli OR et al (1993) Application of the adenosine triphosphate-cell viability assay in human breast cancer chemosensitivity testing: A report on the first results. J Surg Oncol 54:119–125
36. Andreotti PE (1995) Chemosensitivity testing of human tumors using a microplate adenosine triphosphate luminescence assay: Clinical correlation for cisplatin resistance of ovarian carcinoma. Cancer Res 55:5276–5282
37. Cree IA et al (1996) Correlation of the clinical response to chemotherapy in breast cancer with ex vivo chemosensitivity. Anti-Cancer Drugs 7:630–635
38. Cree IA et al (1997) Measurement of cytotoxicity by ATP-based luminescence assay in primary cell cultures and cell lines. Toxicol in Vitro 11:553–556
39. Kurbacher CM et al (1998) Use of an ex vivo ATP luminescence assay to direct chemotherapy for recurrent ovarian cancer. Anti-Cancer Drugs:51–57
40. Cree IA et al (1994) Elucidation of molecular determinants of tumor chemosensitivity by ATP-based luminescence assay. In: Campbell AC, Stanley PE, Kricka LJ (eds) Chemiluminescence and bioluminescence. Wiley, Chichester, pp 407–410
41. Fidler IJ et al (1994) Modulation of tumor cell response to chemotherapy by the organ environment. Cancer Metast Rev. 13:209–222
42. Kern DH et al (1990) High specific prediction of antineoplastic drug resistance with an in vitro assay using suprapharmacologic drug exposures. J Natl Cancer Inst 82 (7):582–588
43. Kern DH et al (1998) Heterogeneity of drug resistance in human breast and ovarian cancer. Cancer J Sci Am 4 (1):41–45
44. Nagourney RA et al (1990) enhancement of anthracycline and alkylator cytotoxicity by ethacrynic acid in primary cultures of human tissues. Cancer Chemother Pharmacol 26:318–322
45. Bosanquet AG et al (1996) Enhanced ex vivo drug sensitivity testing of chronic lymphocytic leukaemia using refined DiSC assay methodology. Leukemia Res 20 (2):143–153

In Vitro Chemosensitivity Testing of Hematological Cancer Patients: Detection of Ornithine Decarboxylase

Uriel Bachrach, Yongchun Wang

U. Bachrach (✉)
Department of Molecular Biology Hebrew University-Hadassah,
Medical School, P.O. Box 12272, Jerusalem, Israel
e-mail: bachur@md2.huji.ac.il

Abstract

The development of reliable methods for the in vitro testing of sensitivity of cancer cells to various drugs has been a longstanding objective in cancer research and treatment. Early attempts to develop individualized chemotherapy were based on clonogenic assays. These attempts failed because of low plating efficiencies. Nonclonogenic assays, such as the MMT test or ATP determinations, are based on metabolic activities and do not reflect the ability of cells to proliferate. To detect proliferation, we selected a universal marker - ornithine decarboxylase (ODC), which is expressed early in the cell cycle and has a short half-life. This marker was detected in hematological cancer cells by quantitative immunohistochemical analyses using an ODC antibody and a FITC-linked second antibody. Drug resistance was detected in five patients, who subsequently died. Lymphocytes from normal individuals were sensitive to all drugs tested, whereas 33 leukemia and lymphoma patients showed different sensitivities to certain drugs. The method also permitted testing of the effect of new drugs on the proliferation of lymphocytes from hematological cancer patients. This test is sensitive, and 100–1,000 cells are required per assay, which can be completed within 2 days. It is very likely that the assay could also be used to test solid tumor patients.

Introduction

Despite many advances in understanding of carcinogenesis, including detection of oncogenes and suppressor genes and measurement of estrogen receptors, the mortality rates from solid tumors remain stubbornly high. Surgery, radiotherapy, and chemotherapy are currently the major means to treat cancer patients. Tumors of the same type show heterogeneity of chemosensitivity, and many patients develop drug resistance, leading to relapse. This heterogeneity of chemosensitivity is unpredictable and may be one explanation for the poor results of chemotherapy. Therefore, many patients are treated with ineffective agents and are exposed to undesired side effects, which are certainly without benefit. Clinicians face a similar problem when patients suffering from infectious diseases need antimicrobial treatment. In this case, drugs are given to the patients after susceptibility assays are performed. It is therefore not surprising that the development of reliable methods for the in vitro testing of sensitivity and/or resistance of cancer cells to various drugs has been a longstanding objective in cancer research and treatment. Attempts to develop individualized chemotherapy started more than 20 years ago (Hamburger and Salmon 1977). Those early studies were based on clonogenic assays, which show the effect of anticancer agents on cell division. These studies gave satisfactory results only when cultured cell lines were tested. On the other hand, poor results were obtained when clonogenic assays were applied to tumor cells isolated from patients. This was mainly due to low plating efficiency; only 1%–2% of the cells are capable of growing in culture (Salmon et al. 1987). In vitro chemosensitivity tests, based on clonogenic assays, failed to meet initial expectations, and subsequent attention was focused on nonclonogenic assays, which were mainly based on the effect of the drugs on the metabolic activity of the tumor cells (Cree and Kurbacher 1997). The MMT (3-[4,5-dimethylthiazol-2-yl]-2,5-diphenyl-tetrazolium bromide) assay was one of the earliest developed nonclonogenic assays (Bellamy 1992). In this assay, which requires relatively large numbers of cells, cell viability is detected by the formation of colored or fluorescent products from substrates added to the cells. Another test, the ATP-tumor chemosensitivity assay (ATP-TCA), is based on the loss of ATP from dead cells (Ahmann et al. 1987). This test has been improved recently with the use of firefly luciferase (Lundin et al. 1986). A commercially available test kit (TCA-100, DCS Innovative Diagnostic Systeme, Hamburg, Germany) permits the standardization of the assay and makes the test relatively easy. The ATP-TCA showed good evaluability (97% in a series of breast cancer biopsies) and has good correlation with clinical outcome of breast (Cree et al. 1996) and ovarian (Kurbacher et al. 1998; Konecny et al. 2000) cancers. The assay requires 20,000 cells per assay and lasts for at least 6 days.

The above-described nonclonogenic assays suffer from a serious drawback: They are based on the effect of the drugs on the metabolic activities of the cells rather than the effect on cell proliferation. It is well known that dead cells, or even cellular extracts, can be active metabolically. The best method would be to grow the tumor cells isolated from patients in vitro in the presence or absence of drugs. As mentioned above, this approach is not practical because of low plating efficiency. It therefore appears that cellular proliferation of primary human tumor cells cannot be determined by in vitro cultures and that other approaches should be explored. In recent studies we suggested (Wang et al. 1999, 2000) the use of a *marker for proliferation* rather than *growing* the cells in cultures. It would be of advantage if the test were fast and if

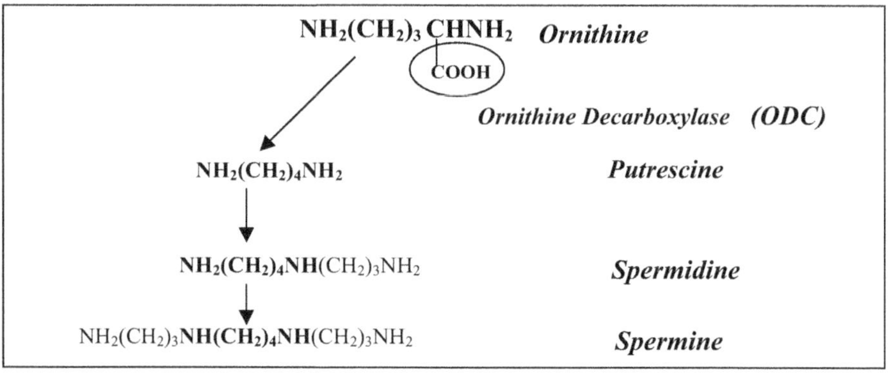

Fig. 1. Ornithine decarboxylase and the biosynthesis of polyamines

the marker could be detected in individual cells, so that tumor cells could be identified and distinguished from normal cells such as fibroblasts.

An ideal marker should meet the following requirements:

1. It should be universal.
2. It should be expressed during the early stages of the cell cycle.
3. It should have a short half-life, so that it would decay rapidly when cell proliferation is arrested.

Ornithine decarboxylase (ODC, E.C. 4.1.1.17) can serve as a marker for proliferation (Russell 1985; Cohen 1998). This enzyme catalyzes the conversion of ornithine into the diamine putrescine (Fig. 1), which is the precursor for the synthesis of the naturally occurring polyamines (Cohen 1998). The polyamines spermidine and spermine play an essential role in growth and proliferation processes. ODC is present in all cells studied, and its induction is mediated by hormones, lectins, and antigens (Russell 1985), which induce transmembrane signals (Flamigni et al. 1999). Additionally, it is expressed early in the cell cycle and has an extremely short half-life (15–20 min), the shortest of any eukaryotic cell (Russell 1985).

Recent studies from our laboratory demonstrated that ODC could indeed serve as a marker for proliferation (Bachrach et al. 1994). Moreover, ODC was used to determine the chemosensitivity of various cultured cells to different anticancer drugs (Assaraf et al. 1994; Shayovits and Bachrach 1995). In those studies, the in vitro chemosensitivity of the cultured cells was assessed by determining the *enzymatic activity* of ODC. This assay requires at least 10^6 cells and does not permit the study of individual cells. To detect ODC in individual cells, an immunohistochemical staining method was used. This method permitted the detection of ODC in individual cultured cells (Shayovits and Bachrach 1994).

The chemosensitivity of lymphocytes from hematological cancer patients was next studied, because of the following considerations:

- Availability of a suspension of cancer cells without surgical intervention
- Possibility of obtaining blood samples for repeated tests
- The test is based on determining the effect of drugs on the proliferation of cancer cells rather than studying the effect on metabolic activities
- The number of cells required is relatively small (100–1,000 cells per assay)
- The test permits the study of individual cells and the identification of cancer cells by morphological studies or by the use of an anticancer antibody
- The test is relatively fast, and results can be obtained within 2 days

The above-described considerations also suggest that the ODC-tumor chemosensitivity assay has a number of advantages over the nonclonogenic assays.

Materials and Methods

Patients

Cancer patients were treated in the Department of Hematology, Shaare Zedek Medical Center, Jerusalem, Israel. Blood samples were obtained from 40 cancer patients and 6 healthy individuals after informed consent.

Tumor Chemosensitivity Assay

The procedure was essentially that described elsewhere (Wang et al. 1999) and can be summarized as follows. To obtain lymphocytes, heparinized fresh blood was mixed with an equal volume of DMEM medium and layered on Ficoll-paque (Pharmacia Biotech, Uppsala, Sweden) at a ratio of 4:1. After centrifugation at 1,500 rpm for 25 min, lymphocytes were collected and washed twice with DMEM medium by centrifugation at 1,200 rpm for 10 min. Lymphocytes were then suspended in complete RPMI 1640 medium (containing 50 U/ml penicillin, 50 μg/ml streptomycin, and 15% autologous plasma) supplemented with 2 μg/ml phytohemagglutinin (Sigma). The stimulated cells were incubated at 37°C in a 5% CO_2 incubator, with or without four anticancer drugs at four or five concentrations. After 24 h, lymphocytes were washed with phosphate-buffered saline by centrifugation at 1,200 rpm for 10 min. Slides were prepared either by dropping the cells on slides coated with L-polylysine (Sigma, 1:10 in double-distilled water) or by using cytospin at 1,500 rpm for 5 min. Slides were dried at room temperature for 2 h and then fixed with cold (–20°C) methanol for 2.5 min. Slides were next rinsed twice with phosphate-buffered saline and incubated with 1% bovine serum for 30 min at room temperature in a humidified box. Slides were then kept overnight at 4°C with rabbit anti-human ODC antibodies (prepared in our laboratory by recombinant DNA technologies). After repeated rinsing, the slides were exposed for 1 h at 37°C to FITC-conjugated Affinipure goat anti-rabbit

IgG antibody (Jackson, West Grove, Pa., USA). Finally, the slides were washed four times with phosphate-buffered saline and covered with a mounting solution (90-5 glycerol, 10% phosphate-buffered saline, pH 10.0, 0.1% sodium azide, and 5% 3,3'-diaminobenzidine). Specimens were examined with a confocal laser scanning microscope, Phoibos 1000 (Sarastro, Sweden) at 370 mV.

The procedure is summarized as follows:

1. Blood samples (2–5 ml) are added to heparin and DMEM medium
2. Samples are layered on Ficoll-paque and lymphocytes are sedimented
3. Lymphocytes are incubated overnight in RPMI 1640 medium, antibiotics, phytohemagglutinins, and autologous plasma in the presence or absence of drugs (4 drugs, 5 dilutions)
4. Sedimented lymphocytes are dropped on slides coated with polylysine
5. Slides are dried at room temperature for 2 h and treated with cold methanol for 2.5 min
6. Slides are incubated with bovine serum albumin for 30 min
7. Slides are incubated overnight with human ODC antibodies
8. Slides are exposed for 1 h to FITC-conjugated goat anti-rabbit antibodies
9. Slides are covered with a mounting solution
10. Slides are examined with a confocal laser microscope, Phoibos 1000

Results and Discussion

Recent studies indicated that two important weapons could be added to our arsenal to combat cancer. One is the prevention of the disease. This can be achieved by improving the environment and by selecting a proper diet. The second is to develop "tailored" cancer therapy, optimized to individual patients. Patients with apparently identical tumor histologies do not always respond identically to the same drug regimen. Therefore, individualized chemotherapy could improve anticancer treatment.

In the present study we have described a newly developed method for individualized tumor chemosensitivity assays. This test is based on measurement of the effect of the drugs on cellular proliferation rather than determination of the effect of the drugs on cellular metabolism, which is the basis of other nonclonogenic assays. Ornithine decarboxylase, which serves as a marker of proliferation, is detected by immunohistochemical methods and a confocal laser microscope. This microscope is not readily available in clinical laboratories, and the work with this instrument is rather laborious. The procedure could be simplified by using a peroxidase-linked second antibody and staining the slides to detect the hydrogen peroxide formed. A cell sorter has also been used to separate and quantitate ODC-containing cells. Attempts are now made to develop an ELISA assay for the immunological detection of cellular ODC.

Some of the results of chemosensitivity assay of hematological cancer patients are depicted in Table 1. The results of the tests were not known to the

Table 1. Results with ornithine decarboxylase chemosensitivity assays

Patients (number)	Results	Reference
Normal controls		
4	Sensitive to all four drugs tested	Wang et al. 1999
2	Sensitive to all four drugs tested	Unpublished
Deceased		
3	Resistant to all four drugs tested	Wang et al. 1999
2	Resistant to all four drugs tested	Unpublished
Chronic myelocytic		
5	Sensitive to various drugs	Wang et al. 1999
3	Sensitive to various drugs	Unpublished
Leukemia, mild cases		
20	Sensitive to some drugs	Wang et al. 1999
5	Sensitive to some drugs	Unpublished
Bone marrow		
1	Resistant to four drugs	Wang et al. 2000
Leukemia		
1	Ara-C, dose response	Unpublished
New compound	Green tea polyphenol	Unpublished

oncologists at the time of making the decision and therefore did not affect the choice of regimen.

It may be seen that lymphocytes of six healthy individuals were sensitive to all four of the anticancer drugs tested. Five patients did not respond to therapy and died. The chemosensitivity assay revealed that their lymphocytes were resistant to all four drugs tested, and they may therefore be regarded as multiple drug-resistant patients. It has been suggested (Von-Hoff et al. 1983), that the real benefit of the in vitro systems may lie in predicting not which drugs to administer but rather which drugs not to administer. The multiple drug-resistant patients are the best examples for that approach. Unlike the patients who died, 33 patients suffered from mild hematological cancers; they responded to chemotherapy, in parallel with the results of the ODC chemosensitivity assays (Table 1).

The ODC-chemosensitivity assay was also applied to bone marrow of a patient suffering from multiple myeloma (Wang et al. 2000). The assay showed (Table 1) that the cells were resistant to four anticancer drugs, and the patient was therefore considered as being multiple drug resistant. The patient died shortly thereafter.

This assay suggests that the ODC cancer chemosensitivity test can also be applied for examining bone marrow. Obviously, more extensive studies should to be carried out confirm the reliability of the assay.

The ODC-cancer chemosensitivity assay can also be used to define the optimal dose for treatment with an anticancer agent. A leukemia patient was treated with Ara-C (Table 1). The result of the assay showed that the dose of the drug used by the clinician was too low and that increasing the concentration of the drug would lead to inhibition of cellular proliferation. Independently, the oncologists increased the concentrations of Ara-C, and, indeed, this caused improvement. This experiment suggests that the method can be used for determining the optimal dose for chemotherapy. Obviously, more extensive studies should to be carried out confirm the reliability of the assay.

Cancer chemosensitivity assays can also be used for in vitro testing of new drugs or their combinations (Cree et al. 1999). In the present study we tested the effect of the green tea polyphenol epigallocatechin gallate (EGCG) on the proliferation of leukemic blast cells (Table 1). It has been shown (unpublished data) that 20 μM EGCG inhibited proliferation as measured by the ODC cancer chemosensitivity assay.

Although individualization of chemotherapy is theoretically attractive, past attempts to provide such information by using clonogenic assays have produced many papers and little progress. The use of nonclonogenic assays, including the ATP-TCA assay, showed promising leads and oncologists started to modify their treatment according to the results of the in vitro assays. The possibility of testing the effect of new drugs and their combinations opens new horizons for cancer chemotherapy. Avoidance of unnecessary suffering, injury, or harm should be considered in oncology decision-making (Smith and Bodurtha 1995). If side effects can be reduced and therapies that are not effective can be excluded, funds can be saved and the anticancer treatment can be improved considerably.

In the present communication we propose the use of a new technology for cancer chemosensitivity assays. We found the assay useful in testing the sensitivity of lymphocytes from hematological cancer patients, but the application of the methodology for testing solid tumors is also conceivable. Even if at the beginning, consistent failures have led many oncologists to abandon in vitro assays, there is no rational alternative in sight (Cree and Kurbacher 1997). Recent studies thus bring the notion of "tailored" cancer therapy for individual patients to near reality.

Conclusions

Despite major advances made in cell biology and oncology, we have not witnessed a striking breakthrough in cancer therapy. The development of "tailored" cancer therapy for individual patients could improve the chance of survival. We have recently developed an in vitro chemosensitivity assay for the prediction of the response of cancer cells to anticancer drugs. This assay is based on the use of ornithine decarboxylase (ODC) as a marker for proliferation. The disappearance of the marker in cells treated with a drug would predict their sensitivity, whereas the persistence of the marker would suggest that the cells are drug resistant. This method differs from most other in vitro cancer chemosensitivity assay by measuring cell proliferation rather than monitoring the effect of drugs on cell metabolism. The presence or absence of the marker was measured by an immunohistochemical method.

When hematological cancer patients were studied, drug resistance was detected in five patients, who subsequently died. Lymphocytes from normal individuals were sensitive to all of the drugs tested, whereas 33 leukemia and lymphoma patients showed different sensitivities to certain drugs. The method was also applied to testing of a bone marrow specimen, and it was also useful for predicting the dose of the drug that would be most effective. In addition, the ODC tumor chemosensitivity assay was used to study the therapeutic potential of new drugs. Thus a green tea polyphenol demonstrated significant anticancer activity. It is our hope that this method will add to the known in vitro chemosensitivity assays, provide a better treatment for cancer patients, and reduce their suffering induced by inappropriate anticancer agents.

References

Ahmann FR, Garewal HS, Schifman R, Celniker A, Rodney S (1987) Intracellular adenosine triphosphate as a measure of human tumor cell viability and drug modulated growth. In Vitro Cell Dev Biol 23:474–480

Assaraf YG, Drori S, Bachrach U, Shaugan-Labay V (1994) Determination of multidrug resistance levels in cultured mammalian cells using ornithine decarboxylase activity. Anal Biochem 216:97–109

Bachrach U, Shayovitz A, Marom Y, Ramu A, Ramu N (1994) Ornithine decarboxylase – a predictor for tumor chemosensitivity. Cell Mol Biol 40:957–964

Bellamy WT (1992) Prediction of response to drug therapy. A review of in vitro assays. Drug 44:690–708

Cohen SS (1998) A guide to the polyamines. Oxford University Press, New York

Cree IA, Kurbacher CM, Untch M, Sutherland LA, Hunter EM, Subedi AM, James EA, Dewer JA, Preece PE, Andreotti PE, Bruckner HW (1996) Correlation of the clinical response to chemotherapy in breast cancer with ex vivo chemosensitivity. Anti-Cancer Drugs 7:630–635

Cree IA, Kurbacher CM (1997) Individualizing chemotherapy for solid tumors – is there any alternative? Anti-Cancer Drugs 8:541–548

Cree IA, Neale MH, Myatt NE, de Takats PG, Hall P, Grant J, Kurbacher CM, Reinhold U, Neuber K, MacKie RN, Chana J, Weaver PC, Khoury GG, Sartori C, Andreotti PE (1999) Heterogeneity of chemosensitivity of metastatic melanoma. Anti-Cancer Drugs 10:437–444

Flamigni F, Facchini A, Capanni C, Stefanelli C, Tantini B. Caldarera CM (1999) p44/42 mitogen-activated protein kinase is involved in the expression of ornithine decarboxylase in leukemia L1210 cells. Biochem J 341:363–369

Hamburger AW, Salmon SE (1977) Primary bioassay of human tumor stem cells. Science 197:461–463

Konecny G, Crohns C, Pegram M, Felber M, Lude S, Kurbacher C, Cree IA, Hepp H, Untch M (2000) Correlation of drug response with ATP tumorchemosensitivity assay in primary stage III ovarian cancer. Gynecol Oncol 77:258–263

Kurbacher CM, Cree IA, Bruckner HW, Brenne U, Kurbacher JA, Muller K, Ackerman T, Gilster TJ, Wilhelm LM, Engel H, Mallmann PK, Andreotti PE (1998) Use of an ex vivo ATP luminescence assay to direct chemotherapy for recurrent ovarian cancer. Anti-Cancer Drugs 9:51–57

Lundin A, Hasenson M, Persson J, Pousette A (1986) Estimation of biomass in growing cell lines by adenosine triphosphate assay. Meth Enzymol 133:27–42

Russell DH (1985) Ornithine decarboxylase: a key regulatory enzyme in normal and neoplastic growth. Drug Metab Rev 16:1–88

Salmon SE, Young L, Scuderi P, Clark B (1987) Antineoplastic effects of tumor necrosis factor alone and in combination with gamma-interferon on tumor biopsies in clonogenic assay. J Clin Oncol 5:1816–1821

Shayovits A, Bachrach U (1994) Immunochemical detection of ornithine decarboxylase in individual cells: potential application for in vitro chemosensitivity assays. J Histochem Cytochem 42:607–611

Shayovits A, Bachrach U (1995) Ornithine decarboxylase: an indicator for growth of NIH 3T3 fibroblasts and their c-Ha-*ras* transformant. Biochem Biophys Acta 1267:107–114

Smith TJ, Bodurtha JN (1995) Ethical considerations in oncology: balancing the interest of patients, oncologists and society. J Clin Oncol 13:2464–2470

Von-Hoff D, Clark GM, Stogdill BJ, Sarosdy MF, O'Brian MT, Casper JT, Mattox DE, Page CP, Cruz AB, Sandbach JF (1983) Prospective clinical trial of human tumor cloning system. Cancer Res 43:1926–1931

Wang Y, Ashkenazi YJ, Bachrach U (1999) In vitro chemosensitivity testing of hematological cancers: immunohistochemical detection of ornithine decarboxylase. Anti-Cancer Drugs 10:797–805

Wang Y, Or R, Bachrach U (2000) Chemosensitivity testing of hematological cancers using ornithine decarboxylase as a marker. Int J Med Biol Environ 28:51–56

2 Tumor Chemosensitivity Assays: Evaluation of In Vitro Results

The Chemosensitivity Profile of Retinoblastoma

Federica Di Nicolantonio, Michael Neale, Zerrin Onadim,
John L. Hungerford, Judith L. Kingston, Ian A. Cree

I.A. Cree (✉)
Translational Oncology Research Centre, Department of Histopathology,
Queen Alexandra Hospital, Portsmouth, PO6 3LY, UK
e-mail: ian.cree@port.ac.uk

Abstract

Retinoblastoma is a rare malignant tumour of the developing retina with an incidence of 1 in 20,000 live births in all human races. Chemotherapy is used in retinoblastoma as adjuvant therapy to prevent the growth of metastases and to treat metastatic disease once this has become clinically apparent. Current regimens are based on empirical drug combinations, and few clinical trials have been conducted because of the rarity of this tumour. Chemosensitivity testing offers a way of testing a large number of agents against tumours. The ATP-based chemosensitivity assay (ATP-TCA) has already helped to design new regimens for melanoma and breast and ovarian cancer. Primary retinoblastoma tumour material was obtained from 10 eyes, 7 of which contained sufficient viable cells for ATP-TCA. The results show very high sensitivity to single agents, particularly cisplatin, doxorubicin and vinca alkaloids. Of the anti-metabolites tested, 5-FU is relatively disappointing (although still active), and gemcitabine shows considerable activity consistent with a cytotoxic effect. The shape of the inhibition curves is interesting. There is a plateau effect with the topoisomerase inhibitors and vinblastine, which is not present with the cisplatin. One tumour was much more resistant than the others tested, particularly to vinblastine but also to the topoisomerase inhibitors, which failed to achieve complete kill at any concentration tested, consistent with a multidrug resistance phenotype. Of the combinations (VAC and VEC), the VAC regimen looks marginally more active in the more resistant of the two cases tested to date. These data confirm that retinoblastoma is a rapidly growing malignancy that is very susceptible to cytotoxic drugs of all types. Chemosensitivity testing provides a practical method of testing new regimens before clinical trials in retinoblastoma patients.

Recent Results in Cancer Research, Vol. 161

Introduction

Retinoblastoma is the most common primary intraocular tumour in children, with an incidence of 1 in 15,000–20,000 live births (Finger et al. 1999). More than 90% of cases are diagnosed before 5 years of age, and presentation of retinoblastoma in adults is rare (Biswas et al. 2000).

Successful treatment of retinoblastoma has traditionally depended on surgery and external beam radiation therapy, associated with significant short- and long-term morbidity (reviewed in Wilson et al. 2001). Recently, multiple studies have been published reporting initial experiences with an association of systemic chemotherapy and focal methods as a primary treatment for this type of cancer (Shields and Shields 1999; Friedman et al. 2000).

Chemotherapy is used in retinoblastoma as adjuvant therapy to control intraocular tumour growth with or without radiation, to prevent the growth of metastases and to treat metastatic disease once this has become clinically apparent (Gallie et al. 1996; Kingston et al. 1996; Gunduz et al. 1998). Current regimens are based on empirical drug combinations derived from neuroblastoma treatments, which have been found to work (Gobie et al. 1990; Kingston et al. 1996). Few clinical trials have been conducted because of the rarity of this tumour and the difficulty of funding such trials.

The current regimens in use tend to use the following four drugs:

- Carboplatin
- Etoposide or doxorubicin
- Vincristine

Carboplatin is a less toxic platinum compound than cisplatin but acts similarly by platination of DNA. The platinum adducts are usually repaired by mismatch repair, deficiency of which is associated with greater sensitivity to this agent (Brown et al. 1997). Etoposide is a podophyllin inhibitor of topoisomerase II, an enzyme responsible for unfolding DNA during transcription and replication. It is associated with an increased risk of leukaemia and is therefore rarely used as a first-line drug for other tumour types (Felix 1998). Doxorubicin is an anthracycline inhibitor of topoisomerase II which has recently been shown also to have some activity against topoisomerase I (Foglesong et al. 1992). Vincristine is a vinca alkaloid, one of a class of drugs which inhibit microtubule assembly and are particularly effective against rapidly cycling cell populations.

Metastasis is rare after adjuvant therapy, but potentially devastating. There is a need to design less toxic but equally or more effective regimens with a low risk of mutagenesis which might aid the development of second malignancies (Tucker et al. 1987). This is a particular problem for some alkylating agents (such as cyclophosphamide, which has been used in retinoblastoma) and for etoposide, which is still widely used, although at a dose not expected to cause problems (Shields et al. 1997). Although there is a feeling that more retinal tumours may develop in patients treated with chemotherapy (C.L.

Shields, personal communication), there is as yet no evidence of an increase in second malignancies in retinoblastoma patients.

Chemosensitivity testing offers a way of testing a large number of agents against tumours. The ATP-based chemosensitivity assay (ATP-TCA) method does not require the generation of cell lines, unlike the single previously published study of chemosensitivity testing in retinoblastoma (Chan et al. 1989, 1991). ATP-TCA has already helped to design new regimens for melanoma and breast and ovarian cancer (Myatt et al. 1997; Kurbacher et al. 1998; Cree and Kurbacher 1997; Cree et al. 1999). It can also be used to examine the relationship between chemosensitivity and molecular mechanisms of resistance and sensitivity (Petty et al. 1994; Satherley et al. 2000).

Materials and Methods

Tumours

Material from ten untreated primary retinoblastomas [2 M:8 F, patient median age 5 months (range 2–36 months)] and one skin metastasis from a primary tumour which was not required for diagnosis was taken by a histopathologist under sterile conditions and transported to the laboratory in cell culture medium (DMEM, Sigma, Poole, UK) with antibiotics (100 U/ml penicillin and 100 µg/ml streptomycin, Gibco BRL, Paisley, UK) at 4°C. Of these samples, only six primary tumours and the metastasis contained sufficient viable cells.

ATP-TCA

Cells were obtained from the tumours by a very gentle enzymatic dissociation, usually 75 µg/ml collagenase for 2 h. Viable tumour-derived cells were separated from dead cells and debris by density centrifugation (Histopaque 1077–1, Sigma), washed, counted and resuspended to 100,000 cells/ml. The cells were used to set up ATP-TCA plates according to Andreotti et al. (1995).

Briefly, cells from enzymatic digestion of solid tumour were placed in 96-well polypropylene microplates at 10,000 cells/well with each drug/combination at six doubling dilutions in triplicate from 200% TDC (test drug concentration) to 6.25% TDC. TDCs were 3 µg/ml for cisplatin (CDDP), 0.5 µg/ml for doxorubicin (DOXO), 16 µg/ml for etoposide (ETO), 45 µg/ml for 5-fluorouracil (5-FU), 12 µg/ml for gemcitabine (GEM) and 0.5 µg/ml for vinblastine (VINB).

The plates were then incubated at 37°C in 5% CO_2 for 6 days. The degree of cell inhibition at the end of this period was assessed by measurement of the remaining ATP in comparison with negative control (no drug, MO) and positive control (maximum inhibitor, MI) rows of 12 wells each. ATP was extracted from the cells and measured by light output in a microplate luminometer (Berthold Diagnostic Systems GmbH) after addition of luciferin-luciferase.

Statistics

The percentage inhibition for each drug concentration was calculated as 1–[(Test–MI)/(MO–MI)]*100 using at Excel 97 spreadsheet (Microsoft). For each drug-concentration curve, the area under the curve ($Index_{AUC}$), the sum of the inhibition at each concentration ($Index_{SUM}$), the 50% inhibitory concentration (IC_{50}) and the 90% inhibitory concentration (IC_{90}) were calculated as previously described (Cree 1998).

Results

The results show very high sensitivity to single agents, particularly cisplatin, doxorubicin and vinca alkaloids (Table 1). Of the anti-metabolites tested, 5-FU is relatively disappointing (although still active), and gemcitabine shows considerable activity consistent with a cytotoxic effect. The shape of the inhibition curves is interesting. There is a plateau effect with the topoisomerase inhibitors and vinblastine which is not present with the cisplatin (Fig. 1).

One tumour (Fig. 2) is much more resistant than the others tested, particularly to vinblastine but also to the topoisomerase inhibitors, which fail to achieve complete kill at any concentration tested. This may represent overexpression of MDR1 by a proportion of the cells present, and it would be helpful to check this with immunohistochemistry.

Of the combinations (VAC and VEC), the VAC regimen looks marginally more active in the more resistant of the two cases tested to date.

Discussion

These data confirm that retinoblastoma is a rapidly growing malignancy that is very susceptible to cytotoxic drugs of all types. Based on other tumour types, all these results show significant activity, although in one case none produced complete ATP inhibition consistent with 100% cell kill. This is prob-

Table 1. Median values for AUCs, $Index_{SUM}$, IC_{90} and IC_{50} measured in seven samples. An $Index_{SUM}$ lower than 300 indicates strong sensitivity in the assay, if >95% inhibition is achieved

Drug	$Index_{AUC}$	IC_{90}	IC_{50}	$Index_{SUM}$
Cisplatin	18,409 (17,626–19,021)	18 (6–72)	4 (3–7)	55 (21–135)
Etoposide	17,939 (17,312–18,399)	48 (5–95)	4 (3–5)	51 (29–99)
Doxorubicin	16,963 (16,697–17,621)	17 (6–94)	4 (3–6)	77 (4–127)
Vinblastine	18,769 (11,739–19,041)	11 (6–293)	4 (3–9)	50 (14–256)
5-FU	14,153 (13,915–14,931)	188 (180–195)	12 (11–13)	218 (212–223)
Gemcitabine	18,386 (15,308–19,287)	20 (6–218)	4 (3–5)	50 (4–148)
VEC	18,806 (17,904–19,207)	6 (6–53)	3 (3–4)	21 (9–78)
VAC	19,033 (18,841–19,225)	6 (–)	3 (–)	17 (7–26)

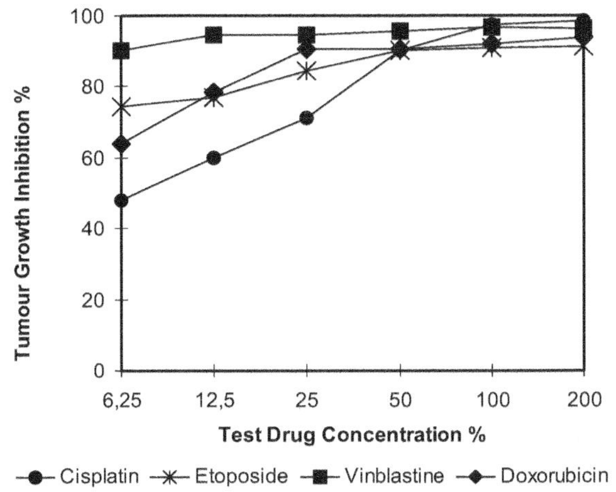

Fig. 1. Example concentration–inhibition curves showing a plateau effect with the topoisomerase inhibitors and vinblastine and not with cisplatin in a retinoblastoma

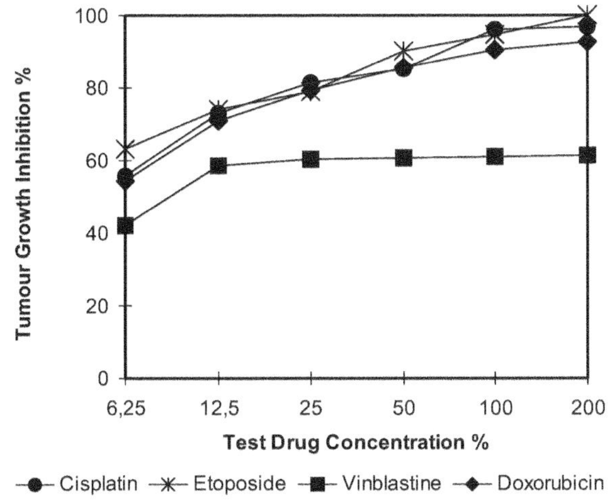

Fig. 2. Example concentration–inhibition curves in a resistant retinoblastoma

ably academic in most patients. The best dose-response effect was seen with cisplatin, which probably indicates that platinum is the most effective drug here. The combination with doxorubicin is likely to be as active as the three-drug combination, and the availability of liposomal preparations (Doxil/Caelyx) should allow high concentrations to be achieved with a lower risk from MDR+ tumours. Addition of an MDR inhibitor in such patients may be more rational than the use of the current three-drug regimen incorporating vincristine.

The major risk to survival in these patients is second malignancy. Etoposide use is associated with haematogenous malignancy and could probably be avoided. The evidence of this study suggests that doxorubicin is equally effective and it does carry lower risk. However, retinoblastoma patients may not behave in the same way as those with other malignancies in this regard, given the propensity for DNA damage to kill rapidly growing cells with Rb mutations.

Drug resistance can occur, and it may arise in several different ways. There is relatively little information on the relative importance of these mechanisms in retinoblastoma, although as a tumour with a relatively simple molecular pathogenesis, it may have much to teach oncology in general. The MDR1/PgP mechanism has been studied in some detail by the Toronto group. Up to 15% of retinoblastomas express the MDR1 drug efflux protein, and there is evidence that resistant cases express MRP (Chan et al. 1997). Cyclosporin, an inhibitor of MDR1, can augment the control of retinoblastoma (Chan et al. 1996), and new inhibitors are in development. Other mechanisms are less well studied: LRP and MRP are alternative drug efflux pump molecules similar to PgP in their function; resistance to DNA-damaging agents could be influenced by anti-apoptotic mechanisms. In retinoblastoma, p53 inactivation and $p21^{Waf1}$ expression have recently been implicated in resistance to apoptosis, as could BCL-2 expression, which also occurs in retinoblastoma (Divan et al. 2001).

Although chemotherapy for retinoblastoma is already very successful, several newer cytotoxic drugs are available with improved side effect profiles and anti-neoplastic activity, including different mechanisms of action. While it would be difficult to justify clinical trials of the large number of different options in retinoblastoma, it would be sensible to explore these options pre-clinically and then conduct a trial against existing practice.

In this study we have shown that ATP-TCA can be used to study the chemosensitivity profile of retinoblastoma samples despite the small numbers of cells available. The results show that this is a very chemosensitive tumour, in keeping with its high growth fraction and the observed clinical efficacy of the drugs tested. Similar data have been produced by Gertjan Kaspers' group in Amsterdam with the MTT assay (Kaspers and Veerman, *vide infra*). This suggests that chemosensitivity testing of retinoblastoma is feasible and that it can be used to improve understanding of the sensitivity to/resistance of retinoblastoma to chemotherapy and to develop new drug combinations.

References

Andreotti PE, Cree IA, Kurbacher CM, Hartmann DM, Linder D, Harel G, Gleiberman I, Caruso PA, Ricks SH, Untch M, Sartori C, Bruckner HW (1955) Chemosensitivity testing of human tumors using a microplate adenosine triphosphate luminescence assay: Clinical correlation for cisplatin resistance of ovarian carcinoma. Cancer Res 55:5276–5282

Biswas J, Mani B, Shanmugam MP, Patwardhan D, Kumar KS, Badrinath SS (2000) Retinoblastoma in adults: report of three cases and review of the literature. Surv Ophthalmol 44:409–414

Brown R, Hirst GL, Gallagher WM, McIlwrath AJ, Margison GP, van der Zee AG, Anthoney DA (1997) hMLH1 expression and cellular responses of ovarian tumour cells to treatment with cytotoxic anticancer agents. Oncogene 15:45–52

Chan HS, Canton MD, Gallie BL (1989) Chemosensitivity and multidrug resistance to antineoplastic drugs in retinoblastoma cell lines. Anticancer Res 9:469–474

Chan HS, Thorner PS, Haddad G, Gallie BL (1991) Multidrug-resistant phenotype in retinoblastoma correlates with P-glycoprotein expression. Ophthalmology 98:1425–1431

Chan HSL, DeBoer G, Thiessen JJ, Budning A, Kingston JE, O'Brien JM, Koren G, Giesbrecht E, Haddad G, Verjee Z, Hungerford JL, Ling V, Gallie BL (1996) Combining cyclosporin with chemotherapy controls intraocular retinoblastoma without requiring radiation. Clin Cancer Res 2:1499–1508

Chan HS, Lu Y, Grogan TM, Haddad G, Hipfner DR, Cole SP, Deeley RG, Ling V, Gallie BL (1997) Multidrug resistance protein (MRP) expression in retinoblastoma correlates with the rare failure of chemotherapy despite cyclosporine for reversal of P-glycoprotein. Cancer Res 57:2325–2330

Cree IA, Kurbacher CM (1997) Individualising chemotherapy for solid tumours – is there any alternative? Anti-Cancer Drugs 8:541–548

Cree IA (1998) Luminescence-based cell viability testing. In: LaRossa RA (ed) Bioluminescence methods and protocols. Meth Molec Biol 102:169–177

Cree IA, Neale MH, Myatt NE, de Takats PG, Hall P, Grant JG, Kurbacher CM, Reinhold U, Neuber K, MacKie RM, Chana J, Weaver PC, Khoury GG, Sartori C, Andreotti PE (1999) Heterogeneity of chemosensitivity of metastatic cutaneous melanoma. Anti-Cancer Drugs 10:437–444

Divan A, Lawry J, Dunsmore IR, Parsons MA, Royds JA (2001) p53 and p21waf-1 expression correlates with apoptosis or cell survival in poorly differentiated, but not well-differentiated, retinoblastomas. Cancer Res 61:3157–3163

Felix CA (1998) Secondary leukemias induced by topoisomerase-targeted drugs. Biochim Biophys Acta 1400:233–255

Finger PT, Czechonska G, Demirci H, Rausen A (1999) Chemotherapy for retinoblastoma. Drugs 58(6):983–996

Friedman DL, Himelstein B, Shields CL, Shields JA, Needle M, Miller D, Bunin GR, Meadows AT (2000) Chemoreduction and local ophthalmic therapy for intraocular retinoblastoma. J Clin Oncol 18:12–17

Foglesong PD, Reckord C, Swink S (1992) Doxorubicin inhibits human DNA topoisomerase I. Cancer Chemother Pharmacol 30:123–125

Gallie BL, Budning A, DeBoer G, Thiessen JJ, Koren G, Verjee Z, Ling V, Chan HSL (1996) Chemotherapy with focal therapy can cure intraocular retinoblastoma without radiotherapy. Arch Ophthalmol 114:1321–1328

Gobie R, McKenzie J, Kingston JE, et al (1990) Orbital recurrence of retinoblastoma successfully treated by combined therapy. Br J Ophthalmol 74:97–98

Gunduz K, Shields CL, Shields JA, Meadows AT, Gross N, Cater J, Needle M (1998) The outcome of chemoreduction treatment in patients with Reese-Ellsworth group V retinoblastoma. Arch Ophthalmol. 116:1613–1617

Kingston JE, Hungerford JL, Madreperla SA, Plowman PN (1996) Results of combined chemotherapy and radiotherapy for advanced intraocular retinoblastoma. Arch Ophthalmol 114:1339–1343

Kurbacher CM, Cree IA, Bruckner HW, Mallmann P, Andreotti PE (1998) Use of an ex vivo ATP luminescence assay to direct chemotherapy for recurrent ovarian cancer. Anti-Cancer Drugs 9:51–57

Myatt N, Cree IA, Kurbacher CM, Foss AJE, Hungerford JL, Plowman PN (1997) The ex vivo chemosensitivity profile of choroidal melanoma. Anti-Cancer Drugs 8:756–762

Petty RD, Cree IA, Sutherland LA, Hunter EM, Lane DP, Preece PE, Andreotti PE (1994) Expression of the p53 tumour suppressor gene product is a determinant of chemosensitivity. Biophys Biochem Res Comm 199:264–270

Satherley K, De Souza L, Neale MH, Alexander RA, Myatt N, Foss AJE, Hungerford JL, Hickson ID, Cree IA (2000) Relationship between expression of topoisomerase II isoforms and chemosensitivity in choroidal melanoma. J Pathol 192:174–181

Shields CL, Shields JA, Needle M, de Potter P, Kheterpal S, Hamada A, Meadows AT (1997) Combined chemoreduction and adjuvant treatment for intraocular retinoblastoma. Ophthalmology. 104:2101–2111

Shields CL, Shields JA (1999) Recent developments in the management of retinoblastoma. J Pediatr Ophthalmol Strabismus 36(1):8–18

Tucker MA, Meadows AT, Boice JD, Stovall M, Oberlin O, Stone BJ, Birch J, Voute PA, Hoover RN, Fraumeni JF (1987) Leukaemia after therapy with alkylating agents for childhood cancer. J Natl Cancer Inst 78:459–464

Wilson MW, Czechonska G, Finger PT, Rausen A, Hooper ME, Haik BG (2001) Chemotherapy for eye cancer. Surv Ophthalmol 45(5):416–444

Chemosensitivity Testing in Malignant Melanoma

Selma Ugurel, Wolfgang Tilgen, Uwe Reinhold

S. Ugurel (✉)
Department of Dermatology, The Saarland University Hospital,
66421 Homburg/Saar, Germany

Abstract

The prognosis of patients with metastatic melanoma remains poor. In patients with distant metastases only low response rates between 10% and 15% have been achieved by the most effective cytostatics in single-agent therapy leading to a mean 5-year survival rate of less than 5%. More aggressive treatment regimens using multidrug chemotherapy yielded response rates of up to 40% but failed to show a significant benefit in overall survival compared to single-agent therapy. However, complete remissions of metastatic lesions after multidrug cytostatic regimens have been reported in some cases of melanoma patients. To evaluate an in vitro test system providing information on the drug sensitivity profile of melanoma cells, we examined tumor tissue specimens from 31 metastatic melanoma patients with an ATP-based chemosensitivity assay (ATP-TCA) testing eight anticancer drugs alone or in different combinations. Chemosensitivity was assessed using a luciferin-luciferase- based luminescence assay providing individual chemosensitivity indices for each test drug. We found a heterogeneous chemosensitivity in the melanoma tissue samples tested. The highest sensitivity was detected for the combination of treosulfan and gemcitabine, with 76% of the tissue samples revealing high sensitivity and 10% resistance, followed by the combination of paclitaxel and doxorubicine (66%/0%), gemcitabine and cisplatin (55%/21%),and paclitaxel and cisplatin (46%/8%). Our data indicate that the ATP-TCA can be used to select patients who might benefit from an individually adapted cytostatic therapy. On the basis of these results a multicenter trial has recently been initiated to evaluate the feasibility and predictive value of an ATP-TCA directed chemotherapy in metastatic melanoma patients.

Recent Results in Cancer Research, Vol. 161

Introduction

Malignant melanoma is known as a tumor entity of high resistance against chemotherapeutic agents [1, 2]. Clinical trials comparing multidrug chemotherapy with treatment regimens using single agents showed increased response rates but no benefit in overall survival in melanoma patients receiving combinations of cytostatic drugs [3]. Thus, the standard chemotherapy for metastatic malignant melanoma remains single-agent therapy with dacarbazine, resulting in response rates of 10%–15% leading to 5-year survival rates of less than 5% [4]. This poor outcome is not the result of an impaired penetration of dacarbazine into the tumor tissue but has been proposed to be due to intracellular resistance mechanisms intrinsic to melanoma cells [5]. However, cases of metastatic melanoma patients who revealed a complete remission of metastatic lesions after multidrug cytostatic treatment regimens have been reported [6–9], suggesting that a subgroup of melanoma patients might gain a long-term benefit from chemotherapy with anticancer drugs other than dacarbazine. Various efforts have been undertaken to identify these patients and to select them for a treatment regimen individually adapted to their chemosensitivity/chemoresistance profile. First in vitro studies using an agarose-based cell culture system combined with measurement of ^{3}H-thymidine uptake revealed heterogeneous sensitivity to different anticancer drugs in melanoma cells freshly obtained from tissue specimens as well as in established melanoma cell lines [10]. In contrast, Schadendorf et al. found both freshly obtained melanoma cells and long-term cultured melanoma cell lines to be moderately to highly chemoresistant with an agarose-based colony-forming assay [11] or the tetrazolium color reaction (MTT test) [12], respectively. Thereafter, no more studies were performed in the field of chemosensitivity testing in melanoma until 1997, when Myatt et al. described heterogeneous chemosensitivity in tumor cells derived from primary uveal melanoma specimens [13]. In this study, the authors used a newly designed test system, the ATP-based tumor chemosensitivity assay (ATP-TCA) (Fig. 1) [14], which was successfully used later on to predict chemosensitivity in patients with recurrent ovarian cancer [15]. Thereafter, a multicenter study was performed testing a larger panel of specimens obtained from tumor lesions from metastatic melanoma patients [16]. Here, the authors again found a considerable heterogeneity of sensitivity against the different cytostatics tested, whereas completely chemoresistant tumors were only occasionally detected.

Based on these promising results, we performed in vitro chemosensitivity testing in patients with metastatic melanoma using the ATP-TCA, followed by a preliminary number of sensitivity-directed treatment regimens in selected patients. The aim of our study was a first evaluation of the feasibility and predictive value of an individually sensitivity-adapted chemotherapy in patients with advanced metastatic melanoma.

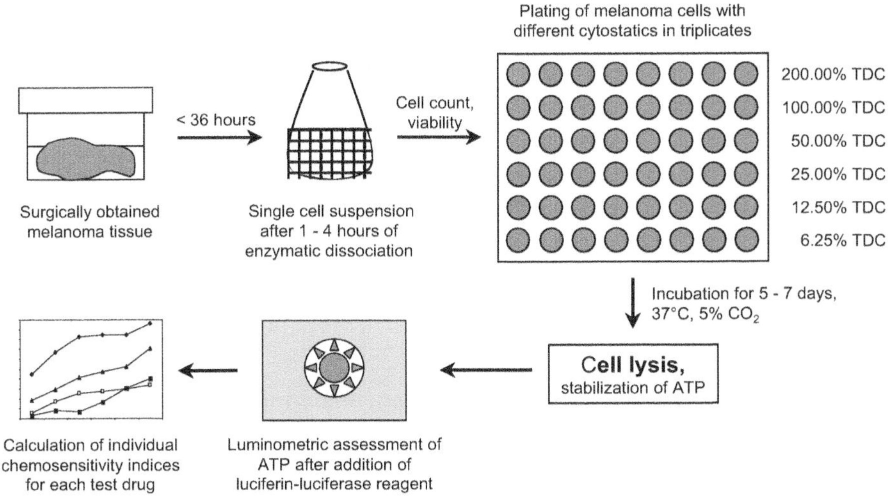

Fig. 1. Principle of chemosensitivity testing using the ATP luminescence method (ATP-TCA). For further details, see "Patients and Methods". TDC, test drug concentration

Patients and Methods

After informed consent was obtained, tumor material was surgically removed from at least one metastatic site of 31 patients with stage IV metastasized malignant melanoma. Clinical staging of patients was performed according to the criteria of the American Joint Committee on Cancer (AJCC) [17], with stage IV consisting of patients with distant metastases. Follow-up was performed in at least 3-month intervals including physical examination, X-ray of the chest, ultrasound of the abdomen and lymph nodes, computer tomography of the brain, scintigraphy of the skeleton, and blood chemistry. Twenty-four patients received treatment before chemosensitivity testing according to therapy protocols of the Dermatologic Cooperative Oncology Group (DeCOG) including cytostatic (dacarbacine, cisplatinum, temozolomide, vincristine) and immunomodulatory (interferon-α) agents in different combinations and schedules.

In vitro chemosensitivity testing of surgically obtained tumor tissue samples was performed with a nonclonogenic ATP-based assay (ATP-TCA, DCS Innovative Diagnostic Systems, Hamburg, Germany) [14]. Briefly, at least 1 cm^3 of tumor material was minced and thereafter enzymatically dissociated. The obtained single-cell suspension was depleted of red blood cells and cellular debris by Ficoll-Hypaque density gradient centrifugation and thereafter assessed for cell viability and tumor cell count. Thereafter, cells were incubated in polypropylene round-bottom 96-well plates (2×10^4 cells/well) with or without different cytostatic agents including temozolomide, dacarbazine, cisplatin, doxorubicin, vindesine, paclitaxel, gemcitabine and treosulfan at six different dilutions (6.25%–200%) of the test drug concentrations (TDC) shown in Ta-

Table 1. Cytostatic drugs used in the ATP-TCA

Drug	TDC[a] (μg/ml)
Temozolomide	20.0
Dacarbazine (DTIC)	20.0
Cisplatin	3.8
Doxorubicin	0.5
Vindesine	0.5
Paclitaxel	13.6
Gemcitabine	12.5
Treosulfan	20.0

[a]TDC, test drug concentration.

ble 1. The individual TDC for each cytostatic drug was determined previously [14] by reference to known pharmacokinetic and response data. After 5–7 days of incubation at 37°C, 5% CO_2 and 100% humidity, the cells were lysed and the ATP content of each well was measured by a luciferin-luciferase-based luminescence assay with a Dynatech ML1000 luminometer. Individual sensitivity indices for each test drug or drug combinations were calculated from the obtained data curves by summing up the percentages of tumor growth inhibition for each drug concentration tested (6.25, 12.5, 25, 50, 100, 200) followed by the subtraction of 600. A sensitivity index of 600 indicates unrestrained tumor cell growth and minimal drug sensitivity, whereas a sensitivity index of 0 reflects a complete tumor growth inhibition and maximal drug sensitivity. Moreover, the chemosensitivity of the test samples was classified as shown in Table 2 .

Results

Heterogeneous Chemosensitivity of Melanoma Tissue Specimens

As shown in Table 3, we found heterogeneous sensitivity to different cytostatic drugs in tumor tissue samples from 31 stage IV metastasized melanoma patients with the ATP-TCA. Overall, chemoresistance was strongest for dacarba-

Table 2. Classification of chemosensitivity testing results of the ATP-TCA

	Tumor growth inhibition at 200% TDC[a]	Tumor growth inhibition at 25% TDC
High sensitivity	>95%	>70%
Moderate sensitivity	>95%	50–70%
Low sensitivity	>95%	<50%
	<95%	>50%
Resistant	<95%	<50%

[a]TDC, test drug concentration.

Table 3. Chemosensitivity testing in 31 metastasized melanoma patients with ATP-TCA

Cytostatics	Resistant	Low sensitivity	Moderate sensitivity	High sensitivity	Mean sensitivity index[a]
Temozolomide	8/10 (80%)	2/10 (20%)	0/10 (0%)	0/10 (0%)	538.9
Dacarbazine (DTIC)	17/18 (94%)	0/18 (0%)	0/18 (0%)	1/18 (6%)	498.2
Cisplatin	16/29 (55%)	6/29 (21%)	1/29 (3%)	6/29 (21%)	353.4
Doxorubicin	12/31 (39%)	5/31 (16%)	6/31 (19%)	8/31 (26%)	309.7
Vindesine	19/31 (61%)	6/31 (19%)	1/31 (3%)	4/31 (13%)	401.2
Paclitaxel	2/20 (10%)	8/20 (40%)	4/20 (20%)	6/20 (30%)	284.9
Gemcitabine	13/19 (68%)	4/19 (21%)	2/19 (11%)	0/19 (0%)	320.9
Treosulfan	5/27 (19%)	9/27 (33%)	3/27 (11%)	10/27 (37%)	242.2
Treosulfan+Gemcitabine	3/29 (10%)	0/29 (0%)	4/29 (14%)	22/29 (76%)	146.8
Paclitaxel+Cisplatin	2/26 (8%)	7/26 (27%)	5/26 (19%)	12/26 (46%)	231.3
Gemcitabine+Cisplatin	6/29 (21%)	3/29 (10%)	4/29 (14%)	16/29 (55%)	210.0
Vindesine+Cisplatin	2/9 (22%)	4/9 (44%)	2/9 (22%)	1/9 (11%)	313.6
Paclitaxel+Doxorubicin	0/18 (0%)	3/18 (17%)	3/18 (17%)	12/18 (66%)	227.7
Gemcitabine+Vindesine	10/17 (59%)	5/17 (29%)	1/17 (6%)	1/17 (6%)	388.0
Temozolomide+Vindesine+Cisplatin	2/8 (25%)	1/8 (13%)	3/8 (38%)	2/8 (25%)	330.3

[a]Data are means from individual chemosensitivity indices for each test drug or drug combination, which were calculated by summing up the tumor growth inhibition for each drug concentration tested followed by the subtraction of 600. A sensitivity index of 600 indicates unrestrained tumor cell growth and minimal drug sensitivity, whereas a sensitivity index of 0 reflects a complete tumor growth inhibition and maximal drug sensitivity.

zine (DTIC), with 94% of the samples revealing resistance and 6% high sensitivity, followed by temozolomide (80%/0%) and gemcitabine (68%/0%). The test samples revealed higher sensitivity to combinations of two cytostatics than to single drugs. The highest chemosensitivity was found for the combination of treosulfan and gemcitabine, with 76% of the samples revealing high sensitivity and 10% resistance, followed by the combination of paclitaxel and doxorubicine (66%/0%), gemcitabine and cisplatin (55%/21%), and paclitaxel and cisplatin (46%/8%).

Different Chemosensitivity Profiles of Melanoma Tissue Samples Taken at Different Time Points or from Different Metastatic Sites of the Same Patient

Tumor material surgically obtained from a subcutaneous metastatic lesion of a 67-year-old female melanoma patient with multiple lung and liver metastases was subjected to in vitro chemosensitivity testing with the ATP-TCA method. The patient was pretreated with three cycles of dacarbazine, leading to a >50% progression of the metastatic lesions. Chemosensitivity testing was per-

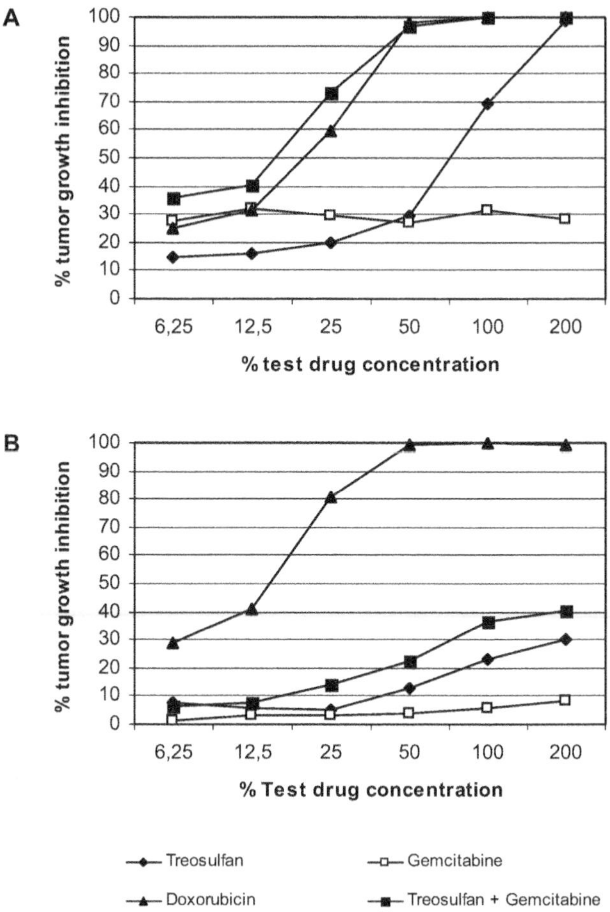

Fig. 2A, B. Original data curves obtained with ATP-TCA indicating the individual chemosensitivity profiles of the tumor samples tested. Each plot shows the corresponding testing results with four representative cytostatics on a stage IV melanoma patient's tumor material obtained before (**A**) and after (**B**) four cycles of combined chemotherapy with treosulfan and gemcitabine. For further details, see Table 4

formed with the intention of selecting a second-line cytostatic regimen with a high probability of clinical response. The ATP-TCA results showed the patient's tumor material to be highly sensitive to the combination of treosulfan and gemcitabine (Table 4, Fig. 2A). After the sensitivity profile, a combined chemotherapy with treosulfan (3.5 g/m^2 i.v. on days 1 and 8) and gemcitabine (1,000 mg/m^2 i.v. on days 1 and 8) was started and the first follow-up examination after two therapy cycles revealed a stabilization of the disease. After two more cycles, a >50% progression of the metastatic lesions was detected and again tumor material from a subcutaneous metastasis was tested for chemosensitivity. The retesting by ATP-TCA revealed a chemosensitivity pro-

Table 4. Chemosensitivity testing in a metastasized melanoma patient before and after four cycles of combined cytostatic therapy with treosulfan and gemcitabine

Cytostatics	Testing before therapy Test result	Sensitivity index	Testing after four therapy cycles Test result	Sensitivity index
Temozolomide	Resistant	470	Resistant	588
Cisplatin	Resistant	566	Resistant	432
Vindesine	Resistant	185	Resistant	151
Doxorubicin	Moderate sensitivity	348	High sensitivity	351
Paclitaxel	Moderate sensitivity	161	Resistant	353
Gemcitabine	Resistant	424	Resistant	528
Treosulfan	Low sensitivity	352	Resistant	515
Treosulfan+Gemcitabine	High sensitivity	157	Resistant	472
Paclitaxel+Cisplatin	Low sensitivity	206	Low sensitivity	350
Paclitaxel+Doxorubicin	High sensitivity	160	High sensitivity	162
Gemcitabine+Vindesine	Resistant	355	Resistant	410
Gemcitabine+Cisplatin	Resistant	341	Resistant	329

The individual chemosensitivity index for each test drug or drug combination was calculated by summing up the tumor growth inhibition for each drug concentration tested followed by the subtraction of 600. A sensitivity index of 600 indicates unrestrained tumor cell growth and minimal drug sensitivity, whereas a sensitivity index of 0 reflects a complete tumor growth inhibition and maximal drug sensitivity. Both tumor tissue samples were obtained surgically from subcutaneously localized metastases. The patient was treated with treosulfan and gemcitabine, resulting in a stable disease after the first two therapy cycles followed by a progressive disease after two more cycles. For further details, see "Patients and Methods."

file similar to the first one, except for slight changes toward higher chemoresistance for the drugs paclitaxel and treosulfan and a change toward higher sensitivity for doxorubicin (Table 4, Fig. 2B). In contrast, the sensitivity for the combination of treosulfan and gemcitabine changed from highly sensitive to resistant, corresponding to the situation of the patient.

A 40-year-old female patient suffering from metastasized melanoma presented with rapidly growing renal, intramuscular, and lymph node metastases. The patient was treated surgically with the intention of curing the disease. The tumor material obtained from the renal and intramuscular metastases was tested for chemosensitivity with ATP-TCA. The tumor samples differed strongly to moderately in their chemosensitivity to the cytostatic drugs cisplatin, doxorubicin, treosulfan, and some combinations using these drugs, whereas the sensitivity to temozolomide, vindesine, paclitaxel, and gemcitabine showed only slight differences (Table 5, Fig. 3).

Preparation of tumor material obtained from axillary lymph node dissection of a 72-year-old female melanoma patient with pulmonary and lymph node metastases revealed one metastatic mass consisting of a melanotic and an amelanotic part. Both parts were separately subjected to chemosensitivity testing with ATP-TCA. The test results showed slight differences in sensitivity for the single agent treosulfan and for the combinations treosulfan + gemc-

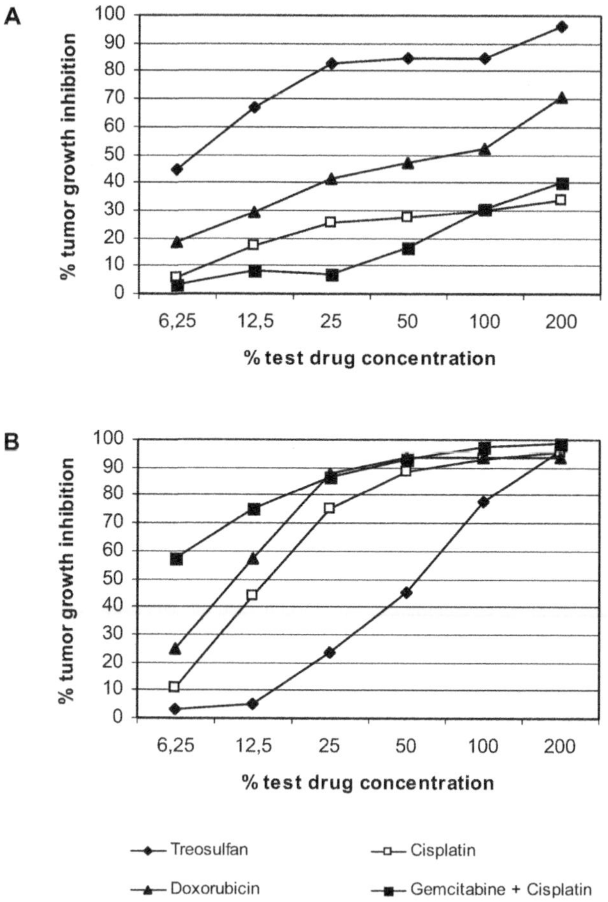

Fig. 3A, B. Original data curves obtained with ATP-TCA indicating the individual chemosensitivity profiles of the tumor samples tested. Each plot shows the corresponding testing results with four representative cytostatics on a stage IV melanoma patient's tumor material obtained in the same surgical procedure from renal (**A**) and intramuscular (**B**) metastases. For further details, see Table 5

itabine, paclitaxel + cisplatin, and gemcitabine + cisplatin between the two differently pigmented tumor parts (Table 6, Fig. 4).

Discussion

Chemosensitivity testing in melanoma is of great interest because of the poor response rates achieved by standard chemotherapy with dacarbazine. A reliable in vitro testing system is needed that reveals precise information about the drug sensitivity profile of melanoma tissue specimens combined with a considerable correlation to in vivo therapy responses in melanoma patients. The ATP-TCA has been approved in prospective studies to fulfill these re-

Table 5. Chemosensitivity testing of tumor specimens from two different metastatic sites of a melanoma patient

Cytostatics	Renal metastasis		Intramuscular metastasis	
	Test result	Sensitivity index	Test result	Sensitivity index
Temozolomide	Resistant	339	Resistant	328
Cisplatin	Resistant	467	High sensitivity	193
Vindesine	Resistant	341	Resistant	148
Doxorubicin	Resistant	576	High sensitivity	515
Paclitaxel	High sensitivity	135	High sensitivity	106
Gemcitabine	Resistant	301	Resistant	319
Treosulfan	High sensitivity	140	Low sensitivity	363
Treosulfan+Gemcitabine	High sensitivity	122	Moderate sensitivity	228
Paclitaxel+Cisplatin	Moderate sensitivity	135	High sensitivity	69
Paclitaxel+Doxorubicin	High sensitivity	121	High sensitivity	80
Gemcitabine+Vindesine	Resistant	586	Resistant	447
Gemcitabine+Cisplatin	Resistant	488	High sensitivity	91

The individual chemosensitivity index for each test drug or drug combination was calculated by summing up the tumor growth inhibition for each drug concentration tested followed by the subtraction of 600. A sensitivity index of 600 indicates unrestrained tumor cell growth and minimal drug sensitivity, whereas a sensitivity index of 0 reflects a complete tumor growth inhibition and maximal drug sensitivity. Both tumor tissue samples were obtained in one surgical procedure. For further details, see "Patients and Methods."

Table 6. Chemosensitivity testing of tumor specimens from two differently pigmented regions of a melanoma patient's lymph node metastasis

Cytostatics	Melanotic part		Amelanotic part	
	Test result	Sensitivity index	Test result	Sensitivity index
Temozolomide	Resistant	581	Resistant	552
Cisplatin	Resistant	459	Resistant	438
Vindesine	Resistant	468	Resistant	576
Doxorubicin	Low sensitivity	497	Low sensitivity	515
Paclitaxel	Moderate sensitivity	238	Moderate sensitivity	171
Gemcitabine	Resistant	473	Resistant	316
Treosulfan	Low sensitivity	248	Moderate sensitivity	200
Treosulfan+Gemcitabine	Moderate sensitivity	196	High sensitivity	124
Paclitaxel+Cisplatin	Moderate sensitivity	226	High sensitivity	182
Paclitaxel+Doxorubicin	High sensitivity	159	High sensitivity	104
Gemcitabine+Vindesine	Resistant	370	Resistant	366
Gemcitabine+Cisplatin	Low sensitivity	318	Moderate sensitivity	212

The individual chemosensitivity index for each test drug or drug combination was calculated by summing up the tumor growth inhibition for each drug concentration tested followed by the subtraction of 600. A sensitivity index of 600 indicates unrestrained tumor cell growth and minimal drug sensitivity, whereas a sensitivity index of 0 reflects a complete tumor growth inhibition and maximal drug sensitivity. For further details, see "Patients and Methods."

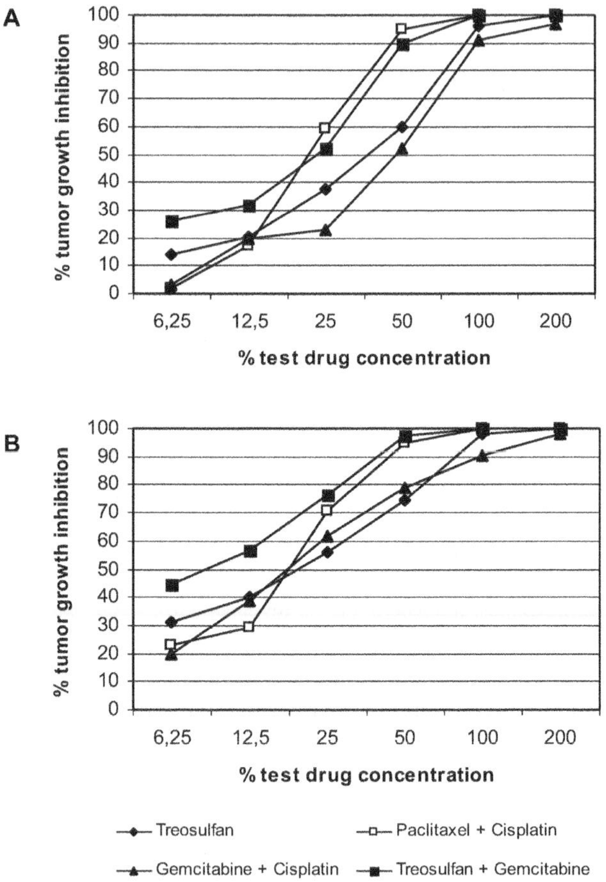

Fig. 4A, B. Original data curves obtained with ATP-TCA indicating the individual chemosensitivity profiles of the tumor samples tested. Each plot shows the corresponding testing results with four representative cytostatics on a stage IV melanoma patient's tumor material obtained from the melanotic part (**A**) and the amelanotic part (**B**) of a lymph node metastasis. For further details, see Table 6

quirements by showing strong predictive value for the response to different chemotherapy regimens in metastasized breast cancer [18] and recurrent ovarian cancer [15]. Moreover, the ATP-TCA has been shown to be a method of high reproducibility, with intra- and interassay variations <15%, high sensitivity, linearity and precision of assessment by luminometry, and an approved selective growth of malignant cells due to a special culture medium [14]. First studies in melanoma with ATP-TCA showed heterogeneous chemosensitivity of the specimens tested but yet allowed no correlation to the clinical responses of the patients tested [13, 16, 19].

Our results obtained in metastasized melanoma patients with the ATP-TCA confirm the previously described heterogeneous chemosensitivity of melanoma tissue specimens. The assay has proved in our hands to be a feasible and reliable method with a success rate of >90% (a success rate of 87% was reported previously [14]). As previously described [16], combinations of anticancer drugs revealed higher sensitivities in melanoma than single agents; the most effective combination was treosulfan and gemcitabine followed by paclitaxel and doxorubicin. Confirming previous data [16], only low in vitro sensitivity was found for dacarbazine and its derivative temozolomide. Although dacarbazine is a prodrug and requires microsomal activation by cytochrome P450, which in vivo takes place in the liver, an in vitro activity similar to that of temozolomide, whose activity is not dependent on enzymatic activation, has been reported [16]. Therefore, both agents were used in the present study, showing no significant differences in their poor rates of sensitivity.

In regard to a first preliminary evaluation of the correlation of in vitro drug sensitivity with in vivo therapy response, the number of patients treated with a sensitivity-directed chemotherapeutic regimen is still too low to draw any significant conclusions. Nevertheless, an observation of far-reaching importance was the poor response of patients pretreated with cytostatics shortly before chemosensitivity testing, which was the case in more than 75% of the patients tested in this study. Treatment with cytostatics is known to induce multidrug resistance mechanisms in melanoma cells [20, 21], promoting not only high resistance against the anticancer drug already given to the patient but also inducing cross-resistances against other cytostatics.

To evaluate the feasibility of an individually selective sensitivity-directed chemotherapy based on the results of pretherapeutic in vitro chemosensitivity testing with ATP-TCA, we initiated a multicenter prospective first-line phase II trial in 110 stage IV metastatic melanoma patients. In light of the results of this study, randomized trials comparing a sensitivity-directed chemotherapy after ATP-TCA results with standard cytostatic treatment, e.g., dacarbazine single-agent therapy, are needed.

References

1. Serrone L, Hersey P (1999) The chemoresistance of human malignant melanoma: an update. Melanoma Res 9:51–58
2. Helmbach H, Rossmann E, Kern MA, Schadendorf D (2001) Drug-resistance in human melanoma. Int J Cancer 93:617–622
3. Middleton MR, Lorigan P, Owen J, Ashcroft L, Lee SM, Harper P, Thatcher N (2000) A randomized phase III study comparing dacarbazine, BCNU, cisplatin and tamoxifen with dacarbazine and interferon in advanced melanoma. Br J Cancer 82:1158–1162
4. Serrone L, Zeuli M, Sega FM, Cognetti F (2000) Dacarbazine-based chemotherapy for metastatic melanoma: thirty-year experience overview. J Exp Clin Cancer Res 19:21–34
5. Joukhadar C, Klein N, Mader RM, Schrolnberger C, Rizovski B, Heere-Ress E, Pehamberger H, Strauchmann N, Jansen B, Muller M (2001) Penetration of dacarbazine and its active metabolite 5-aminoimidazole-4-carboxamide into cutaneous metastases of human malignant melanoma. Cancer 92:2190–2196
6. Iqbal M, Marshall E, Green JA (2000) Ten-year survival in advanced malignant melanoma following treatment with interferon and vindesine. Ann Oncol 11:483–485

7. Metzger U, Rothlin M, Burger HR, Largiader F (1997) Long-term complete remission of melanoma liver metastases after intermittent intra-arterial cisplatin chemotherapy and surgery. Eur J Surg Oncol 23:270–274
8. Petit T, Borel C, Rixe O, Avril MF, Monnier A, Giroux B, Weil M, Khayat D (1996) Complete remission seven years after treatment for metastatic malignant melanoma. Cancer 77:900–902
9. Oliver V, Aliaga A, Lopez Lopez JJ, Perez E, Ponchon A, Bizzari JP, Cour V (1993) Long-term complete remissions in patients with disseminated melanoma treated by fotemustine and dacarbazine. Eur J Cancer 29:287
10. Marshall ES, Finlay GJ, Matthews JH, Shaw JH, Nixon J, Baguley BC (1992) Microculture-based chemosensitivity testing: a feasibility study comparing freshly explanted human melanoma cells with human melanoma cell lines. J Natl Cancer Inst 84:340–345
11. Schadendorf D, Worm M, Algermissen B, Kohlmus CM, Czarnetzki BM (1994) Chemosensitivity testing of human malignant melanoma. A retrospective analysis of clinical response and in vitro drug sensitivity. Cancer 73:103–108
12. Schadendorf D, Jurgovsky K, Worm M, Czarnetzki BM (1994) In vitro sensitivity of human melanoma cells to chemotherapeutic agents and interferons. Melanoma Res 4:243–249
13. Myatt N, Cree IA, Kurbacher CM, Foss AJ, Hungerford JL, Plowman PN (1997) The ex vivo chemosensitivity profile of choroidal melanoma. Anticancer Drugs 8:756–762
14. Andreotti PE, Cree IA, Kurbacher CM, Hartmann DM, Linder D, Harel G, Gleiberman I, Caruso PA, Ricks SH, Untch M, Sartori C, Bruckner HW (1995) Chemosensitivity testing of human tumors using a microplate adenosine triphosphate luminescence assay: clinical correlation for cisplatin resistance of ovarian carcinoma. Cancer Res 55:5276–5282
15. Kurbacher CM, Cree IA, Bruckner HW, Brenne U, Kurbacher JA, Muller K, Ackermann T, Gilster TJ, Wilhelm LM, Engel H, Mallmann PK, Andreotti PE (1998) Use of an ex vivo ATP luminescence assay to direct chemotherapy for recurrent ovarian cancer. Anticancer Drugs 9:51–57
16. Cree IA, Neale MH, Myatt NE, de Takats PG, Hall P, Grant J, Kurbacher CM, Reinhold U, Neuber K, MacKie RM, Chana J, Weaver PC, Khoury GG, Sartori C, Andreotti PE (1999) Heterogeneity of chemosensitivity of metastatic cutaneous melanoma. Anticancer Drugs 10:437–444
17. American Joint Committee on Cancer (1977) Staging manual. Lippincott, Philadelphia
18. Cree IA, Kurbacher CM, Untch M, Sutherland LA, Hunter EM, Subedi AM, James EA, Dewar JA, Preece PE, Andreotti PE, Bruckner HW (1996) Correlation of the clinical response to chemotherapy in breast cancer with ex vivo chemosensitivity. Anticancer Drugs 7:630–635
19. Neale MH, Myatt N, Cree IA, Kurbacher CM, Foss AJ, Hungerford JL, Plowman PN (1999) Combination chemotherapy for choroidal melanoma: ex vivo sensitivity to treosulfan with gemcitabine or cytosine arabinoside. Br J Cancer 79:1487–1493
20. Kern MA, Helmbach H, Artuc M, Karmann D, Jurgovsky K, Schadendorf D (1997) Human melanoma cell lines selected in vitro displaying various levels of drug resistance against cisplatin, fotemustine, vindesine or etoposide: modulation of proto-oncogene expression. Anticancer Res 17:4359–4370
21. Ichihashi N, Kitajima Y (2001) Chemotherapy induces or increases expression of multidrug resistance-associated protein in malignant melanoma cells. Br J Dermatol 144:745–750

Human Melanoma: Drug Resistance

Heike Helmbach, Pranav Sinha, Dirk Schadendorf

D. Schadendorf (✉)
Klinische Kooperationseinheit für Dermatoonkologie (DKFZ)
an der Universitäts-Hautklinik Mannheim, Universität Heidelberg,
68135 Mannheim, Germany
e-mail: d.schadendorf@dkfz-heidelberg.de

Abstract

Advanced malignant melanoma has a poor prognosis since chemotherapy is mostly ineffective because, in part, of the intrinsic and/or extrinsic resistance of melanoma cells to systemic treatment with antineoplastic agents. The reasons for the chemoresistant phenotype are currently unknown. The relevance of well-analyzed drug resistance mechanisms in melanoma such as intracellular and extracellular transport, drug resistance by induction of certain enzyme systems, and altered drug-target interaction is reviewed. It has been shown that most anticancer drugs kill susceptible cells through induction of apoptosis. Therefore, the significance of apoptotic deficiency caused by alteration in the apoptotic pathway is discussed in relation to specific molecules and apoptotic mechanisms like death-receptors, the Bcl-2 family, and the Hsp family of proteins. The complexity of the molecular variants involved in signal transduction along apoptotic pathways suggests that the cell may possess a variety of possibilities for regulating apoptosis and generating apoptosis deficiency. Thus apoptosis and apoptosis deficiency should be analyzed to understand the mechanisms of melanoma resistance.

Introduction

Human melanoma, a malignancy that develops through the malignant transformation of melanocytes, is a major medical problem characterized by rapidly growing incidence and mortality rate. During the past decade the incidence of melanoma has increased steadily. The age-adjusted incidence rate is about 6–10 per 100,000 individuals in Germany and 12 per 100,000 individuals in the United States and is threefold higher in some geographic areas such as Australia (Ross and Balch 1991). If melanoma is not recognized in time, the survival rate decreases rapidly in correlation with tumor thickness. Dissemi-

Recent Results in Cancer Research, Vol. 161

nated melanoma shows survival rates of less than 5% over 5 years (McGovern et al. 1985). Thorough surgical removal of the tumor is the only curative treatment for malignant melanoma. Systemic therapy for advanced melanoma, both adjuvant therapy and treatment of disseminated (stage IV) disease, remains unsatisfactory, with response rates lower than 30% in vivo and in vitro. Regimes including treatment with dacarbacine are still the most common therapy forms for metastatic melanoma. Nevertheless, only in a minority of patients is a long-lasting response achieved and the overall survival is rather short (Middleton et al. 2000b). Chemotherapy is extremely ineffective and unsatisfactory for treating malignant melanoma because of the drug resistance that is characteristic of this disease and is either intrinsic at onset or develops during chemotherapy (Helmbach et al. 2001). With use of an in vitro soft agar culture system to predict tumor cell sensitivity in well-established human melanoma cell lines, a high degree of resistance was found against all cytostatic drugs studied. This suggests the presence of intrinsic cellular mechanisms that confer drug resistance (Schadendorf et al. 1994). In vitro analysis confirmed that exposure of human melanoma cells to cytostatic drugs induced increasing drug-resistance in a dose-dependent manner (Kern et al. 1997). The underlying cellular resistance mechanisms involved in chemoresistance of melanoma have not yet been clarified (reviewed in Helmbach et al. 2001; Serrone and Hersey 1999). Alternative treatment methods based on immunological principles are presently being developed but have not reached the stage where they could be applied routinely in clinical practice. Thus chemotherapy will continue to be the primary treatment method and urgently needs to be improved. This could be achieved if the mechanisms conferring drug resistance could be identified and examined to develop strategies for counteracting them. Resistance may be primary (intrinsic), e.g., the tumor cells do not respond from the beginning of the therapy, or it may be secondary (extrinsic or acquired), e.g., the tumor initially responds to therapy but eventually tumor growth resumes and relapses occur. It is likely that the biochemical mechanisms involved in primary and secondary resistance are largely similar, but few details of the mechanisms are available.

Drug Resistance Mechanisms

Drug Resistance Mediated by Altered Transport

The phenomenon of drug efflux by a nonspecific carrier is one of the best-investigated mechanisms of drug-resistance. The classic *"multidrug resistance (MDR)"* arises from P-glycoprotein-dependent export of cytostatic substances out of the cell by a transmembrane 170-kDa protein. The P-glycoprotein (Pgp) is coded by the *mdr*-1 gene on chromosome 7q21 and belongs to the ATP binding cassette (*ABC*) transporter family. It catalyzes the energy-dependent export of a number of structurally different substances such as anthracycline, epipodophyllotoxins and vinca-alkaloids (overview in Gottesman and

Pastan 1993). Expression of Pgp in primary and metastatic lesions of melanoma as well as in melanoma cell lines was analyzed by several groups, but no significant melanoma-specific Pgp-upregulation could be detected. Moreover, no correlation could be found between Pgp status and the response to chemotherapy in melanoma patients or drug-sensitivity testing. Therefore, Pgp cannot be regarded as a major common feature mediating drug resistance in human melanoma cells (Schadendorf et al. 1995).

Another transport-protein that plays a role in MDR ("non Pgp-MDR") is the "*multidrug resistance-related protein, MRP*" (Kavallaris 1997), which is a 190-kDa transmembrane glycoprotein also belonging to the ABC transporter superfamily; they also act as energy-dependent efflux pumps to decrease the intracellular concentration of cytostatic agents. The family of MRPs consists of at least six members. MRP1 and MRP2 share a similar substrate spectrum despite differences in cellular localization and kinetic properties (Konig et al. 1999). MRP1 is frequently expressed in melanoma; however, no significant upregulation in response to chemotherapy in melanoma cell lines, melanoma tissues, and melanocytes was detectable (Schadendorf et al. 1995b). Other investigators have associated the MRP1 expression with resistance toward a specific class of antibiotic drugs such as daunorubicine and doxorubicine but not to other cytostatic agents in melanoma (Berger et al. 1997). MRP2 was found in various epithelial malignant tumors and may contribute to their resistance to antitumor drugs but has not been analyzed in detail in melanoma. MRPs can transport unconjugated drugs and drugs that are conjugated to glutathione, a process catalyzed by glutathione-*S*-transferase (GST) (Borst et al. 2000). Whether other MRP family members are involved in drug resistance is unknown.

Drug Resistance Mediated by Altered Detoxification

Another form of drug resistance in tumor cells arises from the intracellular detoxification of anticancer agents via *glutathione metabolism* and is accompanied by an increased glutathione level as well as increased activity of associated enzymes GST, reductase, and peroxidase in tumor cells (Zhang et al. 1998). Glutathione (GSH) is a nonprotein thiol that can interact with the reactive site of a drug. The conjugate, which is less active and more water soluble, is extruded from the cell with transporter proteins called GS-X. Resistance toward various cytostatic substances (alkylating agents, e.g., cisplatin, BCNU, adriamycin, daunorubicin) has been associated with an increase in the expression of GST or related enzymes, especially in ovarian and gastrointestinal tumor lines. The GST/GSH system is involved in adaptation to oxygen stress resulting from melanogenesis, and only a few studies have analyzed the role of the GST/GSH system in drug resistance in melanoma cells. Although high glutathione concentration could be measured in some melanoma cells (Benathan et al. 1992), no correlation was found between alteration in GST/GSH metabolism and drug sensitivity in melanoma (Schadendorf et al. 1995a).

Drug Resistance Mediated by Altered Drug-Target Interaction

Topoisomerase II is a nuclear enzyme essential for the transcription and recombination of DNA as well as segregation of chromatids during mitosis. In mammalian cells, two isoforms of topoisomerase II, Topo IIα and Topo IIβ, exist as homodimers. Topoisomerase II represents a primary intracellular target of many topoisomerase-inhibiting anticancer drugs, including etoposide. Quantitative and qualitative alteration of target enzymes has been implicated in the development of resistance toward these drugs. One of the mechanisms that has been found to contribute to drug resistance is mediated by decreased activity of topoisomerase II (Beck et al. 1993). Only very few studies have investigated the relevance of topoisomerase II regarding drug resistance in melanoma. Recent studies demonstrated an increase of topoisomerase activity in association with resistance to doxorubicine and etoposide (Lage et al. 2000) in melanoma cells. Mutant topoisomerase II has also been correlated with etoposide resistance in a melanoma cell line (Campain et al. 1995). Therefore, alteration of topoisomerase-activity might be involved in mediating resistance to specific drugs in melanoma.

Drug Resistance Mediated by Altered DNA Repair

In the past few years, increasing evidence has been provided that DNA damage induced by cytostatic drugs is compensated and counteracted by corresponding modulation of DNA repair mechanisms. Therefore, increased DNA repair, a mechanism for protection of normal cells and essential for their survival, might inhibit cell death in drug-treated tumor cells. In a recent study it was demonstrated that DNA-mismatch repair (MMR) deficiency results in drug -resistance by impairing the ability of cells to repair DNA damage (Fink et al. 1998). It has also been demonstrated that decreased nuclear mismatch-repair protein expression is associated with a drug-resistant phenotype in melanoma cell lines (Lage et al. 1999). Increased DNA repair could also be demonstrated in fotemustine- and cisplatin-resistant human melanoma cells (Rünger et al. 2000). An upregulation of O^6-methylguanine-DNA methyltransferase (MGMT), an enzyme involved in DNA repair of DNA damage caused by alkylation, was associated with a fotemustine-resistant phenotype in melanoma cells (Lage et al. 1999). However, previous studies could not prove the association between MGMT concentration in tumors before treatment and sensitivity of tumors to the methylating agent temozolomide in melanoma patients (Middleton et al. 1998). In contrast, other studies of the same group demonstrated improved survival of patients with tumors expressing low levels of MGMT after treatment with temozolomide (Middleton et al. 2000a). The relationship between MGMT levels, activity, and response to chemotherapy with alkylating agents in melanoma patients still requires further investigation.

Drug Resistance via Modulation of the Apoptotic Pathway

A number of studies have implicated apoptosis (programmed cell death) as an important mechanism by which chemotherapeutic agents kill susceptible cells (Houghton 1999; Kaufmann and Earnshaw 2000; Sellers and Fisher 1999). Apoptosis is a type of cell death involving characteristic morphological and biochemical changes that proceeds in part via aggregation and multimerization of upstream death effector molecules that sequentially activate a cascade of caspases (Rathmell and Thompson 1999). Tremendous progress has been made in understanding apoptosis as a result of molecular identification of the key components of this intracellular suicide program (reviewed in Budihardjo et al. 1999; Rathmell and Thompson 1999). There are currently two well-characterized caspase-activating cascades that regulate apoptosis (Fig. 1). The extrinsic pathway is initiated by a cell surface death receptor that recruits adapter molecules like FADD and initiator caspases (caspase-8/FLICE). This is followed by activation of effector caspases (e.g., caspase-3/-7) (Scaffidi et al. 1998). The intrinsic pathway, in contrast, is initiated by mitochondrial release of cytochrome *c* that binds to Apaf-1 and thereby induces conformational changes of this apoptotic protein followed by recruitment of pro-caspase-9 to the complex (Zou et al. 1997). The subsequent autocatalysis of pro-caspase-9 is followed by activation of effector caspases (Li et al. 1997; Zou et al. 1999) and induction of specific endonucleases resulting in DNA fragmentation (Liu

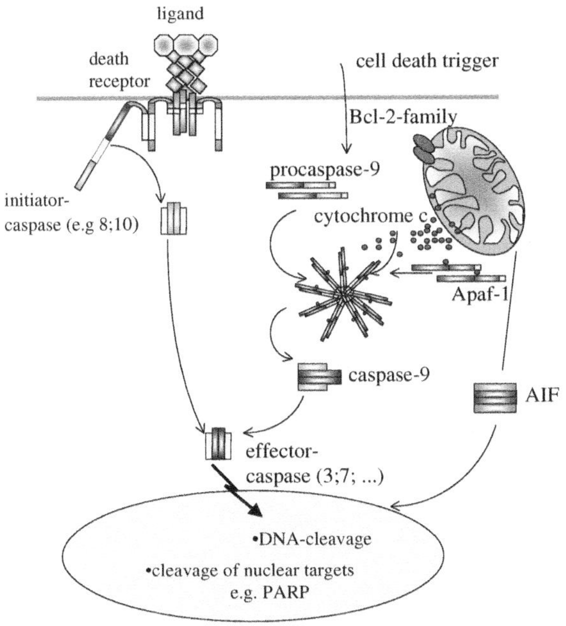

Fig. 1. The apoptotic pathway, illustrating the extrinsic and intrinsic pathway, either launched by death receptor ligands or by changes in the mitochondrial integrity, respectively (for details see text)

et al. 1997). Other apoptogenic molecules are also released from the mitochondria along with cytochrome *c*: AIF (apoptosis-inducing factor) and Smac (secondary mitochondria-derived activator of caspase, also called DIABLO). AIF directly translocates to the nucleus and triggers caspase-independent nuclear changes (Daugas et al. 2000; Du et al. 2000). Smac activates apoptosis by neutralizing the inhibitory activity of IAPs (inhibitory apoptotic proteins) that associates with and inhibit caspases (Du et al. 2000). The translocation of these proteins from the mitochondria is controlled by Bcl-2 and Bcl-2-related proteins (Kroemer and Reed 2000). It has been suggested that resistance to anticancer drugs is caused by inhibition or dysregulation of apoptosis (Eliopoulos et al. 1995; Los et al. 1997). Anticancer agents induce cell death by several different ways, for example, by upregulation of p53, by induction of the ceramide pathway, by the activation of death receptor/ligand systems, by affecting Bcl-2-like proteins, and/or by compromising the redox or energy balance (Bennett 1999; Fulda et al. 1998; Jarvis et al. 1996; Reed 1995). These are endogenous effectors that are involved in the physiologic control of apoptosis and also mediate mitochondrial permeabilization, a process by which proapoptotic factors are released into the cytosol to relay the apoptotic signal transduction. The following key processes seem to be involved in preventing apoptosis that is supposed to be induced by chemotherapy:

p53 plays a crucial role in apoptosis. Wild-type p53 function is required for apoptosis after contact with anticancer drugs in vitro, most likely by controlling transcriptional regulation of target genes such as Bcl-2 and Bax (Miyake et al. 1998; Petty et al. 1998). Overexpression of wild-type p53 was observed in metastatic, but not primary, melanoma (Hartmann et al. 1996). Mutations in the p53 gene were found in 25%–30% of metastatic melanoma but not in benign lesions (Hartmann et al. 1996). Furthermore, it has been demonstrated that melanoma cell lines expressing wild-type p53 exhibit a two to threefold higher response to anticancer agents than the response in cell lines with mutant p53, which leads to G1 arrest and downregulation of Bcl-2 and Pgp (Li et al. 2000; Li et al. 1998). Another very common specific gene defect in human melanoma are activated *ras* mutations (reviewed in Serrone and Hersey 1999). The incidence of ras gene mutations is approximately 15% and among these N-ras mutations are most common (69%) (Ball et al. 1994). In experiments using a melanoma mouse xenotransplantation model a correlation between the expression of activated N-ras and a reduction in drug-induced apoptosis was detected, thus indicating that N-ras plays a role in drug resistance in human melanoma (Jansen et al. 1997). However, the exact mechanism by which the activated ras oncogene is involved in drug resistance remains unclear and requires further examination.

The extrinsic pathway of apoptosis is triggered by ligation of *death receptors* belonging to the TNF receptor superfamily. Many studies have analyzed the expression of death receptors in primary melanoma, metastases, melanoma cell lines, and melanocytes. Downregulation or loss of CD95/Fas receptor has been found in a variety of malignancies including melanoma, and, as a result, these melanoma cells exhibit resistance to CD95L/Fas-ligand triggering

(Thomas and Hersey 1998; Ugurel et al. 1999). In addition, mutations in the death domain of CD95/Fas have also been described in melanoma (Shin et al. 1999). A recent study investigated the role of soluble CD95 (sCD95) and soluble CD95L (sCD95L) in the response of human melanoma to chemotherapy in vivo (Mouawad et al. 2000). This group reported that patients with little or no clinical response to various drugs (cisplatin, recombinant interleukin-2, and interferon-α) exhibited a significant increase of sCD95 and sCD95L in the plasma after drug treatment, whereas no changes in sCD95/sCD95L levels in the plasma of responders were observed. Interestingly, sCD95/sCD95L levels were already elevated in all untreated patients in comparison to healthy donors.

A defect in cytochrome *c* release in melanoma cell lines was described by others (Raisova et al. 2000). This phenomenon correlates with resistance to CD95/Fas-induced and ceramide-mediated apoptosis. These data suggest that alterations of mitochondrial processes in tumor cells might also lead to drug resistance. Various studies demonstrated that, in contrast to the CD95-receptor, the TRAIL-receptor 2 (TRAIL-R2) is widely expressed in melanoma. Furthermore, melanoma cell lines were shown to undergo apoptosis on exposure to recombinant TRAIL very readily, whereas melanocytes did not demonstrate such a high TRAIL sensitivity. In addition, abundant expression of a cellular inhibitor of death receptor signaling named FLICE inhibitory protein (FLIP) was shown to contribute to apoptotic resistance in melanoma cells on contact with death-receptor-ligands (Griffith et al. 1998; Zhang et al. 1999).

The mitochondrial response of apoptotic triggering is strictly regulated by pro- and antiapoptotic members of the *Bcl-2 family*. The Bcl-2 family comprises at least 16 pro- and antiapoptotic proteins. It has been shown that the ratio of pro- to antiapoptotic proteins during the apoptotic process prearranges the signal transduction. The protooncogene Bcl-2, a 26-kDa protein originally identified because of its deregulated expression in follicular B-cell lymphomas, is capable of inhibiting many forms of apoptosis (Reed 1995). The precise underlying mechanisms are still under investigation. Nevertheless, Bcl-2 seems to alter the response to anticancer agents by interfering with the induction of apoptosis, a pathway triggered by many cytostatic drugs including alkylating agents, topoisomerase inhibitors, antimetabolites, and others. Human melanoma primary tumors express Bcl-2 in 90% of all cases (Selzer et al. 1998). The high expression of Bcl-2 has been correlated with a decreased survival of patients and resistance to chemotherapy in human melanoma and other tumors (Grover and Wilson 1996; Reed 1999). It has been observed that a decrease in Bcl-2 levels or the inhibition of Bcl-2 activity leads to an increase in apoptosis or at least an increase in the responsiveness of cells to apoptotic stimuli.

In a recent study the expression of antiapoptotic Bcl-2 and proapoptotic Bax in the drug-resistant human melanoma cell line MeWo has been observed by Western blot (Fig. 2). In sensitive cells cisplatin and fotemustine induced a significant Bcl-2 reduction and Bax increase, indicating the involvement of these proteins in drug-induced apoptosis (Fig. 2A, E). The constitutive expres-

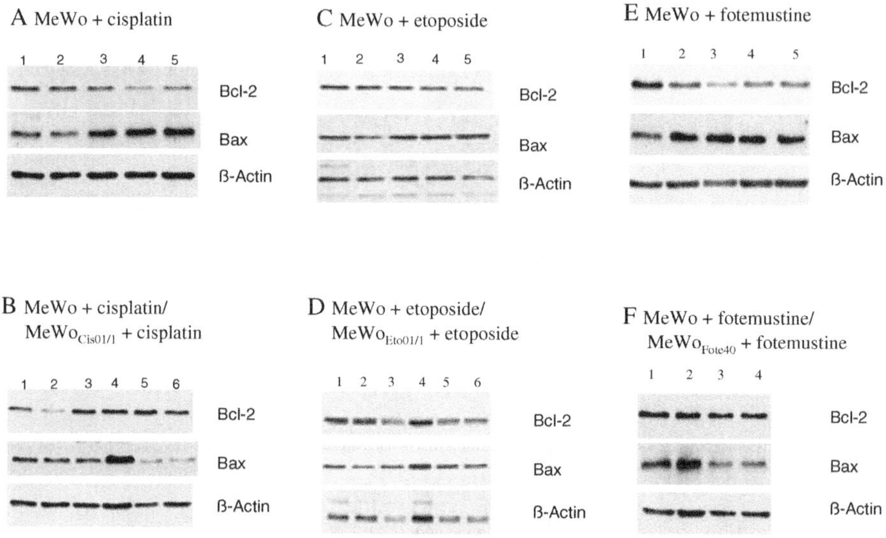

Fig. 2A–F. Members of the Bcl-2 family are known to regulate the translocation of several apoptotic proteins at the external mitochondrial membrane. Analysis of Bcl-2 and Bax-α by immunoblot of sensitive MeWo melanoma cells untreated (lane 1) and treated for 24 h, 48 h, 72 h, and 96 h (lanes 2–5) with cisplatin (**A**), etoposide (**C**), and fotemustine (**E**) as well as in cisplatin-MeWo$_{Cis01/1}$ untreated (lanes 3, 5) and treated (lanes 4, 6) (**B**), etoposide-MeWo$_{Eto01/1}$ untreated (lanes 3, 5) and treated (lanes 4, 6) (**D**), and fotemustine-resistant MeWo$_{Fote40}$ untreated (lanes 3, 5) and treated (lanes 4, 6) (**F**) MeWo melanoma cells after exposure with their drug of resistance. We compared untreated sensitive cells (lane 1), treated sensitive cells (lane 2), untreated (lane 3) and treated (lane 4) low resistant, and untreated (lane 5) and treated (lane 6) highly resistant cells. Cisplatin induced a 30% reduced Bcl-2 expression in sensitive cells, whereas Bax expression was increased about 40% (**A**). The regulation of Bcl-2 proteins was less definitive (about 10%) in resistant cells (**B**). The constitutive expression was elevated in low-resistant (~30%) (**B**, lane 3) and highly cisplatin-resistant cells (~70%) (**B**, lane 5), whereas the constitutive expression of Bax is reduced mainly in highly resistant cells (~40%). The regulation of Bcl-2 and Bax after etoposide-exposure (**C**) is less definitive: 10% Bcl-2 reduction and Bax increase. Fotemustine induced a clear reduced Bcl-2 (~35%) and increased Bax expression (~45 %) (**E**). Although Bcl-2 expression is not significantly different in fotemustine-sensitive and -resistant cells, Bax expression is 20% reduced in resistant MeWo cells (**F**, lane 3) compared with sensitive cells (lane 1)

sion of Bcl-2 in cisplatin-resistant cells was increased up to 70%, whereas the expression of Bax was shown to be reduced by 40% (Fig. 2B). This emphasizes again the relevance of the balance of these proteins in cisplatin-induced apoptosis and suggests that a imbalance may lead to drug resistance. Whereas fotemustin resistance was mainly associated with a reduction of constitutive Bax expression by ~20%, Bcl-2 expression was not significantly affected (Fig. 2F). In contrast, etoposide-resistant cells exhibited a slightly increased Bcl-2 expression compared with sensitive cells but showed no differences in the Bax expression. In all cases apoptosis was associated with a reduced Bcl-2-to-Bax ratio whereas resistance was associated with an increased Bcl-2-to-Bax ratio, which was more than 2 in cisplatin-resistant cells. By RNase protection assay (RPA) we could not confirm these differences on mRNA level (Fig. 3). The re-

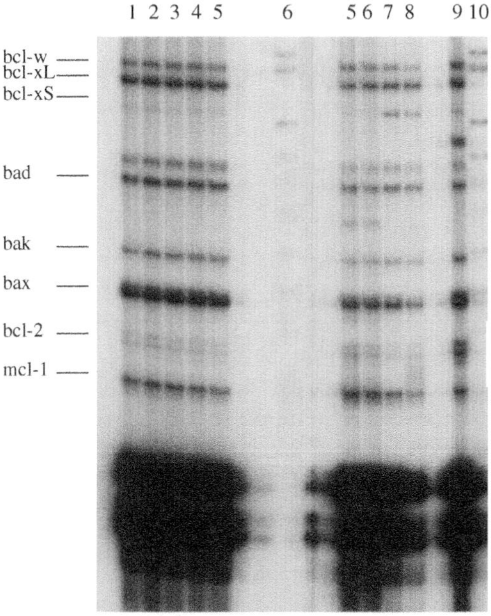

Fig. 3. Analysis of mRNA expression of Bcl-2 family members by RNase protection assay. The presence of transcripts of bcl-w, bcl-xL, bcl-xS, bad, bak, bax, bcl-2, and mcl-1 was analyzed with the hApo-2c multi-probe template set (Pharmingen, Hamburg, Germany). In this template set L32 and glyceraldehyde-3-phosphate dehydrogenase (GAPDH[1]) are included as internal controls. Probe synthesis, hybridization, and RNase treatment were performed with the RiboQuant Multi-Probe RNase Protection Assay System according to the manufacturer's instructions (Pharmingen). We compared untreated sensitive MeWo melanoma cells (lane 1) and sensitive cells treated with cisplatin 0.1 μg/ml (lane 2) and 1 μg/ml (lane 3) as well with etoposide 0.1 μg/ml (lane 4) and 1 μg/ml (lane 5). The constitutive expression of Bcl-2 family members was also observed in cisplatin-resistant $MeWo_{Cis01}$ and $MeWo_{Cis1}$ cells (lanes 5, 6) as well as in etoposide-resistant $MeWo_{Eto01}$ and $MeWo_{Eto1}$ cells (lanes 7, 8). We also checked mRNA of B-cell lymphoma cell line SKW6.4 (lane 9) as a control. Lane 6 and lane 10 present the probe. Exposure to cisplatin or etoposide did not induce different expression of any bcl-2 member tested. Considering L32 and GAPDH mRNA expression, no differential expression in sensitive and resistant cells could be observed

sults demonstrate the involvement of the dysregulation of Bcl-2 and Bax expression in the drug resistance mechanisms in melanoma cells and suggest that the degree and the exact justification is drug dependent.

A recent study demonstrated that the combination of Bcl-2 antisense oligonucleotide G-3139 (Genta) and dacarbacine improved chemosensitivity of human melanoma xenografts grown in SCID mice (Jansen et al. 1998). This has successfully been translated into a clinical phase I/IIa study in which 6 of 14 treated patients showed an antitumor response associated with low Bcl-2 levels and increased apoptosis in melanoma biopsies (Jansen et al. 2000). Currently, a worldwide prospective randomized controlled trial is being performed with metastatic melanoma to demonstrate the effectiveness of this novel treatment approach.

Caspase proteases are the key effector molecules of death processes. Every mammalian cell contains a set of different caspases that suitably equip it for apoptotic death. Caspases can be controlled by several ways, e.g., by processing and activation of upstream molecules (like FADD or Apaf-1) and furthermore by a variety of inhibitors that directly interact with proteases. One of the most prominent gene products associated with a wide variety of human melanoma is survivin. This protein is a member of the inhibitor of apoptosis (IAP) family that directly inhibits caspases. Antisense oligonucleotides directed against this molecule were shown to induce spontaneous apoptosis in melanoma in vitro (Grossman et al. 1999), suggesting that therapeutic targeting of survivin might also be beneficial in patients with recurrent or metastatic melanoma. Although the specific role of survivin in drug resistance of melanoma has not been analyzed, there are strong reasons for assuming that caspase inhibitors can be considered as therapeutic tools in drug-resistant melanoma.

Recent investigations of *Apaf-1* expression in human melanoma were able to demonstrate downregulation of Apaf-1 in metastatic melanoma in comparison with primary tumor cells and melanocytes. This negative Apaf-1 expression was associated with consistent drug resistance and defects in the execution of the typical apoptotic program in response to p53 activation (Soengas et al. 2001). These results are in contrast to our own data obtained in the above-described cell system, which did not exhibit differential Apaf expression in sensitive and drug-resistant MeWo melanoma cells (unpublished observation).

In a recent study, cisplatin- and etoposide-resistant human melanoma cells demonstrated reduced apoptotic activities. This was represented by a deficiency of caspase activation. Moreover, etoposide resistance was associated with a greatly reduced dose-dependent cytochrome *c* release in response to drug treatment followed by a dramatic decrease in activation of the downstream apoptotic cascade. Cisplatin resistance in these melanoma cells was associated with an only slightly reduced cytochrome *c* release, initiating a pathway that finally resulted in effector-caspase-activation and DNA fragmentation but not activation of caspase-9. These results indicate that the modulation of the apoptotic pathways demonstrated by human melanoma cells is drug dependent and plays a significant role in the development of the drug-resistant phenotype (Helmbach et al. 2002).

One of the major protein groups found to be overexpressed in certain chemoresistant melanomas is the group of *chaperones* (Fig. 4). These proteins are well known to facilitate the correct folding of newly synthesized proteins (Bukau and Horwich 1998). Recent findings suggest a role in regulation of apoptosis signaling for chaperone and chaperone-like proteins. The proteins are found in nearly every cellular compartment, and they can be classified based on molecular weight into several major groups: the Hsp90, Hsp70, and Hsp60 families and the family of small Hsps. Recently, it was recognized that Hsps also regulate apoptosis. Hsp70 and Hsp27 are antiapoptotic, whereas Hsp60 and Hsp10 are proapoptotic. Hsps function at multiple points in the apoptotic signaling pathway (Fig. 2). Hsp27 and Hsp70 have been shown to inhibit ap-

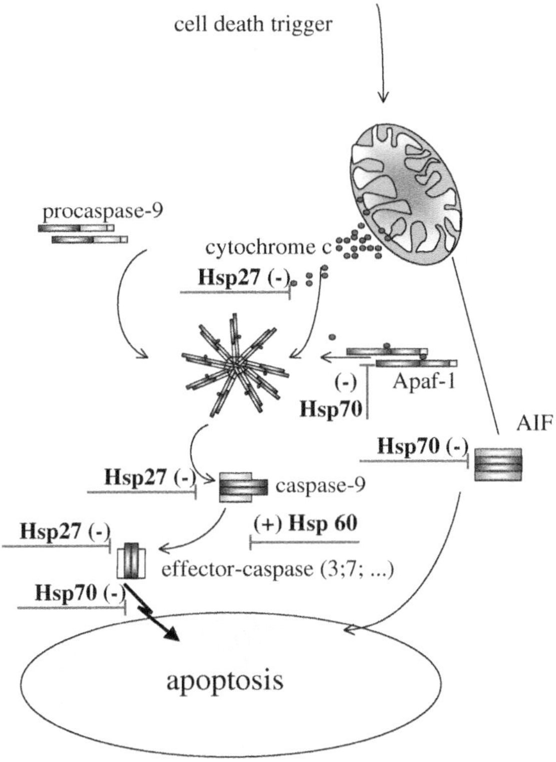

Fig. 4. Proposed apoptosis regulatory function of Hsps in the intrinsic pathway. Hsp27 binds to cytochrome c (Bruey et al. 2000) and Hsp70 and Hsp90 bind to Apaf-1 in all cases, resulting in the inhibition of apoptosome formation and thereby prevention of caspase-9 maturation (Pandey et al. 2000; Saleh et al. 2000). Additional further negative influence of Hsp27 and Hsp70 has also been described. (Pandey et al. 2000)

optosis (Garrido et al. 1998; Mehlen et al. 1996; Creagh and Cotter 1999; Jaattela et al. 1998; Mosser et al. 2000). Both proteins have been repeatedly demonstrated to inhibit apoptosis induced by different chemotherapeutics, especially drugs such as anthracyclines and etoposide that target topoisomerase II enzymes. In apoptosis induced by the anticancer drug etoposide activation of caspase-9, but not cytochrome *c* release, is inhibited by Hsp27. Thus Hsp27 may exert its effect on the apoptosome (Garrido et al. 1999). Heat shock proteins can accelerate apoptosis, as well. For example, Hsp90, Hsp60, and Hsp10 may work in a proapoptotic fashion. They copurify with caspase-3 from Jurkat cells and enhance its activation (Xanthoudakis et al. 1999). Hsp 90 has been implicated in the induction of apoptosis in response to TNF in combination with cycloheximide. This may be linked to the blockage of an unknown apoptotic inhibitor. Thus heat shock proteins regulate apoptosis on different levels and by multiple mechanisms. High expression of Hsps, namely Hsp70 and Hsp27, in breast, endometrial, or gastric cancer has been associated with metastasis, poor prognosis, and resistance to chemotherapy. A recent comparative study on chemosensitive and -resistant human melanoma cell lines using functional proteomics could demonstrate an increased expression of the small stress protein Hsp27 in cisplatin-, etoposide-, fotemustine- and vindesine-resistant cells. Furthermore, the Hsp70/Hsx70 variants were differentially upregulated in the same drug-resistant lines. It is worth noting that the expression is not dose dependent. Thus Hsx70 expression is more moderate in chemoresistant melanoma cell lines treated with low concentrations of the cytostatic drug. Furthermore, proteome analysis revealed downregulation of Hsp90 in cisplatin- and fotemustine-resistant cells (Scriha et al. 2002).

A recent study showed the involvement of the *proteasome subunit β type 3* in the development of drug resistance in resistant melanoma cell lines. The proteasome is a multienzyme complex that degrades proteins targeted for destruction by the ubiquitin pathway. This association with resistance is supported by the effect of proteasome inhibitors that induced apoptosis and inhibited proliferation in different cell lines. This effect was independent of p53 mutations and induction of p21 and p27 pathway.

Furthermore, the γ-form of 14-3-3 protein was found to be overexpressed in chemoresistant melanoma cells. This family of proteins is supposed to regulate apoptotic signal transduction by sequestering (proto)oncogene products and other proteins by binding their phosphoserine motifs. 14-3-3-Deficient cells have been shown to be unable to maintain cell cycle arrest after DNA damage with cytotoxic drugs. These cells died without DNA repair as they entered mitosis. These processes were associated with failure of sequestering mitosis initiating proteins, such as cyclins. Chemoresistance has also been shown to be regulated by dephosphorylation/phosphorylation processes. Phosphorylated molecules are known to show a reduced activity. In this way, phosphorylated proapoptotic BAD is sequestered by the 14-3-3 protein, preventing its binding to Bcl-x_L and leading to the inactivation of its proapoptotic function (Scriha et al. 2002).

Conclusion and Future Perspectives in Research and Treatment

Various mechanisms of drug resistance have been considered in light of their functional variations at different action levels and their specific relation to certain chemotherapeutic agents (Fig. 5). Several studies confirmed that mechanisms conferring drug resistance in hematological tumors are operative in the same way in solid tumors such as melanoma. Thus comprehensive analysis must be performed in the future to gain a better understanding of drug resistance in human melanoma. Apoptosis is widely considered to be one of the most important mechanisms by which cytostatic agents kill tumor cells. Therefore, deficiency in the apoptotic cascade should lead to a drug-resistant phenotype. The apoptotic pathway is still under intensive investigation, and analysis of apoptosis deficiency as a relevant mechanism of drug resistance has only just begun. The substantial amount of data generated in several stud-

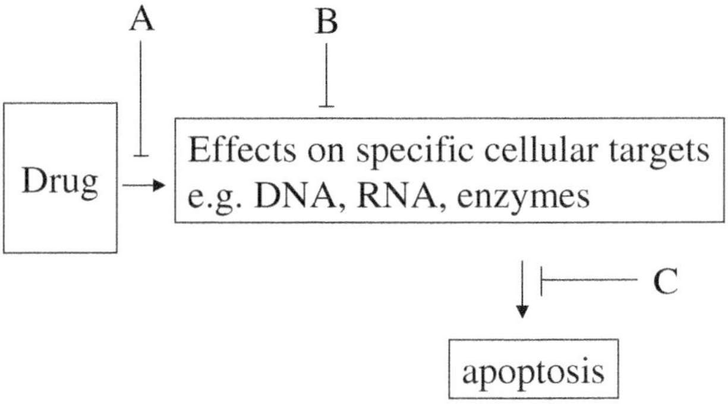

A: Drug-specific Mechanisms
preventing drug-target interaction and subsequent effects
- drug-efflux
- drug-modulation (e.g. detoxification)
- target-modulation

B: Effect-specific Mechanisms („Counter acting principles")
compensating effects preventing cell death
- DNA-repair
- upregulation of target-molecules
- downregulation of activating enzymes

C: Cell Death-specific mechanisms
inhibition of apoptosis
- upregulation of anti-apoptotic molecules
- downregulation pro-apoptotic factors
- altered mitochrondial release
- mutations in p53 or ras

Fig. 5. A hypothetical concept for specificity of drug resistance mechanisms in human melanoma dependent on the chemotherapeutic agent and the tumor entity. In the first phase, drug effect-specific mechanisms may intervene drug-target interaction by drug removal, by transport mechanisms and detoxification or target modulation (A). Other mechanisms reverse and compensate drug effects before the cell death cascades are initiated (B). Another possible drug resistance mechanism is alteration of apoptotic pathways leading to apoptosis deficiency and prevention of cell death (C)

ies, mentioned in this review, points to the complex network of the apoptotic regulation. Furthermore, it is also reasonable to assume that various resistance mechanisms that have not yet been discovered do exist. Several molecular biological approaches have been employed to identify these unknown mechanisms possibly associated with a drug-resistant phenotype. By applying CGH (comparative genomic hybridization) analysis to drug-resistant and -sensitive melanoma cells, a large number of additional acquired genetic imbalances have been detected (Nessling et al. 1999). Furthermore, differential gene expression in drug-sensitive and drug-resistant melanoma cells could be demonstrated by means of *differential display reverse transcription-polymerase chain reaction* (DDRT-PCR). This technique has led to the identification of several known and unknown genes that have not been associated with tumor drug resistance so far (Grottke et al. 2000). Functional assays for both approaches are needed to confirm the relevance of the identified molecules in conferring drug resistance in melanoma cells. In light of the evidence gained so far it seems that the lethality of malignant melanoma is due to a large extent to the ability of these tumor cells to resist chemotherapy, and any further knowledge gained on the nature of this resistance would improve the prospects of melanoma therapy. Identification of target molecules conferring resistance and a better understanding of signal transduction leading to tumor cell death would allow the development of strategies to overcome drug resistance. First steps have been taken in this direction. Many more are needed.

Acknowledgements. The authors acknowledge Dr. Hermann Lage for critical reading of the manuscript. This work was supported by grants of Deutsche Forschungsgemeinschaft (DFG, Scha 422/7-3) and Forschungsfond Klinikum Mannheim. This work was also supported by a grant 10-1628-La4 of the Deutsche Krebshilfe.

References

Ball NJ, Yohn JJ, Morelli JG, Norris DA, Golitz LE, Hoeffler JP (1994) Ras mutations in human melanoma: a marker of malignant progression. J Invest Dermatol 102(3):285–290

Beck WT, Danks MK, Wolverton JS, Granzen B, Chen M, Schmidt CA, Bugg BY, Friche E, Suttle DP (1993) Altered DNA topoisomerase II in multidrug resistance. Cytotechnology 11(2):115–119

Benathan M, Alvero Jackson H, Mooy AM, Scaletta C, Frenk E (1992) Relationship between melanogenesis, glutathione levels and melphalan toxicity in human melanoma cells. Melanoma Res 2(5–6):305–314

Bennett MR (1999) Mechanisms of p53-induced apoptosis. Biochem Pharmacol 58(7):1089–1095

Berger W, Hauptmann E, Elbling L, Vetterlein M, Kokoschka EM, Micksche M (1997) Possible role of the multidrug resistance-associated protein (MRP) in chemoresistance of human melanoma cells. Int J Cancer 71(1):108–115

Borst P, Evers R, Kool M, Wijnholds J (2000) A family of drug transporters: the multidrug resistance-associated proteins. J Natl Cancer Inst 92(16):1295–1302

Bruey JM, Ducasse C, Bonniaud P, Ravagnan L, Susin SA, Diaz-Latoud C, Gurbuxani S, Arrigo AP, Kroemer G, Solary E, Garrido C (2000) Hsp27 negatively regulates cell death by interacting with cytochrome *c*. Nat Cell Biol 2(9):645–652

Budihardjo I, Oliver H, Lutter M, Luo X, Wang X (1999) Biochemical pathways of caspase activation during apoptosis. Annu Rev Cell Dev Biol 15:269–290

Bukau B, Horwich AL (1998) The Hsp70 and Hsp60 chaperone machines. Cell 92(3):351–366

Campain JA, Slovak ML, Schoenlein PV, Popescu NC, Gottesman MM, Pastan I (1995) Acquisition of multiple copies of a mutant topoisomerase II alpha allele by chromosome 17 aneuploidy is associated with etoposide resistance in human melanoma cell lines. Somat Cell Mol Genet 21(6):451–471

Creagh EM, Cotter TG (1999) Selective protection by hsp 70 against cytotoxic drug-, but not Fas-induced T-cell apoptosis. Immunology 97(1):36–44

Daugas E, Susin SA, Zamzami N, Ferri KF, Irinopoulou T, Larochette N, Prevost MC, Leber B, Andrews D, Penninger J, Kroemer G (2000) Mitochondrio-nuclear translocation of AIF in apoptosis and necrosis. FASEB J 14(5):729–739

Du CY, Fang M, Li YC, Li L, Wang XD (2000) Smac, a mitochondrial protein that promotes cytochrome *c*-dependent caspase activation by eliminating IAP inhibition. Cell 102(1):33–42

Eliopoulos AG, Kerr DJ, Herod J, Hodgkins L, Krajewski S, Reed JC, Young LS (1995) The control of apoptosis and drug resistance in ovarian cancer: influence of p53 and Bcl-2. Oncogene 11(7):1217–1228

Fink D, Aebi S, Howell SB (1998) The role of DNA mismatch repair in drug resistance. Clin Cancer Res 4(1):1–6
Fulda S, Susin SA, Kroemer G, Debatin KM (1998) Molecular ordering of apoptosis induced by anticancer drugs in neuroblastoma cells. Cancer Res 58(19):4453–4460
Garrido C, Bruey JM, Fromentin A, Hammann A, Arrigo AP, Solary E (1999) HSP27 inhibits cytochrome *c*-dependent activation of procaspase-9. FASEB J 13(14):2061–2070
Garrido C, Fromentin A, Bonnotte B, Favre N, Moutet M, Arrigo AP, Mehlen P, Solary E (1998) Heat shock protein 27 enhances the tumorigenicity of immunogenic rat colon carcinoma cell clones. Cancer Res 58(23):5495–5499
Gottesman MM, Pastan I (1993) Biochemistry of multidrug resistance mediated by the multidrug transporter. Annu Rev Biochem 62:385–427
Griffith TS, Chin WA, Jackson GC, Lynch DH, Kubin MZ (1998) Intracellular regulation of TRAIL-induced apoptosis in human melanoma cells. J Immunol 161(6):2833–2840
Grossman D, McNiff JM, Li F, Altieri DC (1999) Expression and targeting of the apoptosis inhibitor, survivin, in human melanoma. J Invest Dermatol 113(6):1076–1081
Grottke C, Mantwill K, Dietel M, Schadendorf D, Lage H (2000) Identification of differentially expressed genes in human melanoma cells with acquired resistance to various antineoplastic drugs. Int J Cancer 88(4):535–546
Grover R, Wilson GD (1996) Bcl-2 expression in malignant melanoma and its prognostic significance. Eur J Surg Oncol 22(4):347–349
Hartmann A, Blaszyk H, Cunningham JS, McGovern RM, Schroeder JS, Helander SD, Pittelkow MR, Sommer SS, Kovach JS (1996) Overexpression and mutations of p53 in metastatic malignant melanomas. Int J Cancer 67(3):313–317
Helmbach H, Kern MA, Rossmann E, Renz K, Schadendorf D (2002) Drug-resistance towards etoposide and cisplatin in human melanoma cells is associated with different modulations of apoptotic pathways. J Invest Dermatol 118:923–932
Helmbach H, Rossmann E, Kern MA, Schadendorf D (2001) Drug-resistance in human melanoma. Int J Cancer 93(5):617–622
Houghton JA (1999) Apoptosis and drug response. Curr Opin Oncol 11(6):475–481
Jaattela M, Wissing D, Kokholm K, Kallunki T, Egeblad M (1998) Hsp70 exerts its anti-apoptotic function downstream of caspase-3-like proteases. EMBO J 17(21):6124–6134
Jansen B, Schlagbauer Wadl H, Brown BD, Bryan RN, van Elsas A, Muller M, Wolff K, Eichler HG, Pehamberger H (1998) bcl-2 antisense therapy chemosensitizes human melanoma in Scid mice. Nat Med 4(2):232–234
Jansen B, Schlagbauer Wadl H, Eichler HG, Wolff K, van Elsas A, Schrier PI, Pehamberger H (1997) Activated N-ras contributes to the chemoresistance of human melanoma in severe combined immunodeficiency (SCID) mice by blocking apoptosis. Cancer Res 57(3):362–365
Jansen B, Wacheck V, HeereRess E, Schlagbauer Wadl H, Hoeller C, Lucas T, Hoermann M, Hollenstein U, Wolff K, Pehamberger H (2000) Chemosensitisation of malignant melanoma by BCL2 antisense therapy. Lancet 356(9243):1728–1733
Jarvis WD, Grant S, Kolesnick RN (1996) Ceramide and the induction of apoptosis. Clin Cancer Res 2(1):1–6
Kaufmann SH, Earnshaw WC (2000) Induction of apoptosis by cancer chemotherapy. Exp Cell Res 256(1):42–49
Kavallaris M (1997) The role of multidrug resistance-associated protein (MRP) expression in multidrug resistance. Anticancer Drugs 8(1):17–25
Kern MA, Helmbach H, Artuc M, Karmann D, Jurgovsky K, Schadendorf D (1997) Human melanoma cell lines selected in vitro displaying various levels of drug resistance against cisplatin, fotemustine, vindesine or etoposide: modulation of proto-oncogene expression. Anticancer Res 17(6d):4359–4370
Konig J, Nies AT, Cui Y, Leier I, Keppler D (1999) Conjugate export pumps of the multidrug resistance protein (MRP) family: localization, substrate specificity, and MRP2-mediated drug resistance. Biochim Biophys Acta 1461(2):377–394
Kroemer G, Reed JC (2000) Mitochondrial control of cell death. Nat Med 6(5):513–519

Lage H, Christmann M, Kern MA, Dietel M, Pick M, Kaina B, Schadendorf D (1999) Expression of DNA repair proteins hMSH2, hMSH6, hMLH1, O^6-methylguanine-DNA methyltransferase and *N*-methylpurine-DNA glycosylase in melanoma cells with acquired drug resistance. Int J Cancer 80(5):744–750

Lage H, Helmbach H, Dietel M, Schadendorf D (2000) Modulation of DNA topoisomerase II activity and expression in melanoma cells with acquired drug resistance. Br J Cancer 82(2):488–491

Li G, Bush JA, Ho VC (2000) p53-dependent apoptosis in melanoma cells after treatment with camptothecin. J Invest Dermatol 114(3):514–519

Li G, Tang L, Zhou X, Tron V, Ho V (1998) Chemotherapy-induced apoptosis in melanoma cells is p53 dependent. Melanoma Res 8(1):17–23

Li P, Nijhawan D, Budihardjo I, Srinivasula SM, Ahmad M, Alnemri ES, Wang X (1997) Cytochrome c and dATP-dependent formation of Apaf-1/caspase-9 complex initiates an apoptotic protease cascade. Cell 91(4):479–489

Liu X, Zou H, Slaughter C, Wang X (1997) DFF, a heterodimeric protein that functions downstream of caspase-3 to trigger DNA fragmentation during apoptosis. Cell 89(2):175–184

Los M, Herr I, Friesen C, Fulda S, Schulze Osthoff K, Debatin KM (1997) Cross-resistance of CD95- and drug-induced apoptosis as a consequence of deficient activation of caspases (ICE/Ced-3 proteases). Blood 90(8):3118–3129

McGovern VJ, Balch CM, Wilton GW (1985) Cutaneous Melanoma: Clinical Management and Treatment Results Worldwide. J.B. Lippincott, Philadelphia, PA, pp 29–42

Mehlen P, Schulze-Osthoff K, Arrigo AP (1996) Small stress proteins as novel regulators of apoptosis. Heat shock protein 27 blocks Fas/APO-1- and staurosporine-induced cell death. J Biol Chem 271(28):16510–16514

Middleton MR, Lee SM, Arance A, Wood M, Thatcher N, Margison GP (2000a) O^6-methylguanine formation, repair protein depletion and clinical outcome with a 4 hr schedule of temozolomide in the treatment of advanced melanoma: results of a phase II study. Int J Cancer 88(3):469–473

Middleton MR, Lorigan P, Owen J, Ashcroft L, Lee SM, Harper P, Thatcher N (2000b) A randomized phase III study comparing dacarbazine, BCNU, cisplatin and tamoxifen with dacarbazine and interferon in advanced melanoma. Br J Cancer 82(6):1158–1162

Middleton MR, Lunn JM, Morris C, Rustin G, Wedge SR, Brampton MH, Lind MJ, Lee SM, Newell DR, Bleehen NM, Newlands ES, Calvert AH, Margison GP, Thatcher N (1998) O^6-methylguanine-DNA methyltransferase in pretreatment tumour biopsies as a predictor of response to temozolomide in melanoma. Br J Cancer 78(9):1199–1202

Miyake H, Hara I, Gohji K, Yamanaka K, Arakawa S, Kamidono S (1998) Enhancement of chemosensitivity in human bladder cancer cells by adenoviral-mediated p53 gene transfer. Anticancer Res 18(4c):3087–3092

Mosser DD, Caron AW, Bourget L, Meriin AB, Sherman MY, Morimoto RI, Massie B (2000) The chaperone function of hsp70 is required for protection against stress-induced apoptosis. Mol Cell Biol 20(19):7146–7159

Mouawad R, Khayat D, Soubrane C (2000) Plasma Fas ligand, an inducer of apoptosis, and plasma soluble Fas, an inhibitor of apoptosis, in advanced melanoma. Melanoma Res 10(5):461–467

Nessling M, Kern MA, Schadendorf D, Lichter P (1999) Association of genomic imbalances with resistance to therapeutic drugs in human melanoma cell lines. Cytogenet Cell Genet 87(3–4):286–290

Pandey P, Farber R, Nakazawa A, Kumar S, Bharti A, Nalin C, Weichselbaum R, Kufe D, Kharbanda S (2000) Hsp27 functions as a negative regulator of cytochrome *c*-dependent activation of procaspase-3. Oncogene 19(16):1975–1981

Petty R, Evans A, Duncan I, Kurbacher C, Cree I (1998) Drug resistance in ovarian cancer – the role of p53. Pathol Oncol Res 4(2):97–102

Raisova M, Bektas M, Wieder T, Daniel P, Eberle J, Orfanos CE, Geilen CC (2000) Resistance to CD95/Fas-induced and ceramide-mediated apoptosis of human melanoma cells is caused by a defective mitochondrial cytochrome c release. FEBS Lett 473(1):27–32

Rathmell JC, Thompson CB (1999) The central effectors of cell death in the immune system. Annu Rev Immunol 17:781–828

Reed JC (1995) Bcl-2: prevention of apoptosis as a mechanism of drug resistance. Hematol Oncol Clin North Am 9(2):451–473

Reed JC (1999) Dysregulation of apoptosis in cancer. J Clin Oncol 17(9):2941–2953

Ross MI, Balch CM (1991) The current management of cutaneous melanoma. Adv Surg 24:139–200

Rünger TM, Emmert S, Schadendorf D, Diem C, Epe B, Hellfritsch D (2000) Alterations of DNA repair in melanoma cell lines resistant to cisplatin, fotemustine, or etoposide. J Invest Dermatol 114(1):34–39

Saleh A, Srinivasula SM, Balkir L, Robbins PD, Alnemri ES (2000) Negative regulation of the Apaf-1 apoptosome by Hsp70. Nat Cell Biol 2(8):476–483

Scaffidi C, Fulda S, Srinivasan A, Friesen C, Li F, Tomaselli KJ, Debatin KM, Krammer PH, Peter ME (1998) Two CD95 (APO-1/Fas) signaling pathways. EMBO J 17(6):1675–1687

Schadendorf D, Herfordt R, Czarnetzki BM (1995) P-glycoprotein expression in primary and metastatic malignant melanoma. Br J Dermatol 132(4):551–555

Schadendorf D, Jurgovsky K, Kohlmus CM, Czarnetzki BM (1995a) Glutathione and related enzymes in tumor progression and metastases of human melanoma. J Invest Dermatol 105(1):109–112

Schadendorf D, Makki A, Stahr C, van Dyck A, Wanner R, Scheffer GL, Flens MJ, Scheper R, Henz BM (1995b) Membrane transport proteins associated with drug resistance expressed in human melanoma. Am J Pathol 147(6):1545–1552

Schadendorf D, Worm M, Algermissen B, Kohlmus CM, Czarnetzki BM (1994) Chemosensitivity testing of human malignant melanoma. A retrospective analysis of clinical response and in vitro drug sensitivity. Cancer 73(1):103–108

Scriha P, Poland J, Kohl S, Schnölzer M, Helmbach H, Hütter G, Lage H, Schadendorf D (2002) Study of the development of chemoresistance in melanoma cell lines using proteomics. J Invest Dermatol (in revision)

Sellers WR, Fisher DE (1999) Apoptosis and cancer drug targeting. J Clin Invest 104(12):1655–1661

Selzer E, Schlagbauer Wadl H, Okamoto I, Pehamberger H, Potter R, Jansen B (1998) Expression of Bcl-2 family members in human melanocytes, in melanoma metastases and in melanoma cell lines. Melanoma Res 8(3):197–203

Serrone L, Hersey P (1999) The chemoresistance of human malignant melanoma: an update. Melanoma Res 9(1):51–58

Shin MS, Park WS, Kim SY, Kim HS, Kang SJ, Song KY, Park JY, Dong SM, Pi JH, Oh RR, Lee JY, Yoo NJ, Lee SH (1999) Alterations of Fas (Apo-1/CD95) gene in cutaneous malignant melanoma. Am J Pathol 154(6):1785–1791

Soengas MSPC, Polsky D, Mora J, Esteller M, Optiz-Araya X, McCombie R, Hermann JG, Gerald WL, Lazebnik YA, Cordon-Cardo C, Lowe SW (2001) Inactivation of the apoptosis effector Apaf-1 in malignant melanoma. Nature 409(11):207–211

Thomas WD, Hersey P (1998) TNF-related apoptosis-inducing ligand (TRAIL) induces apoptosis in Fas ligand-resistant melanoma cells and mediates CD4 T cell killing of target cells. J Immunol 161(5):2195–2200

Ugurel S, Seiter S, Rappl G, Stark A, Tilgen W, Reinhold U (1999) Heterogenous susceptibility to CD95-induced apoptosis in melanoma cells correlates with bcl-2 and bcl-x expression and is sensitive to modulation by interferon-gamma. Int J Cancer 82(5):727–736

Xanthoudakis S, Roy S, Rasper D, Hennessey T, Aubin Y, Cassady R, Tawa P, Ruel R, Rosen A, Nicholson DW (1999) Hsp60 accelerates the maturation of pro-caspase-3 by upstream activator proteases during apoptosis. EMBO J 18(8):2049–2056

Zhang K, Mack P, Wong KP (1998) Glutathione-related mechanisms in cellular resistance to anticancer drugs. Int J Oncol 12(4):871–882

Zhang XD, Franco A, Myers K, Gray C, Nguyen T, Hersey P (1999) Relation of TNF-related apoptosis-inducing ligand (TRAIL) receptor and FLICE-inhibitory protein expression to TRAIL-induced apoptosis of melanoma. Cancer Res 59(11):2747–2753

Zou H, Henzel WJ, Liu X, Lutschg A, Wang X (1997) Apaf-1, a human protein homologous to C. elegans CED-4, participates in cytochrome c-dependent activation of caspase-3 [see comments]. Cell 90(3):405–413

Zou H, Li Y, Liu X, Wang X (1999) An APAF-1.cytochrome c multimeric complex is a functional apoptosome that activates procaspase-9. J Biol Chem 274(17):11549–11556

Cisplatin, Doxorubicin and Paclitaxel Induce *mdr1* Gene Transcription in Ovarian Cancer Cell Lines

Thomas Schöndorf, Rainer Neumann, Carolin Benz, Martina Becker, Marion Riffelmann, Uwe-Jochen Göhring, Judith Sartorius, Carl-Heinz Wirsing von König, Martina Breidenbach, Markus M. Valter, Markus Hoopmann, Federica Di Nicolantonio, Christian M. Kurbacher

T. Schöndorf (✉)
Department of Gynecology and Obstetrics, University of Cologne, Kerpener Straße 34, 50931 Köln, Germany
e-mail: thomas.schoendorf@medizin.uni-koeln.de

Abstract

The clinical observation of the multidrug resistance (MDR) phenotype is often associated with overexpression of the *mdr1* gene, in particular with respect to ovarian cancer. However, until now the *mdr1*-inducing potential of commonly used antineoplastics has been only incompletely explored. We performed short-term cultures of six ovarian cancer cell lines (MZOV4, EFO27, SKOV3, OAW42, OTN14, MZOV20) exposed to either blank medium or cisplatin, doxorubicin or paclitaxel at concentrations related to the clinically achievable plasma peak concentration. A highly specific quantitative real-time RT-PCR was used to detect the *Mdr1* transcripts. *Mdr1* mRNA contents were calibrated in relation to coamplified GAPDH mRNA. *Mdr1* mRNA was detectable in each cell line. In 13 out of 18 assays (72%) the specific anticancer drug being tested induced *mdr1* transcription. No decrease in *mdr1* mRNA concentration was observed. Our data suggest that *mdr1* induction by antineoplastics is one of the reasons for failure of ovarian cancer therapy but may vary individually.

Introduction

Ovarian cancer is one of the main causes of death related to gynecological malignancy: Nearly 65% of ovarian cancer patients will die from their disease within 5 years [8]. Although ovarian carcinomas are considered highly responsive to cytotoxic treatment, they rapidly develop chemoresistance [6]. Thus the multidrug resistance (MDR) phenotype of ovarian tumor cells is one of the major obstacles to the therapy of ovarian cancer [12].

On the molecular level, increased expression of the *mdr1* gene is the best-studied mechanism for the MDR phenotype [6]. The *mdr1* gene encodes the p170 glycoprotein, a transmembrane protein that eliminates toxic agents from the intracellular compartment and thus confers resistance to a wide variety of natural products. However, insufficient information is available concerning the regulation of the *mdr1* gene during the clinical course of a cancer patient undergoing antineoplastic chemotherapy. In ovarian cancer as well as in other neoplasms, p170 overexpression leads to the MDR phenotype and indicates a worse prognosis [8, 18].

Consequently, intensified research efforts are needed to obtain more basic data with respect to *mdr1* gene regulation in ovarian cancer [17]. The design of these studies should take into account techniques with increased sensitivity. Recently, *mdr1* gene amplification was excluded as a cause for *mdr1* overexpression in ovarian cancer [19]. Thus, in this tumor entity, p170 overexpression is more likely a result of increased transcription/translation of the *mdr1* gene. The study presented here was designed to explore whether antineoplastics are capable of inducing the *mdr1* gene. We therefore employed a *mdr1* mRNA detection assay using real-time PCR, which is more sensitive than in any other study performed so far. With this assay system the *mdr1*-inducing potency of commonly applied anticancer drugs was investigated.

Materials and Methods

Tumor Cell Culture

The ovarian cancer cell lines were kind gifts from L.G. Poels (Nijmegen, The Netherlands) (OTN14) and V. Möbus (Ulm, Germany) (MZOV4, MZOV20) or were obtained from DSMZ (Braunschweig, Germany) and DKFZ (Heidelberg, Germany). Tumor cells were grown in AIM V medium supplemented with 10% fetal calf serum, 2 mM L-glutamine, 100 IE/ml penicillin and 100 µg/ml streptomycin at 100 cells/µl (37°C, humidified 95% air-5% CO_2 atmosphere). Cells were exposed for 3 days to either blank medium (control) or the different antineoplastic agents: doxorubicin (DOX) 0.5 µg/ml, *cis*-diamino-dichloro-platinum(II) (CDDP) 3.8 µg/ml, and paclitaxel (PCT) 13.6 µg/ml. The cytostatics assayed referred to either the clinical peak plasma concentration (PPC) after administration of an intravenous standard dose (DOX, CDDP) or the equivalent of the area under the plasma elimination curve (PCT). Each assay was performed in triplicate.

Quantitative Real-Time RT-PCR

Cells were harvested by centrifugation (5 min, 8,000 *g*), washed in phosphate-buffered saline (PBS), and resuspended in lysis buffer. Total RNA was extracted with the RNeasy kit (Qiagen, Hilden, Germany) according to the manufacturer's instructions and quantified with the RiboGreen RNA quantification kit (MoBiTec, Göttingen, Germany).

A *mdr1*-specific 411-bp sequence was amplified in the presence of an intrinsic fluorescein-labeled *mdr1* probe. The TaqMan EZ RT-PCR Kit (GAPDH mRNA, Applied Biosystems, Weiterstadt, Germany) was used as an internal control. The mdr/GAPDH biplex-qu-RT-PCR contained 5 ng of RNA, 300 μM dATP, dCTP, and dGTP, 600 μM dUTP, 60 nM reference dye, each primer at 200 nM, each probe at 100 nM, 0.01 U/μl AmpErase UNG, and 0.1 U/μl r*Tth* DNA polymerase in TaqMan EZ buffer (50 mM bicine, 115 mM K-acetate, 0.01 mM EDTA, 40% glycerol, 3 mM Mn-acetate, pH 8.2) in a final volume of 50 μl. Quantitative real-time RT-PCR was performed by reverse transcription for 30 min at 30°C, denaturation for 10 min at 95°C and 40 cycles of 15 s at 95°C, and annealing and elongation for 1 min at 60° C. Resulting fluorescence was detected at each PCR cycle by the ABI 7700 Sequence Detection System (Applied Biosystems) automatically. Each *mdr1* or GAPDH signal, respectively, was quantified by the specific threshold cycle number (C_T).

Results

All ovarian cancer cell lines investigated were successfully analyzed. For GAPDH and *mdr1* expression, both single quRT-PCR and biplex-quRT-PCR revealed similar absolute results, indicating reproducibility and reliability of the assay. The expression of the *mdr1* gene was indicated as a quotient of *mdr1* C_T/GAPDH C_T. The quantitative real-time RT-PCR was performed in triplicate to validate the test. For each RT-PCR the assay system produced comparable results with acceptable variation: The quotients ranged from 0.60 to 0.88 and the intra-assay deviation did not exceed 0.08.

Summarizing all control experiments of the six cell lines, the *mdr1* C_T/GAPDH C_T quotient was 0.66±0.04. Therefore, quotients of 0.62–0.70 represent a “normal” distribution and are equivalent to *mdr1* expression rates ranging between 94% and 106% in relation to the control. For further analyses, each blank medium control was set at 100%.

As summarized in Table 1, all cell lines displayed increased *mdr1* gene expression in response to some of the cytostatics. In none of the assays was downregulation of *mdr1* gene expression detected. In four out of six (66%) ovarian cancer cell lines, treatment with CDDP or DOX increased *mdr1* expression to an average of 118% of the control, ranging from 109% to 133% (CDDP) or 107% to 130% (DOX), respectively. PCT-induced *mdr1* expression was detected in five out of six (83%) ovarian cancer cell lines. The degree of PCT-induced *mdr1* mRNA augmentation ranged between 109% and 119% with a mean of 114%.

Discussion

The unsatisfactory clinical results in refractory ovarian cancer are likely traced back to an increase in expression of the *mdr1* gene [8, 11]. Further-

Table 1. Relative increase of mdr1 gene expression induced by cytostatics in ovarian cancer cell lines. Tumor cells were grown overnight with either blank medium (control) or commonly applied anticancer therapeutics. For better comparison, each control was set as 100%. Increased mdr1 expression values exceeding the "normal" distribution are indicated in bold numbers. For each value, the standard deviation is indicated

	OTN14	EFO27	MZOV4	MZOV20	SKOV3	OAW42
Cisplatin	**121**±4.3	105±1.6	**109**±0.5	**109**±2.9	101±5.7	**133**±4.6
Doxorubicin	**130**±7.2	106±4.6	**107**±0.5	101±0.5	**108**±0.8	**128**±6.2
Paclitaxel	**113**±4.0	**113**±2.8	**119**±2.3	**109**±1.3	99±1.2	**119**±3.4

more, an increase of *mdr1* mRNA is a highly predictive determinant of patients' survival [16]. Accordingly, the impact of *mdr1* expression is a major concern in basic research of the molecular biology of ovarian cancer. We thus designed a study concerning the *mdr1* mRNA increase induced by a particular anticancer drug itself, thereby investigating the role of the *mdr1* gene in the development of drug resistance.

It is reported that anticancer drugs are able to induce *mdr1* transcription [4]. Resistance against doxorubicin or paclitaxel is mediated by the *mdr1* gene in OAW42 cells [13]. Accordingly, chemoresistant ovarian cancers display high *mdr1* mRNA levels [14]. Exposure to DOX results in a fast and dramatic increase of *mdr1* gene expression in human sarcoma in vivo [1]. Consequently, and in contrast to earlier data [5, 9, 10, 22], the predictive value of *mdr1* expression has recently been shown [2]. A study performed with both primary and recurrent native ovarian carcinomas revealed that the increased *mdr1* mRNA levels may not be maintained for a longer interval [20].

In 1999, Robert hypothesized that the *mdr1* gene might be expressed at very low levels in all tumors, including ovarian cancer [17]. New basic research involving new strategies with increased sensitivity is required to investigate the role of the *mdr1* gene in development of the MDR phenotype of ovarian cancer precisely and thus to unravel the aforementioned controversial studies. Here, an assay is presented to determine the *mdr1* expression rate with a high specificity and sensitivity, which is easily incorporated into clinical routine. This study shows a detectable *mdr1* mRNA presence in all cancer cell lines, confirming the hypothesis of low but persistent *mdr1* mRNA levels in ovarian cancer [17]. Furthermore, a drug-induced augmentation of the *mdr1* transcription rate was observed in 72% of the experiments and no decrease occurred. This also holds true for CDDP exposure, although this drug is known not to be a *mdr* target but capable of selecting multidrug-resistant ovarian cancer cells exhibiting high *mdr1* levels [21]. Our data and those of the earlier studies suggest that a particular drug induces *mdr1* transcription and, consequently, supports its own extrusion out of the tumor cell. However, the response rates indicate that the extent of this phenomenon is variable and should be investigated for each single tumor separately.

Nevertheless, the assay presented here performed with native cancer cells may be useful in identifying patients who will definitely benefit from a regimen of a common chemotherapy combined with a *mdr1*-inhibiting drug. Clinical trials have been presented recently with encouraging results [3, 7, 15], but they lack a molecular definition of the tumors.

Acknowledgements. This work was supported by the "Köln Fortune Program," Faculty of Medicine, University of Cologne, Germany.

References

1. Abolhoda A, Wilson AE, Ross H, Danenberg PV, Burt M, Scotto KW (1999) Rapid activation of MDR1 gene expression in human metastatic sarcoma after in vivo exposure to doxorubicin. Clin Cancer Res 5:3352–3356
2. Baekelandt MM, Holm R, Nesland JM, Trope CG, Kristensen GB (2000) P-glycoprotein expression is a marker for chemotherapy resistance and prognosis in advanced ovarian cancer. Anticancer Res 20:1061–1067
3. Baekelandt M, Lehne G, Trope CG, Szanto I, Pfeiffer P, Gustavsson B, Kristensen GB (2001) Phase I/II trial of the multidrug-resistance modulator valspodar combined with cisplatin and doxorubicin in refractory ovarian cancer. J Clin Oncol 19:2983–2993
4. Beck JF, Bohnet B, Brugger D, Dietl J, Scheper RJ, Bader P, Niethammer D, Gekeler V (1998) Expression analysis of protein kinase C isozymes and multidrug resistance associated genes in ovarian cancer cells. Anticancer Res 18:701–705
5. Codegoni AM, Broggini M, Pitelli MR, Pantarotto M, Torri V, Mangioni C, D́Incalci M (1997) Expression of genes of potential importance in the response to chemotherapy and DNA repair in patients with ovarian cancer. Gynecol Oncol 65:130–137
6. Fracasso PM (2001) Overcoming drug resistance in ovarian carcinoma. Curr Oncol Rep 3:19–26
7. Fracasso PM, Brady MF, Moore DH, Walker JL, Rose PG, Letvak L, Grogan TM, McGuire WP (2001) Phase II study of paclitaxel and valspodar (PSC 833) in refractory ovarian carcinoma: a gynecologic oncology group study. J Clin Oncol 19:2975–2982
8. Friedlander ML (1998) Prognostic factors in ovarian cancer. Sem Oncol 25:305–314
9. Goff BA, Ries JA, Els LP, Coltrera MD, Grown AM (1998) Immunophenotype of ovarian cancer as predictor of clinical outcome: evaluation at primary surgery and second-look procedure. Gynecol Oncol 70:378–385
10. Joncourt F, Buser K, Altermatt H, Bacchi M, Oberli A, Cerny T (1998) Multiple drug resistance parameter expression in ovarian cancer. Gynecol Oncol 70:176–182
11. Kavallaris M, Leary JA, Barrett JA, Friedlander ML (1996) MDR1 and multidrug resistance associated protein (MRP) gene expression in epithelial ovarian tumors. Cancer Lett 102:7–16
12. Lehne G (2000) P-glycoprotein as a drug target in the treatment of multidrug resistance cancer. Curr Drug Targets 1:85–99
13. Masanek U, Stammler G, Volm M (1997) Messenger RNA expression of resistance proteins and related factors in human ovarian carcinoma cell lines resistant to doxorubicin, taxol and cisplatin. Anticancer Drugs 8:189–198
14. Moran E, Cleary I, Larkin AM, Nic Amhlaoibh R, Masterson A, Scheper RJ, Izquierdo MA, Center M, ÓSullivan F, Clynes M (1997) Co-expression of MDR-associated markers, including P-170, MRP and LRP and cytoskeletal proteins, in three resistant variants of the human ovarian carcinoma cell line, OAW42. Eur J Cancer 33:652–660
15. Peck RA, Hewett J, Harding MW, Wang YM, Chauturvedi PR, Bhatnagar A, Ziessmann H, Atkins F, Hawkins MJ (2001) Phase I and pharmacokinetic study of the novel MDR1 and MRP1 inhibitor biricodar administered alone and in combination with doxorubicin. J Clin Oncol 19:3130–3141

16. Penson RT, Oliva E, Skates SJ, Glyptis T, Fuller Jr, AF, Goodmann A, Nikrui N, Seiden MV (2000) Expression of multidrug resistance-1 (MDR-1) correlates with paclitaxel response in ovarian cancer (OVCA) patients. Proc ASCO 19:399a.
17. Robert J (1999) Multidrug resistance in oncology: Diagnostic and therapeutic approaches. Eur J Clin Invest 129:536–545
18. Schneider J, Jimenez E, Marenbach K, Marx D, Meden H (1998) Co-expression of the MDR1 gene and HSP27 in human ovarian cancer. Anticancer Res 18:2967–2971
19. Schöndorf T, Scharl A, Kurbacher CM, Bien O, Becker M, Neumann R, Kolhagen H, Rustemeyer J, Mallmann P, Göhring U-J (1999) Amplification of the *mdr1*-gene is uncommon in recurrent ovarian carcinomas. Cancer Lett 146:195–199
20. Tewari KS, Kyshtoobayeva AS, Mehta RS, Yu IR, Burger RA, DiSaia PJ, Fruehauf JP (2000) Biomarker conservation in primary and metastatic epithelial ovarian cancer. Gynecol Oncol 78:130–136
21. Yang X, Page M (1995) P-glycoprotein expression in ovarian cancer cell line following treatment with cisplatin. Oncol Res 7:619–624
22. Yokoyama Y, Sato S, Fukushi Y, Sakamoto T, Futagami M, Saito Y (1999) Significance of multi-drug-resistant proteins in predicting chemotherapy response and prognosis in epithelial ovarian cancer. J Obstet Gynaecol Res 25:387–394

3 Clinical Relevance of Tumor-Directed Therapy

Chemosensitivity Testing as an Aid to Anti-Cancer Drug and Regimen Development

Ian A. Cree

Translational Oncology Research Centre, Department of Histopathology, Queen Alexandra Hospital, Portsmouth, PO6 3LY, UK
e-mail: ian.cree@port.ac.uk

Abstract

The ATP-based chemosensitivity assay has proved particularly useful for the evaluation of new anti-cancer agents and combinations. The majority of our publications in this area have concentrated on topoisomerase inhibitors. Comparison of mitoxantrone with doxorubicin convinced us that these two agents were not completely cross-resistant and led to the design of the mitoxantrone + paclitaxel regimen which is now in clinical practice. Re-assessment of treosulfan in uveal melanoma led to the design of a new regimen combining this alkylating agent with gemcitabine, again with rapid introduction of this combination to clinical practice. The assay has recently been used to examine the concentration-activity curve to determine which tumours might benefit from liposomal preparations capable of delivering 4–16 times the standard dose without cardiotoxicity. Assay-directed use of Caelyx is producing encouraging results, and we are now examining this drug in combination with others. We recently showed that XR5000, a combined inhibitor of topoisomerase I and II, was effective against melanoma as well as ovarian cancer, but at concentrations which were unlikely to be achieved in patients. These data confirm our suggestion that use of the assay could reduce the time to introduction of new anti-cancer drugs and the cost of this process.

Introduction

Medical oncology is a discipline that is based on empiricism. Clinical trials are designed for any new drug based first on an assessment of its safety/toxicity (phase I), then to determine its likely efficacy (phase II), and then to assess its ability to treat patients in comparison with existing treatment (phase III). However, for this to work, patients with a particular form of cancer are assumed to be identical, and treated accordingly with the same drugs, when it is patently clear that they are heterogeneous. The major difference between trials in oncology and in infectious disease is that there is usually no idea of whether the tumour cells are susceptible to the drug in question, whereas the reverse is true for bacterial infection, where microbiological assessment of sensitivity is one of the entry criteria. This ensures that expensive clinical trials of any new drug are only performed in patients who can benefit and targets them to those clinical conditions where the new agent is likely to produce the greatest benefit.

In a review paper published 2 years ago, Christian Kurbacher and I put forward an alternative to the current system, which would use the ATP-based chemosensitivity assay (ATP-TCA) to guide the introduction of new agents to oncology, very much as is already done for infectious disease (Cree and Kurbacher 1999). Several companies have taken up the challenge and have sponsored small studies that have allowed us to assess new agents. Although Dan von Hoff and others have previously used chemosensitivity testing to help guide decision-making in the pharmaceutical industry, the ATP-based assay has considerable advantages in terms of reproducibility and sensitivity compared with other assay types (Andreotti et al. 1995; Cree and Kurbacher 1997; Cree 1998).

The ATP-TCA has also proven useful for the design and testing of new combinations of drugs for use in cancer patients. In the past, this has usually been an empirical process in which the oncologist takes two or more drugs active in a particular tumour and combines them, testing the new regimen in a phase II study. The rationale for combining the two agents is often poorly explained, and in most countries only institutional review board approval is needed for such experimentation in human subjects. The ATP-TCA offers a way to combine drugs and test their effect against patient-derived tumour cells before going near a patient. This is a better approach than similar studies in cell lines, which rarely approximate the behaviour of tumour-derived cells (Andreotti et al. 1994; Di Nicolantonio et al. unpublished data).

Topoisomerase Inhibitors

Topoisomerases unravel DNA to allow transcription and replication. They are therefore present in all cells, and most tumour cells express high levels of topoisomerase activity. Topoisomerases are divided into two main groups – those that cut one DNA strand (topoisomerase I) and those that cut both strands (topoisomerase II). Both allow the DNA to uncoil before the cut ends are rejoined. Topoisomerase II comes as two distinct isoforms coded by genes on chromosomes 17 (topoisomerase IIa) and 3p (topoisomerase IIb). Topoisomerase IIb is constitutively expressed, whereas topoisomerase IIa is regulated, as is topoisomerase I.

Several anti-cancer drugs work as topoisomerase inhibitors. Camptothecin-derived drugs inhibit topoisomerase I (topotecan, irinotecan). Etoposide is a direct inhibitor of topoisomerase II, binding to the enzyme, whereas anthracyclines (e.g. doxorubicin) bind to the minor groove of DNA.

The first indication that the ATP-TCA might be important to drug development was a comparison of doxorubicin and mitoxantrone, a structurally distinct anthracycline, in breast cancer (Kurbacher et al. 1996). As expected, both drugs showed activity against breast cancer, but despite the fact that both work by inhibiting topoisomerase II, there was a lack of complete cross-resistance (Fig. 1). This important observation has allowed patients treated with one anthracycline (usually doxorubicin or the closely related epirubicin) to be successfully retreated with the other drug (usually mitoxantrone).

Caelyx

All anti-cancer drugs are toxic to some degree, and anthracyclines are cardiotoxic in addition to their anti-proliferative activity. This has limited their use significantly. Early results from the ATP-TCA (Hunter et al. 1993) showed a concentration-response curve for anthracyclines that did not achieve 100% inhibition at achievable dose levels (100% TDC) in most tumours. The idea that one could target doxorubicin to tumours and achieve higher intra-tumoural concentrations by encapsulating the drug in liposomes was therefore of considerable interest. In fact, intra-tumoural concentrations of doxorubicin delivered by PEGylated liposomes (Caelyx/Doxil) have been found to be between 5- and 16-fold higher than can be achieved by standard soluble doxorubicin. As liposomes require tissue lipase to release their contents, the liposomal preparation cannot be used directly in the assay, and we have therefore tested an arbitrarily selected 5x TDC, based on the achievable intra-tumoural concentration, to mimic Caelyx (Neale et al. 2000a). Recent results make us feel that this may be a little high, and that a 3x TDC for doxorubicin may provide a better correlation with outcome in patients receiving Caelyx, but this has yet to be formally analysed.

XR5000

Cells exposed to one topoisomerase I are likely to upregulate topoisomerase IIa and vice versa. This has resulted in a search for combined inhibitors of both topoisomerase I and II, of which XR5000 is one of the first representatives. A test drug concentration was established from pharmacokinetic data, and a number of tumour types were tested (Neale et al. 2000b). The results showed activity of XR5000 against recurrent ovarian cancer, a tumour we expected to show some sensitivity as independent inhibitors of topoisomerase I or II are active in this setting. The surprise was that there was also activity against a subset of melanomas. Unfortunately, in both cases, XR5000 rarely produced sufficient activity for it to be likely to produce a response if used alone, although it might be useful in combination (Neale et al. 2000b).

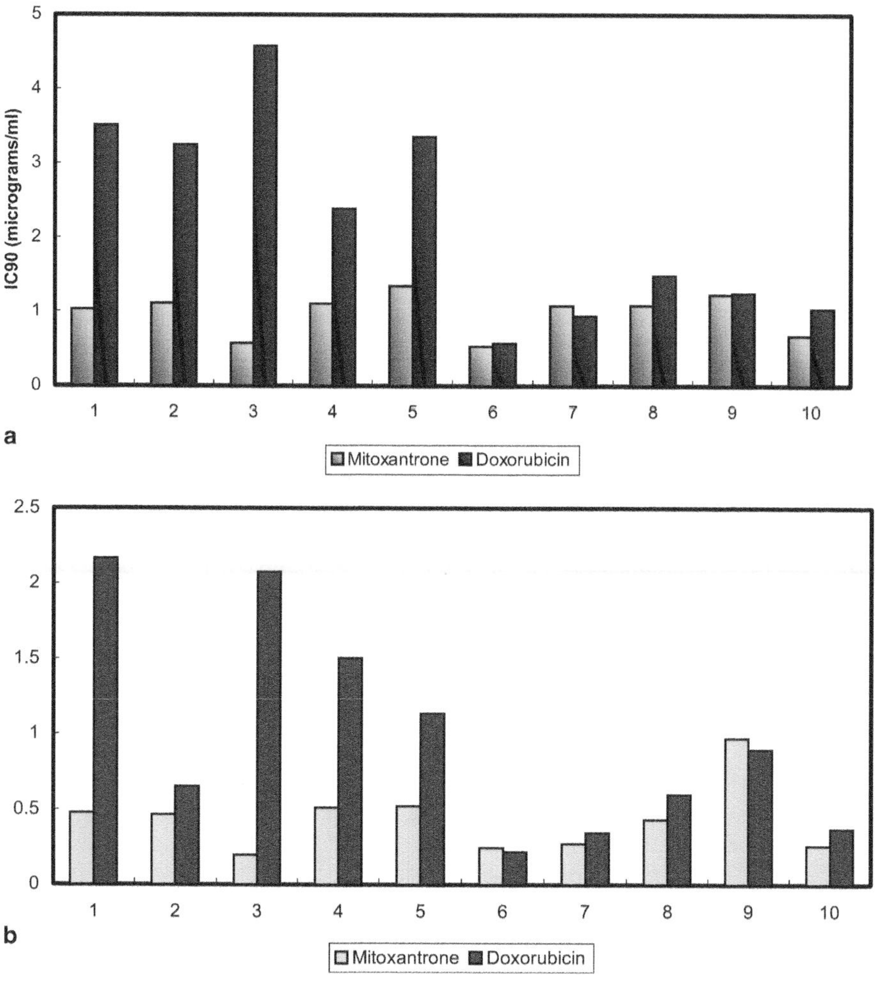

Fig. 1. Comparison of mitoxantrone and doxorubicin in a series of recurrent ovarian tumour specimens for (**a**) IC_{90} and (**b**) IC_{50}. None of the patients had previously received treatment with anthracyclines. High sensitivity is indicated by a low IC_{90}. There is considerable variation, with several patients showing considerably more sensitivity to mitoxantrone than doxorubicin. Note that patient 2 shows similar IC_{50} values for both drugs, but that mitoxantrone has a lower IC_{90} value

Mitoxantrone + Paclitaxel

Few drugs are used alone, and anthracylines have been usefully combined with a large number of different agents, including DNA-damaging agents such as cyclophosphamide or carboplatin. There is also considerable experience combining these drugs with agents that interfere with microtubule function, vinca alkaloids and taxanes. The results from earlier ATP-TCA studies suggested that replacing epirubicin or doxorubicin with mitoxantrone might produce a combination with a taxane, which would be active in some patients previously treated with anthracyclines.

Careful selection of patients for treatment would clearly be important, but at the same time, Christian Kurbacher and his group were beginning to treat patients on the basis of the assay, so this was not a major problem. The results were encouraging (Kurbacher et al. 1997), and this new regimen, developed on the basis of ATP-TCA data is proving very useful, even in patients with recurrent ovarian cancer after first-line taxane treatment (Kurbacher et al. 2001).

Treosulfan + Gemcitabine

Rare tumours (those outside the top 10 common solid tumours) are responsible for around 25% of cancer-related deaths. Drugs are rarely designed specifically for such tumours, as this makes little commercial sense, and clinical trials are often limited. Melanomas of the uveal tract of the eye are the commonest tumours of the eye in caucasian populations and have a 50% 10-year survival. Whereas metastatic cutaneous melanoma is very difficult to treat, uveal melanoma is even worse, and the M.D. Anderson Cancer Center have reported a less than 1% response rate with a range of combinations based on DTIC (Bedikian et al. 1995).

Could the ATP-TCA help? Using the ATP-TCA, we were quickly able to show that uveal melanoma was a very chemoresistant tumour, but that there was heterogeneity of activity for a number of different drugs (Myatt et al. 1997). The best alkylating agent we identified was treosulfan, which alkylates at the O^7 position, rather than the O^6 (Hartley et al. 1999) and is therefore unaffected by O^6 alkyl guanyl transferase activity. However, on its own this drug was clearly unlikely to produce many clinical responses, as it could not achieve 100% inhibition at clinically relevant concentrations. As a result, we looked for ways of modulating its activity. In ovarian cancer, we had previously noted the ability of cytosine analogues such as Ara-C and gemcitabine to modulate cisplatin activity (Kurbacher et al. 1997). The putative mechanism was inhibition of DNA repair (Neale et al. 1999), so we reasoned that it might be sensible to make repair of treosulfan-induced DNA damage for uveal melanoma cells by combining treosulfan with gemcitabine (Fig. 2). The results were spectacular (Neale et al. 1997), and early clinical results in uveal melano-

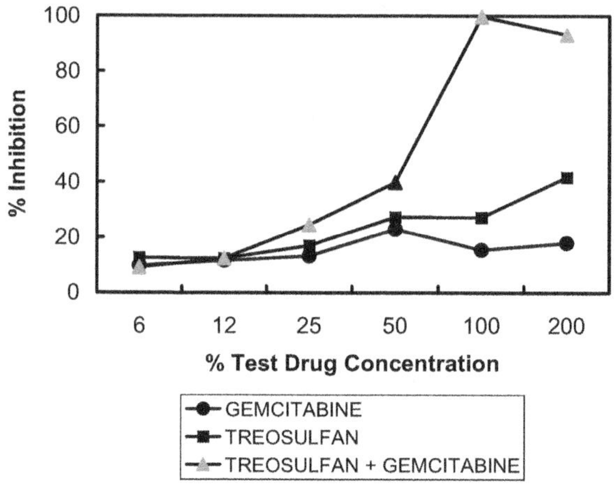

Fig. 2. Results from a patient with uveal melanoma. Treosulfan shows some activity at high concentrations, and gemcitabine does little alone. The combination is much more active at clinically achievable concentrations

ma are encouraging (Cree et al. unpublished data; Ugurel et al., *vide infra*), with one complete response in the first seven patients treated.

Because treosulfan is often used in recurrent ovarian cancer, we were also able to use this combination in other settings, again checking first to ensure that activity in the ATP-TCA warranted this. The results are very good, and this combination is now in widespread use for several different tumour types (Grecu et al. 2001), although there is some debate as to the best regimen to use. We prefer to use treosulfan at 5,000–7,000 mg/m^2 given by i.v. bolus on day 1, with gemcitabine 1,000 mg/m^2 given by rapid (<30 min) infusion after treosulfan on the same day, with a 3-week cycle length. The major toxicity is bone marrow suppression, and GM-CSF is sometimes useful. Reduction of the gemcitabine dose is not a major problem and should be considered in patients who have recently had radiotherapy (which can increase the toxicity of gemcitabine dramatically) or previous chemotherapy with bone marrow suppression.

Future Drug Development

What of the future? The ATP-TCA has shown itself capable of assessing the likely contribution of new drugs to treatment, and for the design of new combinations using new or old drugs. The ability to conduct these tests before patients are treated is particularly attractive, as it ensures that expensive drug trials are not instituted before there is real evidence that patients might benefit.

References

Andreotti PE, Linder D, Hartmann DM, Cree IA, Pazzagli M, Bruckner HW (1994) TCA-100 Tumor chemosensitivity assay: differences in sensitivity between cultured tumor cell lines and clinical studies. Journal of Bioluminescence and Chemiluminescence 9:373–378

Andreotti PE, Cree IA, Kurbacher CM, Hartmann DM, Linder D, Harel G, Gleiberman I, Caruso PA, Ricks SH, Untch M, Sartori C, Bruckner HW (1995). Chemosensitivity testing of human tumors using a microplate adenosine triphosphate luminescence assay: Clinical Correlation for Cisplatin Resistance of Ovarian Carcinoma. Cancer Research 55:5276–5282

Bedikian AY, Legha SS, Mavligit G, Carrasco CH, Khorana S, Plager C, Papadopoulos N, Benjamin RS (1995) Treatment of uveal melanoma metastatic to the liver: a review of the M. D. Anderson Cancer Center experience and prognostic factors. Cancer 76:1665–7160

Cree IA, Kurbacher CM (1997) Individualising chemotherapy for solid tumours – is there any alternative? Anti-Cancer Drugs 8:541–548

Cree IA (1998) Luminescence-based cell viability testing. In: LaRossa RA (ed) Bioluminescence methods and protocols. Meth Molec Biol 102:169 –177

Cree IA, Kurbacher CM (1999) ATP based tumour chemosensitivity testing: assisting new agent development. Anti-Cancer Drugs 10:431–435

Cree IA, Neale MH, Myatt NE, de Takats PG, Hall P, Grant JG, Kurbacher CM, Reinhold U, Neuber K, MacKie RM, Chana J, Weaver PC, Khoury GG, Sartori C, Andreotti PE (1999) Heterogeneity of chemosensitivity of metastatic cutaneous melanoma. Anti-Cancer Drugs 10:437–444

Grecu OM, Kurbacher CM, Mallman P, Bruckner HW, Cree IA (2001) Treosulfan and gemcitabine in heavily pretreated patients with breast and ovarian cancer: laboratory study and clinical pilot trial of the ISCO clinical study group. Proc ASCO 20:187b

Hartley JA, O'Hare CC, Baumgart J (1999) DNA alkylation and interstrand cross-linking by treosulfan. Br J Cancer. 79:264–266

Kurbacher CM, Cree IA, Brenne U, Bruckner HW, Kurbacher JA, Mallmann P, Andreotti PE, Krebs D (1996) Heterogeneity of in vitro chemosensitivity in perioperative breast cancer cells to mitoxantrone versus doxorubicin evaluated by microplate ATP bioluminescence assay. Breast Cancer Res Treatment 41:161–170

Kurbacher CM, Bruckner HW, Cree IA, Kurbacher JA, Wilhelm L, Poch G, Indefrei D, Mallman P, Krebs D, Andreotti PE (1997) Mitoxantrone combined with paclitaxel as salvage therapy for platinum-refractory ovarian cancer: laboratory study and clinical pilot trial. Clin Cancer Res 3:1527–1533

Kurbacher CM, Stier U, Janat M, Cree IA, Bruckner HW (2001) ATP-assay directed chemotherapy for recurrent ovarian cancer: mature results of an ISCO clinical study group trial. Proc ASCO 20:185b

Myatt N, Cree IA, Kurbacher CM, Foss AJE, Hungerford JL, Plowman PN (1997) The ex vivo chemosensitivity profile of choroidal melanoma. Anti-Cancer Drugs 8:756–762

Neale MH, Myatt N, Cree IA, Kurbacher CM, Foss AJE, Hungerford JL, Plowman PN (1999) Combination chemotherapy for choroidal melanoma: ex vivo sensitivity to treosulfan with gemcitabine or cytosine arabinoside. British Journal of Cancer 79:1487–1493

Neale MH, Lamont A, Hindley A, Kurbacher CM, Cree IA (2000a) The ex vivo effect of high concentrations of doxorubicin on recurrent ovarian carcinoma. Anti-Cancer Drugs 11:865–871

Neale MH, Charlton PA, Cree IA (2000b) Ex vivo activity of XR5000 against solid tumours. Anti-Cancer Drugs 11:471–478

Neale MH, Myatt NE, Ghassan G Khoury GG, Weaver P, Lamont A, Hungerford JL, Kurbacher CM, Hall P, Corrie PG, Cree IA (2002) Comparison of the ex vivo chemosensitivity of uveal and cutaneous melanoma. Melanoma Res (in press)

Assay-Assisted Treatment Selection for Women with Breast or Ovarian Cancer

John P. Fruehauf, David S. Alberts

J.P. Fruehauf (✉)
Oncotech Inc., 15501 Redhill Avenue, Tustin, CA 92780, USA
e-mail: johnfruehauf@msn.com

Abstract

Although women suffering from advanced cancer of the breast or ovary are unlikely to be cured, several active agents are available that can prolong their lives. The use of these agents is based on demonstrated benefit in large randomized clinical trials, and the clinical activity of these chemotherapy regimens is initially high, with 60%–70% of patients responding. Unfortunately, their benefit in the second-line setting is often limited, with less than 30% of patients showing significant disease response. Thus some 70% of patients may undergo ineffective treatment during the course of their disease, while still suffering from significant chemotherapy-related toxicity. Having some foreknowledge of a given agent's expected result before its administration would therefore benefit the individual patient. In vitro drug response testing, first developed to assist in the selection of antibiotics for patients with bacterial infections, has recently been demonstrated to accurately predict how cancer patients will respond to chemotherapy. This review discusses the historical development of in vitro testing for cancer patients, some of the pitfalls encountered, and offers an assessment of their current utility. Results of various clinical trials that evaluated correlations between in vitro tumor response and clinical outcomes are described. These data suggest that in vitro drug response assays can accurately predict drug resistance and can identify patients who are more or less likely to benefit from a given agent.

Introduction

Treatment for patients with breast or ovarian cancer has traditionally been based on the selection of active agents and combinations identified by large phase III randomized clinical trials. Clinical trial-based identification of new chemotherapy agents with significant disease specific activity has been a cornerstone of modern oncology, providing statistical validation of their safety and benefit. Perhaps of greatest importance, the impact of new treatment modalities on patient survival can be compared with previously proven treatment regimens. The clinical utility of agents developed through this process has led to significantly improved outcomes for women with advanced stage breast and ovarian cancer. Conventional chemotherapy agents with clinical activity in breast cancer currently include doxorubicin, Doxil, epirubicin, cyclophosphamide, 5-fluorouracil (5-FU), capecitabine, methotrexate, gemcitabine, vinorelbine, paclitaxel, docitaxel, and cisplatin (Esteva et al. 2001; Norton 1999). Chemotherapy has been augmented by advances in hormonal therapy, including selective estrogen receptor antagonists and aromatase inhibitors. Of particular interest is the recent development of synergistic combinations of Herceptin with conventional chemotherapy agents, an approach that integrates rational and empirical treatment approaches. With respect to advanced-stage epithelial ovarian cancer, although platinum-based regimens continue to be the standard of care for first-line treatment, many agents have been found to exhibit comparable second-line activity, including topotecan, vinorelbine, etoposide, Doxil, cyclophosphamide, taxanes, 5-FU, and Hexalen (McGuire et al. 1996; Alberts 1999; Markman and Bookman 2002). However, despite this armamentarium and newer pharmacological strategies, disease progression and patient death are still major problems that largely result from intrinsic and acquired drug resistance. Although current chemotherapy regimens produce clinical response rates for women with breast or ovarian cancer of 60%–70%, 5-year survival rates for these women remains below 50% and cures are rare (Greenlee et al. 2001).

In an attempt to improve treatment response and patient survival, investigators working over the past 50 years have developed in vitro drug response assay systems to determine the potential activity of chemotherapy agents for a given patient before their administration. The central hypothesis underlying this approach is that the drug response profile for each individual patient will differ based on their intrinsic genetic diversity and the development of subclones within tumors that have divergent phenotypes (Goldie and Coldman 1979; Iyer and Ratain 1998). In vitro assays that identify individual differences in tumor drug response make it possible to design patient-specific regimens targeted against each patient's tumor characteristics. By eliminating ineffective agents, the patient is spared toxic treatment without benefit, and the selection of agents active in vitro may increase the probability of response. Although several test systems have emerged that accurately predict patient response in a clinically useful time frame, debate continues about the optimal application of these technologies (Fruehauf and Bosanquet 1993; Chu and DeVita 2001; Cortazar and Johnson 1999). Although this approach has obvious appeal, various technical hurdles have retarded the incorporation of these technologies into standard practice. This review briefly reviews the historical development of in vitro drug response assays and then focuses on recent clinical validation studies that have led to more widespread use of these assays to assist in treatment selection.

Historical Perspective

In vitro drug response assaysoriginated at the beginning of the last century when Louis Pasteur and Paul Ehrlich observed the effects of antimicrobial agents on cultured bacteria (Burger 1988; Pasteur and Joubert 1877). Their pioneering work subsequently led to Fleming's development of penicillin, as well as to the general use of culture and sensitivity testing for antibiotics over the past century (Table 1). It was not until 1953, however, that the first publications appeared by Black and Spear describing the use of an in vitro assay with human tumor biopsy material to evaluate the activity of aminopterin, an early antimetabolite (Black and Spear 1953, 1954). Their assay evaluated the in vitro response of tumor tissue segments composed of both malignant and nonmalignant components to aminopterin exposure. Black and Spear's assay end point was cell viability determined by metabolic conversion in the mitochondria of a tetrazolium dye to a colored product that could be measured spectrophotometrically. These studies eventually led to the development of the MTT assay employed by the NCI to screen newly developed drugs for activity on various cell lines and to direct chemotherapy in the clinic (Grever et al. 1992; Furukawa et al. 2000; Ohie et al. 2000).

Black and Spear's seminal work was significant because it foreshadowed some of the technical hurdles that would confront subsequent investigators. First, their assay end point measured the metabolic activity of both cancer and normal cells, making it difficult to distinguish between drug effects on normal versus cancer components. In addition, because they used tumor segments, the contribution of the malignant component to the end point signal varied from patient to patient, making it difficult to standardize the system and to compare results between patients. Finally, their findings suggested that the accuracy of their system to predict treatment response, the positive predictive value, was not as great as the negative predictive value to predict treatment failure. The overall predictive accuracy of their assay system was below 70%, a value too low for clinical application. On the other hand, the relative advantage of this early in vitro drug response assay to predict drug resistance

Table 1. Historical overview

1877	Pasteur and Joubert described the effects of "chemotherapy" on cultured microbes
1928	Fleming's discovery of penicillin ushers in modern chemosensitivity era
1953	Black and Spear report first in vitro assay for cancer specimens
1956	Marcus and Puck: agar-based assay system selective for malignant cell growth
1977	Salmon and Hamburger report on second-generation human tumor cloning assay
1984	Third-generation thymidine incorporation, DiSC, and ATP assays developed
1984	Southwest Oncology Group: Assay quality controls introduced
1990	Clinical trials indicate that assays predict response
1993	Clinical trials indicate that assay results are significantly associated with survival
2000	Medicare covers in vitro drug resistance assays

better than chemosensitivity has been born out by many other investigators over the ensuing decades (Fruehauf and Bosanquet 1993).

A focused approach to obtain in vitro assay results specific for the malignant component of a tumor began with observations by Puck and Marcus that agarose-based culture systems preferentially supported the growth of transformed cells, whereas the nonmalignant cellular components did not proliferate (Puck and Marcus 1955). Their identification of agar as a selective growth medium for the transformed cells within the tumor led to Hamburger and Salmon's development of the agarose-based human tumor stem cell chemosensitivity assay in the early 1970s (Salmon et al. 1978). This "chemosensitivity" assay was initially met with great enthusiasm, but technical problems prevented its widespread application. Technical pitfalls associated with this system included assay success rates less than 50%, turnaround times of up to 3 weeks, and technical concerns related to the incomplete disaggregation of the tumor into pure single-cell populations required to discern colony formation (Selby et al. 1983). During the late 1970s and early 1980s, advances in scintillation counting technology made it relatively easy to accurately determine tritium-labeled thymidine incorporation in cell culture systems to measure cellular proliferation. Radiolabeled thymidine had been used since the 1960s to assess bacterial proliferation (Brock 1967). Tritiated thymidine uptake as an end point to determine cancer cell response to chemotherapy mirrored results of the clonogenic assay performed in soft agar (Johnson and Glaubiger 1983; Sondak et al. 1984). The merger of agarose-based cultures of cellular clumps with the tritiated thymidine incorporation end point resulted in a third-generation technology capable of determining in vitro drug response in greater than 85% of the cases in as few as 5 days (Sondak et al. 1984). At the same time, alternative end points were developed, including measurement of mitochondrial function (e.g., MTT and ATP assays), membrane integrity [e.g., fluorescent cyto-footprint (FCF)], fluorescein diacetate (FDA), propidium iodine uptake, and differential staining cytotoxicity assays (DiSC) (Kochli et al. 1994; Andreotti et al. 1995; Elledge et al. 1995; Meitner 1991; Weisenthal and Lippman 1985; Bird et al. 1987; Wilbur et al. 1992; Weisenthal 1994; Bosanquet 1991; Bosanquet et al. 1999; Mason et al. 1999). Table 2 shows a comparison of these various assays, and Fig. 1 provides cartoons of the assay schemas.

Assay Technologies

As shown in Table 1, various assay end points have been developed to assess the effects of drugs on cancer cell growth and viability. The advantages or disadvantages of a given end point are related in part to its ease of use, reproducibility, precision, and success rate. Assay end points are generally related to measures of cell proliferation, metabolism, or survival. As depicted in Fig. 1a, the HTCA assay measures the capacity of single malignant cells to divide and form colonies in or on an agar-based matrix. After short-term drug exposure, single cells are plated in or on an agar matrix. Cells that have been

Table 2. Comparison of in vitro drug response assay techniques

Assay type	Culture conditions	Assay end point	Prediction	Cancer cell specificity
ATP	Microtiter plate in defined media (no serum)	ATP content in cultured cells	Sensitivity	Moderate
FCPA	Microorgan culture in cellulose-collagen matrix	Cytosolic esterase formation of fluorescein	Sensitivity	Low
MTT	Microtiter plate in 15% serum-containing media	Succinate dehydrogenase formation of formazan	Sensitivity	Low
DiSC	Cytophobic plates in 15% serum-containing media	Light microscopic reading of nonviable cells	Both	High
HTCA	Agar plates in 15% serum-containing media	Colony formation and counting	Sensitivity	High
^{3}H-uridine	Extracellular matrix strips in 1% serum media	^{3}H-uridine incorporation	Resistance	Moderate
EDR	Agarose suspension culture in 15% serum media	^{3}H-thymidine incorporation	Resistance	High

killed or have undergone damage causing cell cycle arrest fail to form colonies. Colony counts after a 2- to 3-week period is the end point determined in the HTCA. Differential colony formation between untreated controls and treated cells measures drug activity. Agar, the growth substrate, mimics a suspension environment and suppresses the proliferation of nontransformed cells (Puck and Marcus 1955; Hamburger and Salmon 1977). Agar-based culture systems, such as used in the extreme drug resistance (EDR) assay (Fig. 1b), or polypropylene plates employed in the DiSC (Fig. 1c) and ATP assay (Fig. 1d) systems, suppress cellular adherence to a growth surface. Fibroblasts, mesothelial cells, and other stromal cells can proliferate in adherence-based culture systems, adding a non-cancer cell-specific growth signal or component to the end point. In vitro drug response assay results are adversely affected by proliferation of nonmalignant cells that add "noise" to the cancer cell growth signal (Campling et al. 1991; Kitaoka et al. 1997). The growth signal of disaggregated cells obtained from tumor biopsies grown in nonadherent culture conditions is therefore relatively more cancer cell specific than growth in adherent culture systems. The use of low-serum-containing medium is another technique employed to suppress nontransformed cell proliferation. The use of agar or low-serum-containing medium helps ensure that assay end points determined after several days of tissue culture measure cancer cell proliferation or metabolism with minimal contributions from normal cellular components present in each tumor biopsy specimen.

The EDR assay (Fig. 1b) measures the effects of chemotherapy agents to inhibit proliferation of small tumor cell clumps suspended in a low-density layer of agarose that overlays a solid layer of agarose (Sondak et al. 1984). Cell cultures are incubated with drugs for 4 days and pulsed with ^{3}H-thymidine over

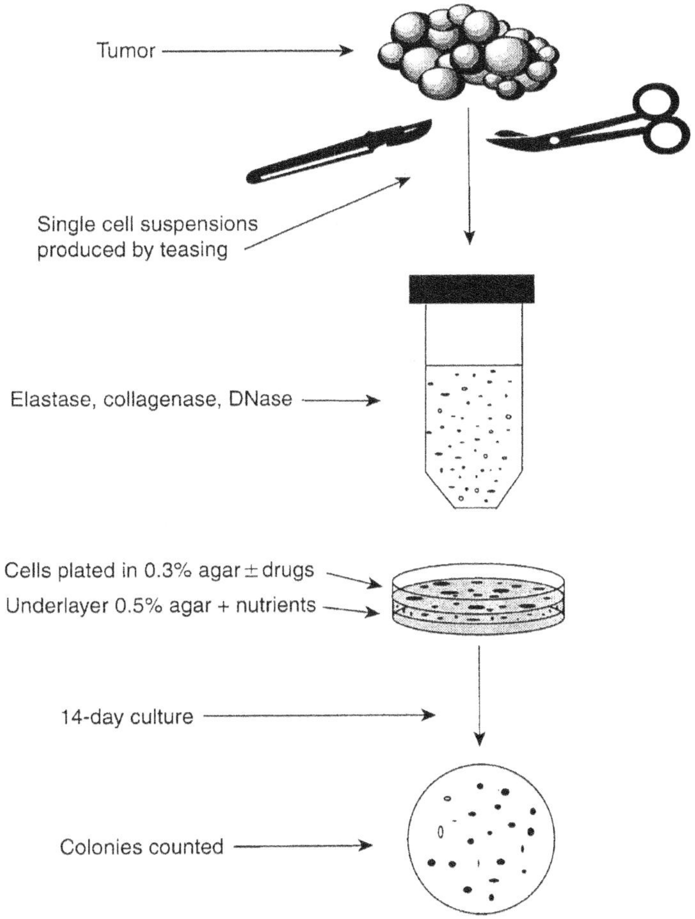

Fig. 1a–f. Comparison of in vitro drug response technologies. **a** Human tumor cloning assay. **b** Extreme drug resistance assay. **c** DiSC assay. **d** MTT assay. **e** ATP assay. **f** Fluorescent cytoprint assay

the last 2 days of the 5-day culture. Radiolabeled thymidine is incorporated into the dividing cells replicating DNA, whereas nonproliferating cells and dead cells fail to incorporate the label. Cells are harvested onto glass fiber filters and lysed with deionized water. The filters trap the labeled macromolecular DNA, whereas unincorporated tritiated thymidine is washed through the filter. Filters and scintillation fluid are added to vials, and radioactive decay is measured in a scintillation counter to determine the amount of DNA synthesis that took place in control and treated tumor cells. ^{3}H-uridine incorporation can also be used to evaluate in vitro drug effects on tumor cell proliferation (Elledge et al. 1995). Tumor cells are constantly exposed to drug during the 5-day period used in the EDR assay, resulting in in vitro drug exposures that are

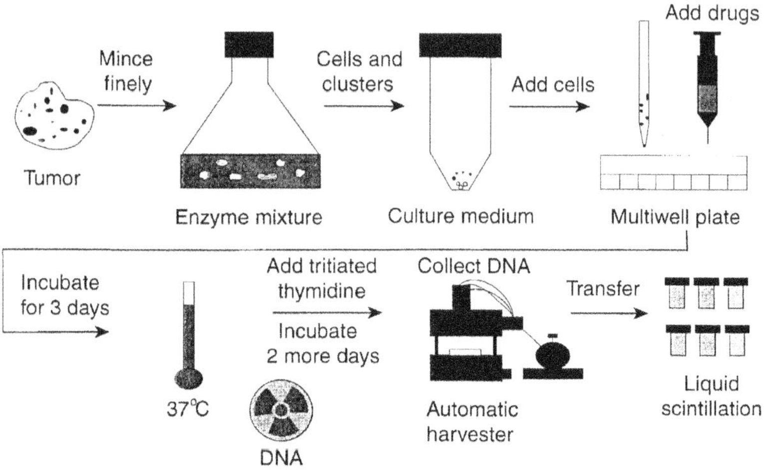

Fig. 1b

Table 3. In vitro versus in vivo drug exposures in the EDR assay*

Drug	Concentration µg/ml	Exposure Time (h)	In vitro C×T	In vivo C×T	Ratio
Doxorubicin 0.1	96	8	1.4	5.8	
5-FU	3	96	288	20.0	14.4
Cisplatin	1	96	33	2.0	16.5
BCNU	10	96	20	1.0	20.0
Melphalan	5	96	20	2.5	8.0

*Fruehauf and Bosanquet

severalfold higher than those achieved clinically after intravenous bolus administration. As shown in Table 3, cisplatin exposure is 16.5-fold higher in the in vitro assay system than when administered intravenously as a bolus (Fruehauf and Bosanquet, 1993). Similar exposures are used in the ATP, DiSC, and MTT assays, whereas short-term drug exposures are used in the HTCA. Longer exposure times with higher areas under the curve (AUC) favor the identification of highly resistant tumor cells that can grow through AUC values in excess of those achieved clinically. Drugs found to be inactive under optimal conditions for activity in vitro are unlikely to be active under suboptimal conditions in vivo. On the other hand, assays that use short-term drug exposures may be more capable of identifying agents with greater sensitivity in vivo. However, as discussed below, this has not been borne out in clinical trials.

The EDR assay and other suspension assay systems measure the growth of tumor aggregates. Plating cells as small organoid clusters allows cells to grow in an environment that recapitulates the in vivo three-dimensional growth pattern. Clustered cells grow better compared with single-cell suspensions,

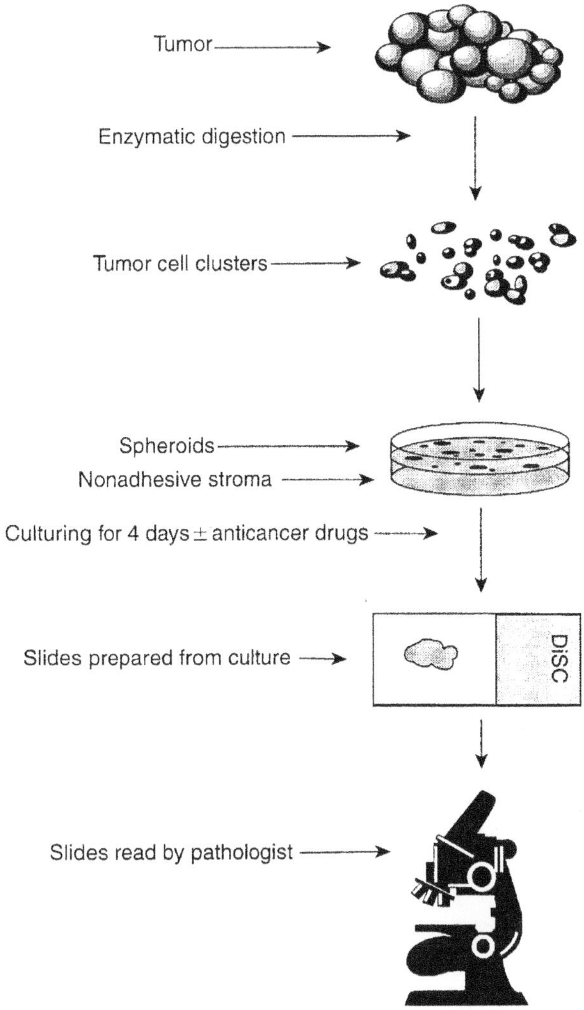

Fig. 1c

improving the assay success rate and shortening the time required for obtaining results. The EDR assay success rate is approximately 85% (Mehta et al. 2001), and the assay takes 5 days. In contrast, the HTCA, which requires that tumors be disaggregated to the single cell level, has a 50% evaluability rate and takes 14 days or longer (Clark and Von Hoff 1984). It has also been reported that three-dimensional cultures demonstrate acquired drug resistance that may not always be detected when cells are grown in monolayers (Graham et al. 1994). The EDR assay has been found to be highly accurate for predicting drug resistance (=97%) (Fruehauf and Bosanquet 1993; Chu and DeVita 2001).

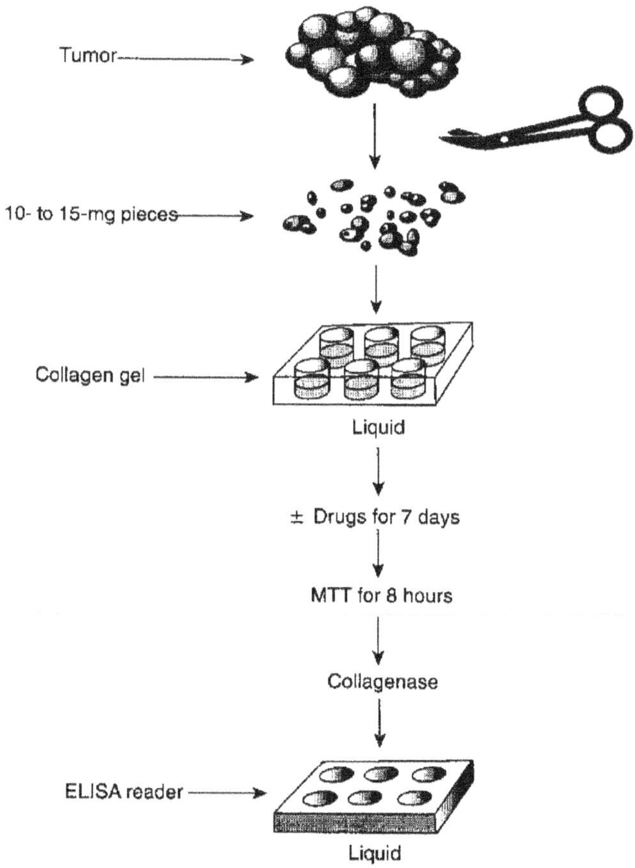

Fig. 1d

Several assays measure the effects of cancer drugs on cellular metabolism. The ATP assay measures the concentration of intracellular ATP in the culture population (Andreotti et al. 1995) (Fig. 1d). ATP is essential for cell viability and DNA replication. Metabolically active cells will produce more ATP, as will cells metabolizing glucose through the citric acid cycle (CAC) linked to aerobic mitochondrial function. In vitro drug effects that inhibit glucose metabolism or mitochondrial function or that cause cell death result in decreased intracellular ATP concentrations. ATP levels in cultured cells are measured by fluorochromes such as luciferin-luciferase that fluoresce after binding to ATP. Loss of cell viability after drug exposure results in decreased cellular ATP levels. The ATP assay uses 96-well round-bottomed polypropylene plates and serum-free media to suppress the proliferation of nontransformed cells. Andreotti et al. studied the growth advantage of the malignant component of 124 biopsies of various types of solid tumors with the ATP assay. Cytological analysis was performed to assess the ratio of malignant to nonmalignant cells be-

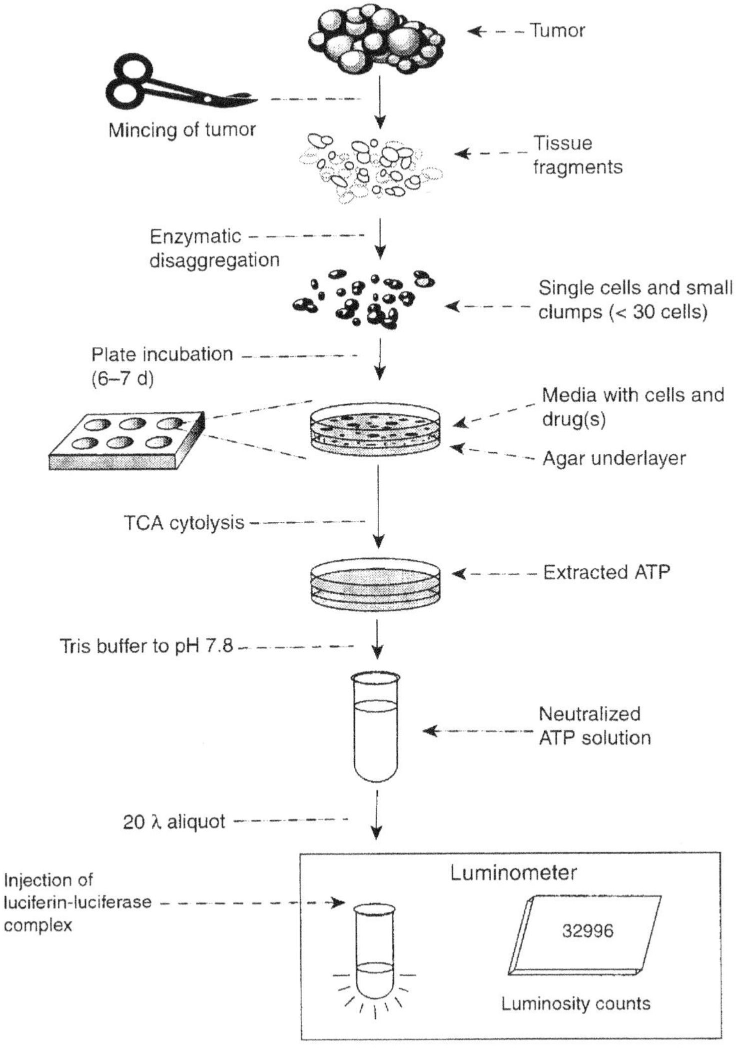

Fig. 1e

fore and after culture. They found that the mean proportion of malignant cells increased from 54% initially to 83% by the end of the 6- to 7-day assay period, with a significant expansion of the malignant population in 98% of the cases evaluated. Several clinical trials in Europe have demonstrated that the ATP assay's predictive reliability favors drug resistance over chemosensitivity (Konecny et al. 2000; Cree et al. 1996; Andreotti et al. 1995).

The MTT assay detects mitochondrial succinate dehydrogenase (SDH) activity as a determinant of mitochondrial function and cell viability (Fig. 1e). SDH is a component of the citric acid cycle, and it generates $FADH_2$ and fu-

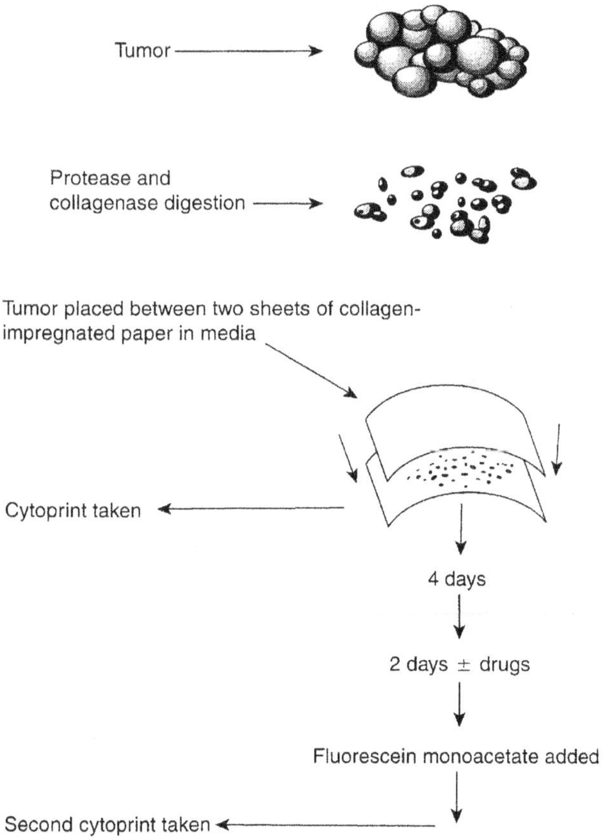

Fig. 1f

marate from succinate and FAD. SDH activity resides on the mitochondrial inner membrane and requires a functioning electron transport system. SDH activity is therefore a measure of mitochondrial and cellular viability. SDH activity is measured by its capacity to convert 3-[4,5-dimethylthiazol-2-yl]-2,5-diphenyltetrazolium bromide (MTT) to a blue crystallized compound that is dissolved in DMSO at the end of the assay. The amount of crystal formation is determined by measuring the optical density of the tissue culture well using a spectrophotometer that measures absorbance at the wavelength absorbed by the blue solution. Tumors can be assessed in the MTT assay as organoids or small fragments grown on collagen gel sponges (Fig. 1d) or as disaggregated cells grown in adherent cultures (Grever et al. 1992; Furukawa et al. 2000; Ohie et al. 2000; Fruehauf et al. 1990). Although the MTT assay works well for cancer cell lines, it is not generally performed with culture conditions that preferentially favor the transformed component of the tumor. The MTT assay signal source stems from all functional mitochondria and therefore does not distinguish between cancer cell and normal stromal cell response to in vitro drug exposures (Fruehauf and Bosanquet 1993).

The fluorescent cytoprint assay (FCPA) is also a metabolic function assay. The FCPA measures the enzyme activity of membrane cytosolic esterases (Fig. 1f) (Rotman et al. 1988; Leone et al. 1991). Esterase activity is related to cell viability and is assayed by monitoring hydrolysis of fluorescein-monoacetate to fluorescein. In the FCPA assay, tumors are disaggregated into small clumps, or "microorgans," which are immobilized between sheets of cellulose-collagen that are subsequently placed onto a grid in tissue culture flasks containing medium. A baseline "fluorescent cytoprint" is recorded by digital photography, and cells are cultured for 24 h before drug exposures. After a subsequent 48-h drug exposure period, cells are rinsed and grown for an additional 48 h in drug-free medium. The second "cytoprint" is obtained, and the difference in fluorescence between the two images is calculated. Computer capture of the images is utilized for an objective comparison. Each culture acts as its own control. Although the "microorgan" structure has the advantage of maintaining the in vivo tumor environment, this assay end point does not distinguish between the fluorescent signal produced by the malignant cells and the nontransformed component of each organoid. Because the malignant component is not enumerated, tumor heterogeneity makes it difficult to compare cases and to discern tumor cell response to treatment from total cellular response. Tumors that have few cancer cells present a particularly troublesome challenge for the FCPA with respect to interpretation.

Clinical Studies in Breast and Ovarian Cancer Correlating In Vitro Assay Results with Response and Survival

The clinical utility of in vitro drug response assays has been evaluated in clinical trials that evaluated the relationship between drug action on a given patient's tumor in vitro and that patient's clinical response to that drug. As shown in Table 4, recent reports have addressed the predictive accuracy of various in vitro drug response technologies for 220 breast cancer cases and 284 ovarian cancer cases. The negative predictive accuracy (NPA) relates to the reliability of the assay to identify ineffective agents that will fail to produce a clinical response, and the positive predictive accuracy (PPA) is a measure of an assay's reliability to identify agents that will cause clinical responses defined as a 50% reduction of measurable tumor size. The NPV for breast cancer cases ranged from 86% to 100%, whereas the PPV ranged from 47% to 91%. For ovarian cancer cases, the NPV ranged from 62% to 100%, whereas the PPV ranged from 58% to 91%. Although these ranges are rather broad, it appears that the negative predictive values were generally higher than the positive predictive values, suggesting that these technologies were better at identifying ineffective agents. This has been a generally accepted axiom for several years based on the clear differences between in vitro models and in vivo pharmacodynamics (see below).

Table 4. Utility of in vitro drug assays to predict clinical response for patients with breast and ovarian carcinomas

Author	Assay type[c]	Tumor	*n*	NPA[a]	PPA[b]
Weisenthal	EDR	Breast	48	100	47
Blackman	FCFA	Breast	47	100	91
Elledge	^{3}H-uridine	Breast	25	94	71
Koechli	ATP	Breast	17	86	90
Xu	MTT	Breast	83	100	77
Alberts	HTCA	Ovarian	44	99	62
Weisenthal	EDR	Ovarian	46	100	58
Taylor	MTT	Ovarian	37	80	61
Blackman	FCFA	Ovarian	72	96	71
Csoka	FCFA	Ovarian	47	100	56
Konecny	ATP	Ovarian	38	89	66

[a]Negative predictive accuracy (%) to identify agents in vitro that will fail to cause a partial or complete tumor response when administered to the patient.

[b]Positive predictive accuracy (%) to identify agents in vitro that will cause a partial or complete tumor response.

[c]Assay types: thymidine, radiolabeled thymidine incorporation in agar; FCP, fluorescent cytoprint; uridine, radiolabeled uridine incorporation; FMCA, fluorometric microculture assay; MTT, methylthiazol diphenyl tetrazolium bromide dye conversion assay; ATP, adenosine triphosphate luminescence assay.

In Vitro Drug Response and Patient Survival

Although it is clear that in vitro drug response assays effectively discriminate between clinically inactive and active agents, this does not necessarily translate to an accurate prediction of patient survival. Various clinical trials have identified agents capable of causing short-term responses without translating clinical response into a survival benefit. Clinical validation of in vitro drug resistance assays requires that they predict poorer survival for patients treated with agents their tumors are resistant to in vitro and improved survival for patients treated with agents their tumors are "sensitive" to in vitro. Table 5 summarizes the results of three recently published studies that demonstrated significantly inferior survival for patients treated with agents found to be inactive in vitro. In the study of Mehta et al., newly diagnosed breast cancer patients were treated with either CMF or AC. Their tumors were studied in the

Table 5. Survival of patients who received assay sensitive versus resistant agents

Author	Tumor type	*n*	Median PFS (months)		*P* value
			Sensitive	Resistant	
Mehta	Breast	96	100	48	0.02
Konecny	Ovary	38	28.5	12.6	0.03
Holloway	Ovary	79	24	6	0.011

EDR assay. If any one of these agents showed in vitro resistance at an intermediate or extreme level, patient progression-free survival was decreased by two-fold. Mehta et al. reported a threefold increased relative risk of death for patients who received agents resistant in vitro based on multivariate analysis adjusted for stage and lymph node status. Konecny et al. and Holloway et al. both reported similar results for newly diagnosed stage III and IV ovarian cancer patients treated with platinum-based chemotherapy after initial cytoreductive surgery. Konecny's study employed the ATP assay, whereas Holloway's study utilized the EDR assay. These two groups independently found that in vitro resistance to either cisplatin or carboplatin was an adverse factor, with significantly reduced progression-free survival seen in patients with tumors that were resistant to platinum in vitro. Konecny et al. found that median time to progression was 2.3-fold shorter for the platinum-resistant group, and Holloway et al. found a 4-fold difference. These recent studies are consistent with others that have evaluated survival differences between patients receiving in vitro resistant versus in vitro sensitive agents, and they suggest that agents found to be inactive in vitro are unlikely to produce clinical responses or improved survival (Fruehauf and Bosanquet 1993).

Assay-Assisted Therapy

Cortazar and Johnson recently summarized results for clinical trials that attempted to determine whether patient survival could be improved by the administration of agents selected by in vitro assays versus physician's choice. They reviewed results for 1,545 cases that were enrolled in "in vitro chemosensitivity" trials. In vitro assays of various types were actually performed in 72% of the cases. The primary technology evaluated was the human tumor cloning assay, which represented 52% of the cases studied, whereas the DiSC assay was performed in 25% of the cases, the MTT assay was performed in 15% of the cases, and the capillary cloning assay accounted for 8% of the cases. Drug resistance assays were not included in their review. Of the 12 peer-reviewed reports analyzed, seven had response data: two for the clonogenic technique, four for the DiSC assay, and one for the capillary cloning assay. Cortazar and Johnson found that response rates for patients treated with the best in vitro regimen was 27%, versus 16% for empiric treatment. With respect to survival outcomes, survival was improved in two of five studies and comparable in three others. They concluded that "patient response rates to in vitro selected chemotherapy were at least as good as those achieved with empiric therapy."

More recently, Kurbacher et al. reported that ATP assay-directed therapy administered to women with platinum-resistant recurrent ovarian cancer versus platinum-sensitive recurrent ovarian cancer resulted in comparable response rates and survival times. With the advent of significantly increased numbers of agents to choose from for both breast and ovarian carcinoma, assay-assisted therapy is a rational approach that provides objectivity to the selection process. The study by Kurbacher et al. provides an impetus for cooperative groups to revisit the issue of assay-directed therapy.

Another assay-directed study was published by Orr et al., who evaluated EDR assay-assisted selection of initial chemotherapy for newly diagnosed ovarian carcinoma cases. After cytoreductive surgery, platinum-based therapy was combined with either paclitaxel or cyclophosphamide depending on which agent showed the lowest level of resistance in the assay. Although no significant difference in survival was noted for the two groups, there was a significant cost savings of approximately $6,000 per patient based on assay utilization. Together, the data summarized in Tables 4 and 5 on treatment response and survival, and the data on assay-directed therapy, suggest that assay-assisted therapy selection may improve survival as well as reduce cost.

Drug Resistance Versus Drug Sensitivity: Two Different Coins

During the 1980s advances in laboratory technologies overcame many of the technical problems of the earlier systems. Advanced assay systems were developed that yielded answers for most cases in a less than a week, making broader clinical applications a real possibility. Significant progress was made to identify issues that prevented tumor growth in vitro, and comparisons were made between the different end points. Results from clinical trials were compared to determine the relative advantages and disadvantages of the different in vitro systems (Weisenthal 1991). Divergent assay end points were generally found to provide comparable predictive accuracy. One particularly notable finding that emerged from these comparisons was that regardless of the assay end points used, in vitro drug response assays were most reliable for accurately identifying drugs that were unlikely to be effective rather than for picking out drugs that would cause tumors to shrink. The negative predictive accuracy was generally on the order of 90%–99%, whereas the positive predictive accuracy was generally on the order of only 50%–70%.

That in vitro drug response tests should vary in their positive and negative predictive reliability is not too surprising when the complexity of drug delivery to the patient's tumor in vivo is considered. Although in vitro assay systems can dependably deliver active drug to the tumor cells in culture, the human side of the equation is far less certain. After intravenous administration, chemotherapy agents are subjected to significant individual differences in biotransformation and biodistribution. Biotransformation differs among patients in part as a function of their enzyme haplotype. Analysis of the impact of single-nucleotide polymorphisms (SNPs) on drug activation and inactivation is an emerging area of pharmacogenetics that may lead to patient-specific drug dosing (Kim et al. 2001). Recent data on SNP has also provided new insight into the genetic basis for why some patients rapidly inactivate drugs and others suffer greater toxicity by virtue of their slower drug metabolism (Roses 2001). Individual differences in drug metabolism that might prevent an active form of the drug from reaching the tumor in vivo cannot be modeled using the current in vitro assay systems. Pharmacodynamic activity ultimately depends on biodistribution of active drug species to the tumor bed through the tumor's blood supply. A great deal of evidence has emerged supporting the notion that tumors of a given type and grade may possess a wide range of microvessel densities. In fact, angiogenesis has become an important new prognostic factor, as well as a new target for cancer treatment (Chen et al. 2001). Unfortunately, individual differences in tumor vascularity are not accounted for by current in vitro drug response assays, adversely impacting on their positive predictive capability. Current in vitro assays lack the capability to account for these critical pharmacodynamic aspects of drug delivery, making it difficult for them to accurately predict in vivo "chemosensitivity." On the other hand, although these pharmacodynamics factors mitigate against accurately predicting that a drug will work, they favor predictions of drug resistance. If the tumor sample is completely resistant after supraoptimal drug exposures in vitro, then suboptimal in vivo delivery resulting from poor tumor vascular supply and/or rapid drug inactivation will most likely result in treatment failure.

Although the Holy Grail may not be at hand for in vitro chemosensitivity, the ability to tailor, or personalize, treatment regimens based on in vitro testing is still a viable approach. In fact, in vitro tests for drug response provide a bridge between the current empirical approach to chemotherapy and the future era that will focus on treatment tailored by biochemical fingerprinting. STI571, Herceptin, Rituximab, and tamoxifen are targeted treatments developed through rational screening programs based on an understanding of cancer cell biology and critical signaling pathways (Sledge 2001). However, even these therapies are not universally effective, and resistance emerges. One reason for the development of drug resistance is that the transformation process is almost universally multifactorial, yielding tumors composed of genetically and biochemically heterogeneous cells containing multiple aberrant pathways. Thus drug resistance will remain a major obstacle until the black box of the cancer phenotype is fully dissected at a proteogenomic level (Houston et al. 1999; Mechetner et al. 1998).

The main advantage of in vitro drug response assays is their determination of the net effect of drug action. Either drugs induce apoptosis or they do not. The measurement of a specific drug target may not account for all of the steps required for drug efficacy. For example, Tamoxifen is expected to be effective as an initial treatment in patients with steroid receptor-positive breast carcinoma. However, coexpression of HER2 can diminish breast cancer sensitivity to Tamoxifen (Houston et al. 1999). Thus a myriad of pathways may be interacting simultaneously to impact on drug entry to a cell, drug movement to its site of action, and the effect of the drug to induce cell death. In vitro tests make it possible to determine whether the process of drug action and cellular response is intact or not. The clinician can take advantage of these findings in two ways. First, because these assays can accurately identify ineffective drugs, such agents can be avoided. Second, although the accuracy of predicting that a drug will work is limited, agents to which the tumor demonstrates low resistance have been found to be more effective than those found to be extremely resistant in vitro. Integration of all pertinent clinical factors together with in vitro data on tumor response to agents defined to be effective for the patient's tumor type may provide the best outcomes for patients with breast or ovarian cancer. Cancer drug development by the cooperative groups should be enhanced by assessing the value of in vitro-assisted chemotherapy selection technologies in combination with proteogenomic techniques that can stratify and assign patients to trials predicted to be of greatest benefit to the individual patient. Such studies may better define the optimal diagnostic criteria for treatment selection and accelerate the approval of new rationally designed agents that may be effective only in small subsets of patients that have developed tumors that bear the appropriate repertoire of drug targets. Integration of in vitro cellular technologies and proteogenomic diagnostics into clinical trials design should be a high priority for the cooperative groups. Assay-assisted treatment selection is now emerging as an important adjunct in the physician's armamentarium.

References

Alberts DS, Salmon SE, Chen HS, Surwit EA, Soehnlen B, Young L, Moon TE (1980) In-vitro clonogenic assay for predicting response of ovarian cancer to chemotherapy. Lancet 2:340–342

Alberts DS (1999) Treatment of refractory and recurrent ovarian cancer. Semin Oncol 26 [Suppl 1]:8–14

Andreotti PE, Cree IA, Kurbacher CM, Hartman DM, Linder D, Harel G, Gleiberman I, Caruso PA, Ricks SH, Untch M, Sartori C, Bruckner HW (1995) Chemosensitivity testing of human tumors using a microplate adenosine triphosphate luminescence assay: Clinical correlation for cisplatin resistance of ovarian carcinoma. Cancer Res 55:5276–5282

Bird MC, Godwin VA, Antrobus JH, Bosanquet AG (1987) Comparison of in vitro drug sensitivity by the differential staining cytotoxicity (DiSC) and colony-forming assays. Br J Cancer 55:429–431

Black MM, Spear FD (1953) Effects of cancer chemotherapeutic agents on dehydrogenase activity of human cancer tissue in vitro. Am J Clin Pathol 23:218–227

Black MM, Spear FD (1954) Further observations on the effects of cancer chemotherapeutic agents on the in vitro dehydrogenase activity of cancer tissue. J Natl Cancer Inst 14:1147–1158

Bosanquet AG (1991) Correlations between therapeutic response of leukaemias and in-vitro drug-sensitivity assay. Lancet 337:711–714

Bosanquet AG, Johnson SA, Richards SM (1999) Prognosis for fludarabine therapy of chronic lymphocytic leukaemia based on ex vivo drug response by DiSC assay. Br J Haematol 106:71–77

Brock TD (1967) Bacterial growth rate in the sea: direct analysis by thymidine autoradiography. Science 155:81–83

Burger A (1988) Drugs and people: medications, their history and origins, and the way they act. University of Virginia Press

Campling BJ, Pym J, Baker HM, Cole SPC, Lam YM (1991) Chemosensitivity testing of small cell lung cancer using the MTT assay. Br J Cancer 63:75–83

Chen QR, Zhang L, Gasper W, Mixson AJ (2001) Targeting tumor angiogenesis with gene therapy. Mol Genet Metab 74:120–127

Chu E, DeVita VT (2001) Principles of cancer management: chemotherapy. In: DeVita VT, Hellman S, Rosenberg S (eds) Cancer: principles and practice of oncology, 6th edn. Lippincott Williams and Wilkins, Philadelphia, chap 17

Clark GM, Von Hoff DD (1984) Quality control of a multicenter human tumor cloning system: the Southwest Oncology Group experience. In Salmon S, Trent JM (eds) Human tumor cloning. Grune and Straton, Orlando, pp 255–265

Cortazar P, Johnson BE (1999) Review of the efficacy of individualized chemotherapy selected by in vitro drug sensitivity testing for patients with cancer. J Clin Oncol 17:1625–1631

Cree IA, Kurbacher CM, Untch M, Sutherland LA, Hunter EM, Subedi AM, James EA, Dewar JA, Preece PE, Andreotti PE, Bruckner HW (1996) Correlation of the clinical response to chemotherapy in breast cancer with ex vivo chemosensitivity. Anticancer Drugs 7:630–635

Elledge RM, Clark GM, Hon J, Thant M, Belt R, Maguire YP, Brown J, Bartels P, Von Hoff DD (1995) Rapid in vitro assay for predicting response to fluorouracil in patients with metastatic breast cancer. J Clin Oncol 13:419–423

Esteva FJ, Valero V, Pusztai L, Boehnke-Michaud L, Buzdar AU, Hortobagyi GN (2001) Chemotherapy of metastatic breast cancer: what to expect in 2001 and beyond. Oncologist 6:133–146

Fruehauf JP, Myers CE, Sinha BK (1990) Synergistic activity of suramin with tumor necrosis factor and doxorubicin on prostate cancer cell lines. J Natl Cancer Inst 82:1206–1209

Fruehauf JP, Bosanquet AG (1993) In vitro determinations of drug response: a discussion of clinical applications. Principles Practice Oncol Updates 7:1–16

Furukawa T, Kubota T, Hoffman RM (2000) Clinical applications of the histoculture drug response assay. Clin Cancer Res 1:305–311

Goldie JH, Coldman AJ (1979) A mathematical model for relating the drug sensitivity of tumors to their spontaneous mutation rate. Cancer Treat Rep 63:1727–1733

Graham CH, Kobayashi H, Stankiewicz KS, Man S, Kapitain SJ, Kerbel RS (1994) Rapid acquisition of multicellular drug resistance after a single exposure of mammary tumor cells to antitumor alkylating agents. J Natl Cancer Inst 86:975–982

Greenlee RT, Hill-Harmon MB, Murray T, Thun M (2001) Cancer statistics, 2001. Ca Cancer J Clin 151:15–36

Grever MR, Schepartz SA, Chabner BA (1992) The National Cancer Institute: cancer drug discovery and development program. Semin Oncol 19:622–638

Hamburger AW, Salmon SE (1977) Primary bioassay of human tumor stem cells. Science 197:461–463

Holloway RW, Mehta RS, Finkler N, Parker RJ, Fruehauf JP (2001) Association between in vitro platinum resistance in the extreme drug resistance assay and clinical outcomes for ovarian cancer patients. Gynecol Oncol 80: Abstract #23

Houston SJ, Plunkett TA, Barnes DM, Smith P, Rubens RD, Miles DW (1999) Overexpression of c-erbB2 is an independent marker of resistance to endocrine therapy in advanced breast cancer. Br J Cancer 79:1220–1226

Iyer L, Ratain MJ (1998) Pharmacogenetics and cancer chemotherapy. Eur J Cancer 34:1493–1499

Johnson GE, Glaubiger DL (1983) Correlation of cellular tritiated thymidine incorporation with soft agar clonogenicity in chemosensitivity testing of human neuroblastoma cells. Cancer Treat Rep 67:163–168

Kim RB, Leake BF, Choo EF, Dresser GK, Kubba SV, Schwarz UI, Taylor A, Xie HG, McKinsey J, Zhou S, Lan LB, Schuetz JD, Schuetz EG, Wilkinson GR (2001) Identification of functionally variant MDR1 alleles among European Americans and African Americans. Clin Pharmacol Ther 70:189–199

Kitaoka A, Muraoka R, Tanigawa N (1997) Improvement of in vitro chemosensitivity assay for human solid tumors by application of a preculture using collagen matrix. Clin Cancer Res 3:295–299

Kochli OR, Sevin BU, Averette HE, Haller U (1994) Overview of currently used chemosensitivity test systems in gynecologic malignancies and breast cancer. Contrib Gynecol Obstet 19:12–23

Konecny G, Crohns C, Pegram M, Felber M, Lude S, Kurbacher C, Cree IA, Hepp H, Untch M (2000) Correlation of drug response with the ATP tumor chemosensitivity assay in primary FIGO stage III ovarian cancer. Gynecol Oncol 77:258–263

Kurbacher CM, Stier U, Janát M-M, Cree IA, Bruckner HW (2001) ATP-assay-directed chemotherapy for recurrent ovarian cancer: mature results of an ISCO clinical study group trial. Proc Am Soc Clin Oncol 20: Abstract 2486

Leone LA, Meitner PA, Myers TJ, Grace WR, Gajewski WH, Fingert HJ, Rotman B (1991) Predictive value of the fluorescent cytoprint assay (FCA): a retrospective correlation study of in vitro chemosensitivity and individual responses to chemotherapy. Cancer Invest 9:491–503

Markman M, Bookman MA (2000) Second-line treatment of ovarian cancer. Oncologist 5:26–35

Mason JM, Drummond MF, Bosanquet AG, Sheldon TA (1999) The DiSC assay. A cost-effective guide to treatment for chronic lymphocytic leukemia? Int J Technol Assess Health Care 15:173–84

McGuire WP, Hoskins WJ, Brady MF, Kucera PR, Partridge EE, Look KY, Clarke-Pearson DL, Davidson M (1996) Cisplatin compared with paclitaxel and cisplatin in patients with stage III and stage IV ovarian cancer. N Eng J Med 334:1–6

Mechetner E, Kyshtoobayeva A, Zonis S, Kim H, Stroup R, Garcia R, Parker RJ, Fruehauf JP (1998) Levels of multidrug resistance (MDR1) P-glycoprotein expression by human breast cancer correlate with in vitro resistance to taxol and doxorubicin. Clin Cancer Res 4:389–398

Mehta RS, Bornstein R, Yu I-R, Parker RJ, McClaren CE, Nguyen KP, Fruehauf JP (2001) Breast cancer survival and in vitro tumor response in the extreme drug resistance assay. Breast Cancer Res Treat 66:225–237

Meitner PA (1991) The fluorescent cytoprint assay: a new approach to in vitro chemosensitivity testing. Oncology (Huntingt) 5:75–81

Norton L (1999) Adjuvant breast cancer therapy: current status and future strategies – growth kinetics and the improved drug therapy of breast cancer. Semin Oncol 26 (1 Suppl 3):1–4

Ohie S, Udagawa Y, Kozu A, Komuro Y, Aoki D, Nozawa S, Moossa AR, Hoffman RM (2000) Cisplatin sensitivity of ovarian cancer in the histoculture drug response assay correlates to clinical response to combination chemotherapy with cisplatin, doxorubicin and cyclophosphamide. Anticancer Res 20:2049–54

Orr JW, Orr P, Kern DH (1999) Cost-effective treatment of women with advanced ovarian cancer by cytoreductive surgery and chemotherapy directed by an in vitro assay for drug resistance. Cancer J Sci Am 5:174–178

Pasteur L, Joubert J (1877) Charbonne et septicemie. CR Acad Sci 85:101–115

Puck TT, Marcus PI (1955) A rapid method for viable titration and clone production with Hela cells in tissue culture: the use of X-irradiated cells to supply conditioning factors. Proc Natl Acad Sci USA 41:432–437

Roses AD (2001) Pharmacogenetics. Mol Genet 10:2261–2267

Rotman B, Teplitz C, Dickinson K, Cozzolino JP (1988) Individual human tumors in short-term micro-organ cultures: chemosensitivity testing by fluorescent cytoprinting. In Vitro Cell Dev Biol 24:1137–1146

Salmon SE, Hamburger AW, Soehnlen B, Durie BGM, Alberts DS, Moon TE (1978) Quantitation of differential sensitivity of human tumor stem cells to anticancer drugs. New Engl J Med 298:1321–1325

Selby P, Buick RN, Tannock I (1983) A critical appraisal of the "human tumor stem cell assay." New Engl J Med 308:129–134

Sevin BU, Perras JP (1997) Tumor heterogeneity and in vitro chemosensitivity testing in ovarian cancer. Am J Obstet Gynecol 176:759–766

Sledge GW Jr (2001) All therapy is targeted therapy: the future of systemic therapy. Clin Breast Cancer 2:94–98

Sondak VK, Bertelsen CA, Tanigawa N, Hildebrand-Zanki SU, Morton DL, Korn EL, Kern DH (1984) Clinical correlations with chemosensitivities measured in a rapid thymidine incorporation assay. Cancer Res 44:1725–1728

Weisenthal LM, Lippman ME (1985) Clonogenic and nonclonogenic in vitro chemosensitivity assays. Cancer Treat Rep 69:615–632

Weisenthal LM (1991) Predictive assays for drug and radiation resistance. In: Masters JRW (ed) Human cancer in primary culture: a handbook. Kluwer, Amsterdam, pp 103–147

Weisenthal LM (1994) Clinical correlations for cell culture assays based on the concept of total tumor cell kill. Contrib Gynecol Obstet 19:82–90

Wilbur DW, Camacho ES, Hilliard DA, Dill PL, Weisenthal LM (1992) Chemotherapy of non-small cell lung carcinoma guided by an in vitro drug resistance assay measuring total tumour cell kill. Br J Cancer 65:27–32

Chemosensitivity Testing in Gynecologic Oncology – Dream or Reality?

M. Untch, N. Ditsch, E. Langer, C. Kurbacher, C. Crohns, G. Konecny, S. Kahlert, I. Bauerfeind, H. Hepp

M. Untch (✉)
Department of Obstetrics and Gynecology, University of München-Großhadern, Marchioninistraße 15, 81377 München, Germany
e-mail: michael.untch@helios.med.uni-muenchen.de

Abstract

Cell culture and animal models have played an essential role in the research of new principles of therapy. Many methods for the individualized testing of therapy sensitivity and resistance have been developed, for example, the clonogenic assay. Presently, the ATP-TCA is commercially available as a testing kit. This review gives an overview of the tumor samples that were tested in the oncologic laboratory in the Department of Obstetrics and Gynecology, Munich Grosshadern between 1993 and 2001. All target parameters show a clear trend in favor of sequential, dose-intensified Epirubicin/Paclitaxel therapy. If this trend remains valid for the total number of patients, a significant impact of this new principle of therapy can be expected. By individualized planning of therapy with ATP-TCA testing, therapy in the individual patient could already be performed by the examination of sensitivity in the preoperative biopsy specimen.

Introduction

Currently, advances in molecular biology are moving very fast. At the moment, we are in a transitional phase, for the findings of molecular biology and genetics have not yet entered the planning of therapy directly but already influence parts of the diagnosis. Richard Klausner, the Director of the National Cancer Institute in the U.S. stated appropriately in the *Journal of the National Cancer Institute* in 1996, in the course of a description of the Cancer Genome Project: "At the moment, all patients are treated with the same drugs. Afterwards, we know that there are different patterns of response to the treatment. We treat essentially different diseases with the same drugs." Currently, one cannot talk of an individualization of therapy. The findings of modern molecular biological research will certainly make individualized therapy possible in

Recent Results in Cancer Research, Vol. 161

Table 1. Advantages and disadvantages of the most frequently used methods for cytostatic testing

Method	Advantages	Disadvantages
HTCA (human tumor clonogenic assay)	Well-researched test	Low rate of availability; questionable whether the stem cell is also biologically active; relatively low predictive significance for sensitivity
	High predictive significance (validity) for resistance	
Kern/Volm (incorporating methods of radioactive marked DNA precursors)	Very rapidly practicable (above all the Volm test)	Primarily only proliferative cells (S-phase) are recorded
	High predictive significance for resistance	Relatively low predictive significance for sensitivity
DiSC (differential staining cytotoxicity assay)	High predictive significance for resistance	Data are almost exclusively from hematologic neoplasia
FCA (fluorescent cytoprint assay)	Tumor integrity is preserved in so-called micro-organs	No control without therapy, uncertainty on the mechanism of cell destruction
CAM (cell-adhesive matrix)	Simplicity of the monolayer system	No sufficient growth inhibition of the nonneoplastic cells by the monolayer system
ATP-CVA (adenosine triphosphate cell viability assay)	Total cell number evaluation	Luminometer necessary
(ATP-TCA/ATP-CSA)	Good sensitivity and specificity	6–7 days of incubation necessary

the future. In the meantime, however, we need practicable solutions, to take into account the heterogeneity of malignant tumor diseases. For that reason, the term "standard therapy" only applies to some of our patients.

Cell culture and animal models have played an essential role in research on new principles of therapy and new substances in the last few decades. For example, the first targeted monoclonal antibody in breast cancer against a defined structural protein (Herceptin, Trastuzumab) first showed its efficacy in the cell culture model [1]. A multitude of methods for individualized testing of therapy sensitivity and resistance have been developed since the 1960s. For example, there is the clonogenic assay, which was described in 1977 for the first time [2].

Table 1 shows an overview of the chemosensitivity assays used so far and their advantages and disadvantages.

Clinical Aspects of Pretherapeutic Testing

The efforts to establish such testing methods in the clinical routine have only produced unsatisfying results within the last 10 years [3].

Nevertheless, predictive testing systems have meanwhile become routine in the planning of therapy for infectious diseases and for the planning of therapy for breast cancer:

1. Antibiogram for targeted antibiotic therapy
2. Hormone receptor measurements for the endocrine therapy of breast cancer

The prediction is about 70% for sensitivity and about 90% for resistance [3, 4]. Although such predictions can also be achieved with the usual chemosensitivity assays in oncology, none of the methods in oncology described so far could be made a routine method. Several reasons are given for this, for example, insufficient reproducibility, technical difficulties, the lack of randomized trials, methodological problems, and insufficient clinical relevance [5, 6].

The requirements of an optimized testing method can be summarized as follows:

1. Simple and reproducible method
2. Exactly defined criteria for the evaluation of the test
3. High rate of culture growth and analysis (over 90% if possible)
4. Use of concentration gradients for at least four to six steps
5. Testing also possible with small amounts of tissue, especially aspirates and effusions
6. Correlation with clinical response

The ATP Chemosensitivity Assay

The ATP-TCA had already been developed in the seventies, when the determination of ATP as a measure of cellular vitality was the focus of attention [7].

In the eighties the ATP testing system was optimized and improved. By now, the ATP-TCA is commercially available as a testing kit (TCA 100: DCS Innovative Diagnostik Systeme, Hamburg, Germany). This test was created according to GMP criteria and is subject to strict quality control. The method is shown in Fig. 1.

After mechanical and enzymatic dissociation, cell suspensions of single cells and tumor particles are produced from solid tumors. Vitality evaluation is performed with the trypan blue dye-exclusion method. One to two million vital tumor cells are distributed in 5–10 μl in 96-well microtiter plates of polypropylene. Untreated controls (references) are compared with triplets treated with cytostatics. The range of concentration is 6.25%–200%. The concentration of 100% approximately corresponds to the plasma peak concentrations achievable in the clinical situation [9–11]. The culture plates are cultivated in incubators at 37°C, water vapor saturation, and 5% CO_2 for 6–7 days. Essen-

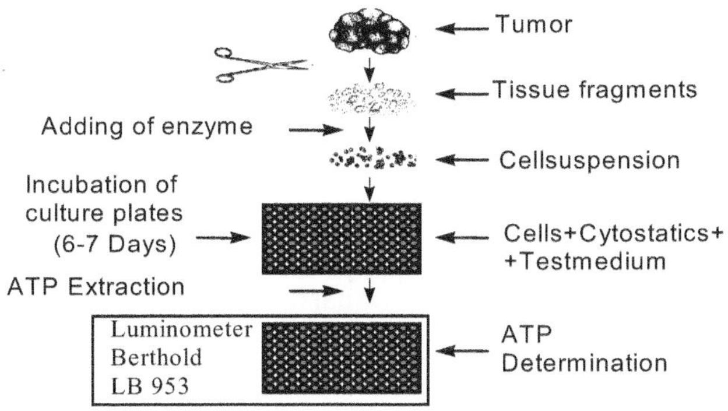

Fig. 1. The method of ATP-TCA

tially, the culture conditions do not depend on the adherence of tumor cells on the vascular walls. Mainly, tumor cells are cultivated; however, nonmalignant cells are also present in the total set as an integral part of the testing system [11, 12].

At the end of the incubation time, ATP is set free by cell lysis and is measured luminometrically. By comparing the triplicate values from the plates treated with cytostatics with the controls, dose-response curves are generated.

The dose-response curve of a tested tumor sample from a 52-year-old female patient with a mammary carcinoma T2, N1, G2 is shown in Fig. 2. Three combinations of cytostatics as well as one single drug have been tested. From the dose-response curve it can be noted that the best combination in this case was the CMF combination. This means that an individualized planning of therapy would be quite possible.

With a computer program the following parameters can be calculated: inhibitory concentration 50 (IC_{50}), inhibitory concentration 90 (IC_{90}), the area under the dose-response curve (AUC), and summation index (SI), with the re-

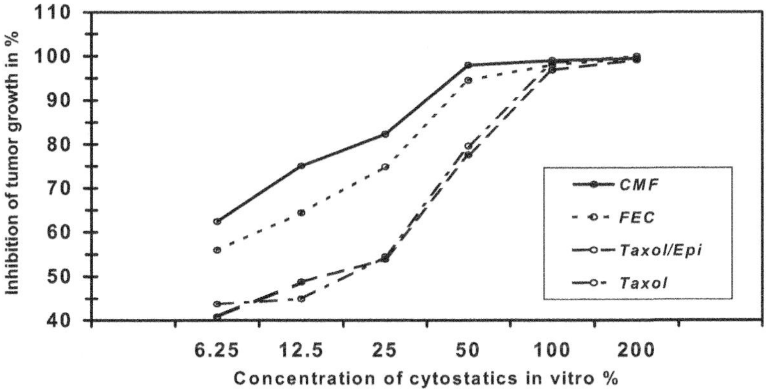

Fig. 2. Dose-response curve of a tumor sample of a patient with breast cancer

Table 2. Overview of the tested tumors

Breast cancer	*n*=555
Ovarian cancer	*n*=375
Endometrial cancer	*n*=44
Cervical cancer	*n*=44
Other tumors (mainly sarcomas)	*n*=45

sponse categories high sensitivity (S), partial sensitivity (P), weak sensitivity (W), and resistance (R) [13].

The examination is subject to strict revision criteria:

1. Only tissue that has clearly been identified as malignant by pathology is tested.
2. Bacterial or yeast contamination, which can occur in approximately 5% of the cases, must be excluded.
3. Interpretable dose-response curves must be obtained.

Clinical Enrollment of ATP-TCA in Gynecologic Oncology

In the last 10 years, the ATP-TCA has been employed mainly in gynecologic oncology. Mainly tumor samples of ovarian cancer and breast cancer have been tested. The Table 2 provides an overview of the tumor samples that have been tested in the oncologic laboratory of the Clinic of Obstetrics and Gynecology, Munich Grosshadern between 1993 and 2001.

The correlation between the result of the test and the clinical response in retrospective analyses has been promising so far [14–16].

Examples

1. The GOG-111-trial defined a new standard combination for the ovarian cancer: Cyclophosphamide/Cisplatin was replaced by Paclitaxel/Cisplatin [17].
   With our ATP-TCA testing system we could predict the results of this clinical trial in the in vitro model with ovarian cancer tissue of operated female patients by 1994 [18].
2. The in vitro response of 83% for the combination Mitoxantron and Paclitaxel in platinum-refractory ovarian cancer could be relatively exactly reproduced in the clinical situation with a remission rate of 79% [19].
3. The prediction of sensitivity and especially of resistance in the prospective situation with the ATP-TCA in ovarian cancer in our department showed

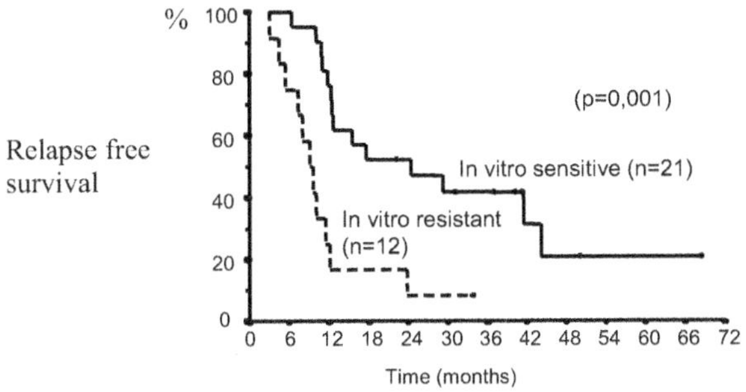

Fig. 3. Correlation of relapse-free survival in 33 primary ovarian cancer cases (16)

an excellent correlation with the clinical response, with a follow-up of 29 months [26].

Figure 3 shows the comparison of relapse-free survival in patients with primary ovarian cancer, whose tumors were tested in vitro with the standard combination at that time, platinum/cyclophosphamide.

The relapse-free survival between in vitro sensitive and in vitro resistant tumors (n=33) is statistically significant (P=0.001).

In a prospective trial in 56 patients with recurrent ovarian cancer, ATP-TCA was employed for therapy planning. A complete remission rate of 36% and a total remission rate of 70% were achieved. The progression-free interval was 11.5 months, and the median overall survival was 21 months (Fig. 4). In particular, patients with platinum-refractory disease could be offered a clinically effective alternative by the in vitro testing [20].

In Fig. 5 the test result of a patient with ovarian cancer with in vitro resistance against Carboplatinum/Cyclophosphamide and in vitro sensitivity for Carboplatinum/Paclitaxel is shown as an example. The Kaplan-Meier curves are shown with a comparison of the survival time between in vitro sensitive and in vitro resistant tumors (n=33). The difference is statistically significant (P=0.066).

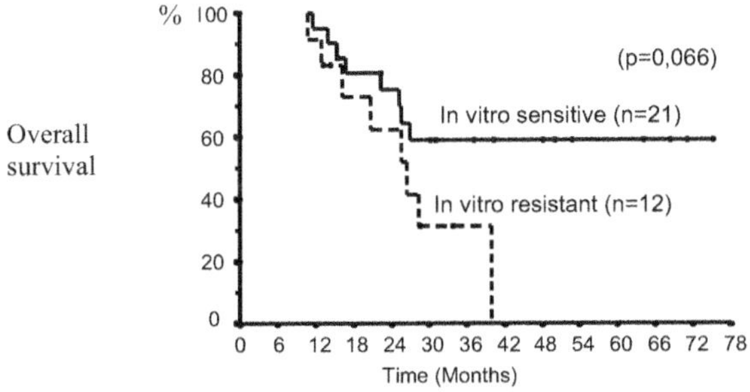

Fig. 4. Overall survival between in vitro sensitive and in vitro resistant tumors (16)

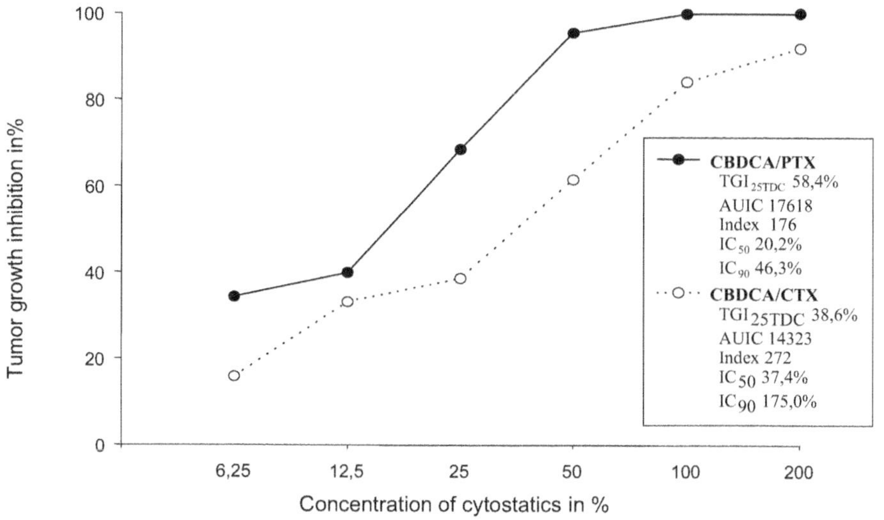

Fig. 5. In vitro sensitivity of a tumor sample for Carboplatinum/Paclitaxel (CBDCA/PTX) and in vitro resistance to Carboplatinum/Cyclophosphamide (CBDCA/CTX). Additionally, AUC (area under the curve), sensitivity index, IC_{50}, and IC_{90} are shown

As a logical consequence of all these results, an international phase III trial in recurrent ovarian cancer has been started. Patients are either treated according to the clinical empirical decision or according to ATP-TCA best response [20].

The main advantage of individualized testing would be the optimization of therapy for the single patient. Kurbacher et al. showed that in ovarian cancer the combination Paclitaxel/Platinum was the most successful regimen in 43% of the cases, but in 23% of the cases it was the "classic" combination Cyclophosphamide/Platinum, in 16% of the cases the combination Cisplatin/Treosulphan, in 8% the combination Cyclophosphamide/Carboplatin, and in 5% of the cases the combination Etoposide/Cisplatin [33].

A comparison of the in vitro sensitivity of the combination Cyclophosphamide/Platin versus Paclitaxel/Platin in primary ovarian cancer in 93 primary ovarian cancer patients showed equal sensitivities of these two combinations in 52% of the cases. In 27% of the cases an in vitro resistance to the Platinum/Cyclophosphamide combination is seen, however, with in vitro sensitivity to the Platinum/Paclitaxel combination. In 21% of the cases resistance to the Platinum/Paclitaxel combination is present, but with sensitivity to the "classic" combination Platinum/Cyclophosphamide. In the present clinical situation this fact is not taken into account, because Platinum/Paclitaxel has been defined as the "new standard" in all primary ovarian cancer after the GOG-111-Trial.

This surely could become an issue of health policy, because savings in the public health system and at the same time individualized optimization of therapy could be made possible by such testing.

The ATP-TCA in Breast Cancer

Breast cancer shows an extremely heterogeneous pattern of response to different drug combinations [21].

Usually, substances from related groups are treated as identical, for example, Doxorubicin, Epirubicin and Mitoxantron as anthracyclines. In the ATP-TCA, however, a different response to these substances in the individual case is present [22].

In advanced breast cancer, good predictions of the in vivo results are possible with the ATP-TCA. Here, the prediction of the response is 83% and the prediction for resistance is 100% [23].

With the help of our in vitro examinations in over 200 breast cancer patients, a good efficacy with mainly synergistic effects of the combination Paclitaxel/Epirubicin could be recognized (Tables 3, 4, 5).

One of the critical and possibly not yet resolved problems of this testing system is "false" positive results. In vitro sensitive tumor samples sometimes do not correlate with the response of the patient in the in vivo situation. Tumor heterogeneity probably plays one of the most important roles here. Mechanisms of resistance development and selection cannot be exactly defined by this testing system. This phenomenon was shown in a first small series of preoperatively treated breast cancer patients. For eight patients, the results of in vitro testing and the preoperative response to the chemotherapy were available. Before treatment, only in one tumor of eight was in vitro resistance to anthracycline present; after treatment resistance to anthracyclines was shown in five of the individual tumors [23].

Table 3. Comparison of Epirubicin versus Paclitaxel on the IC_{50} and IC_{90} levels (n=201)

	Epirubicin	Paclitaxel	*P*
IC_{50}	42.0	37.2	ns (*P*=0.736)
IC_{90}	146.0	113.2	ns (*P*=0.212)

Table 4. Comparison of Epirubicin and Paclitaxel versus Epirubicin/Paclitaxel on the IC_{50} and IC_{90} levels (n=54)

	Epi/Paclitaxel	Epirubicin	*P*
IC_{50}	13.5	42.0	<0.05
IC_{90}	50.8	146.0	<0.05

Table 5. Comparison of Epirubicin and Paclitaxel versus Epirubicin/Paclitaxel on the IC_{50} and IC_{90} levels (n=54)

	Epi/Paclitaxel	Paclitaxel	*P*
IC_{50}	13.5	37.2	<0.05
IC_{90}	50.8	113.2	<0.05

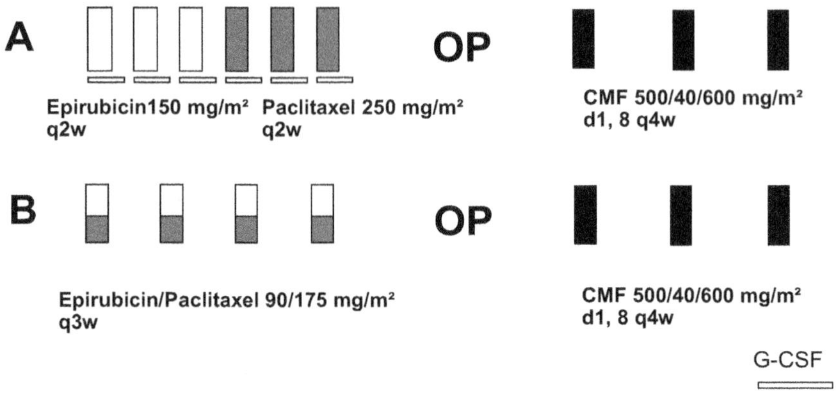

Fig. 6. Preoperative protocol of the AGO. **Arm A**: dose intensified Epirubicin followed by Paclitaxel every 2 weeks; **Arm B**: Epirubicin/Paclitaxel every 3 weeks

Table 6. First results of the preoperative trial of the AGO

	Arm A	Arm B	*P*
Breast-conserving therapy	67%	55%	0.0076
No residual breast tumor	19%	10%	0.030
Axillary node-negative at surgery	51%	42%	0.098

Arm A: dose-intensified Epirubicin followed by Paclitaxel every 2 weeks; Arm B: Standard Arm Epirubicin/Paclitaxel every 3 weeks. Comparisons of breast conservation, node-negative status, and pathohistologic remission in the breast are shown.

The correlation between in vitro sensitivity and response to therapy can ideally be tested in preoperative therapy protocols. Such a protocol is shown in Fig. 6.

After 3 years of recruiting, 452 of 645 breast cancer patients are evaluable for response at the time of surgery. The first results are shown in Table 6.

All target parameters like breast-conserving therapy, node-negative status after preoperative chemotherapy, and no residual tumor in the breast, as well as the pathohistologic complete remission rate, show a clear trend in favor of sequential, dose-intensified Epirubicin/Paclitaxel therapy. If this trend remains valid for the total number of patients, a significant impact of this new principle of therapy can be expected.

By individualized planning of therapy with ATP-TCA testing, therapy in the individual patient could already be performed by the examination of the sensitivity in the preoperative biopsy specimen.

Summary and Discussion

Molecular methods are advancing very fast at the moment for the exact definition of the biological patterns in cancer. However, detailed information for the phenotype of the individual tumor cannot be defined by these methods. In breast cancer the predictive value of such new factors on the protein or gene level are the subject of current examinations, but they are not yet transferable into the clinical routine. Several reasons are responsible for this. As an example, a loss of p53 wild type can be related to chemoresistance. But at the same time, an inhibition of apoptosis is also possible and therefore a therapeutic hypersensitivity by the inhibition of DNA repair mechanisms. Accordingly, in ovarian cancer as well as in breast cancer, it could be shown that neither loss of p53 wild-type function nor bcl-2 overexpression had a clear effect on sensitivity in the ATP-TCA [24, 25].

A change of apoptosis by therapeutic manipulation seems to be more practicable than the pretherapeutic examination of this molecule complex with the aim of therapy prediction [26].

The sensitivity to platinum and alkylating agents is not shown by p53 and bcl-2 status [27]. Here, the chemoresistance is determined by other mechanisms, which we only know partially. The role of the Her2/neu overamplification related to anthracycline sensitivity, especially CMF resistance, in the adjuvant therapy of breast cancer is of great significance [28, 29]. The ATP-TCA examination has shown that Her2/neu-overexpressing breast cancer shows an anthracycline resistance in vivo that can only partially be overcome by concentration increase [30]. This mechanism can be better explained by the partially Her/2-dependent topoisomerase II change that goes together with an anthracycline sensitivity [31].

1. Chemotherapy after individual pretherapeutic testing is an attractive concept from the clinical point of view, but it has neither been verified nor disproved so far.
2. The low cure rate in advanced primary tumors despite high remission rates is a therapeutic challenge. Only unsatisfying results with chemotherapies in relapses, for example, platinum resistance in ovarian cancer relapse, have been recorded so far.
3. The rapid development of agents and the availability of many new substances make a pure clinical evaluation with all indications and in all forms of combinations impossible in the future.
4. So far, in vitro testing has been successfully employed for the recognition of the effects of different new substances. A current example is the direct cytotoxic effect of bisphosphonates on tumor cells in vitro. Green et al. as well as our study group [32] could determine a different, direct cytotoxic effect of bisphosphonates on breast cancer cells and breast cancer tumor samples in vitro after 24-h and 120-h incubation.

Figure 7 shows the different patterns of dose-response mechanisms of four different bisphosphonates (Clodronat, Ibandronat, Pamidronat, Zoledronat) on the T47D breast cancer cell line in vitro. One of the largest prospectively randomized trials for adjuvant therapy with the bisphosphonate Clodronat in breast cancer patients was been presented in December 2001 [34]. Direct cyto-

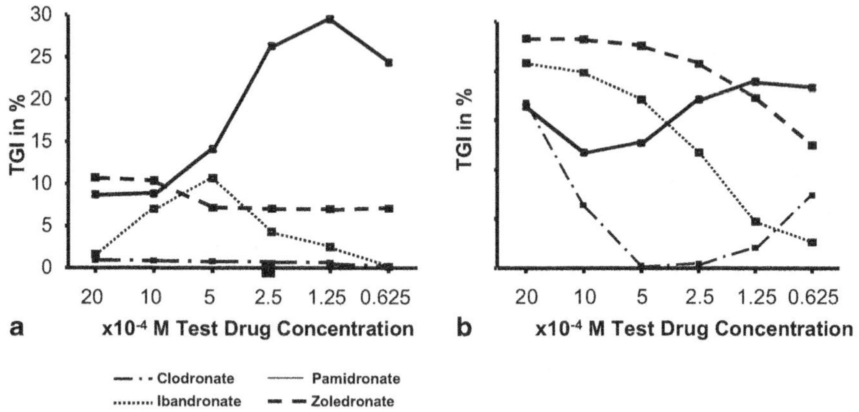

Fig. 7a, b. The dose-response curves of the four different bisphosphonates are shown. Here, a clear dose-effect relationship after 24 h (**a**) and 120 h (**b**) can be recognized

toxic effects with an acceptable range of side effects were shown. Therefore, the adjuvant bisphosphonate therapy might play an increasing role, especially in breast cancer, in the future.

Summary

1. The ATP-TCA meets the requirements of a prospective evaluation.
2. A possible therapy protocol includes biopsy from the primary tumor with ATP-TCA directed therapy compared with a so-called "clinical standard."
3. The early recognition of resistances, especially no response, would have direct therapeutic consequences.
4. Innovative concepts of therapy could consequently be revised, in particular, changed quickly.
5. Chemosensitivity testing is very likely to be realized in oncology, at least as long as clinically valid and practicable molecular genetic models are not established in the routine.

References

1. Pietras RJ, Pegram MD, Finn RS, Maneval DA, Slamon DJ (1998) Remission of human breast cancer xenografts on therapy with humanized monoclonal antibody to HER-2 receptor and DNA-reactive drugs. Oncogene 17(17):2235–2249
2. Hamburger AW, Salmon SE (1977) Primary bioassay of human tumor stem cells. Science 197:161–163
3. Von Hoff SS, Kronmal R, Slamon SE et al. (1991) Selection of cancer chemotherapy for a patient by an in vitro assay versus a clinician. J Natl Cancer Inst 82:110–116

4. Von Hoff DD, Kronmal R, Salmon SE et al. (1991) A Southwest Oncology Group study on the use of a human tumor cloning assay for predicting response in patients with ovarian cancer. Cancer 67:20–27
5. Bellamy WT (1992) Prediction of response to drug therapy of cancer. A review of in vitro assays. Drugs 44:690–708
6. Cortazar P, Jonson BE (1999) Review of the efficacy of individualized chemotherapy selected by in vitro drug sensitivity testing for patients with cancer. J Clin Oncol 17:1625
7. Kangas L, Grönroos M, Nieminen A (1984) Bioluminescence of cellular ATP: a new method for evaluating cytotoxic agents in vitro. Med Biol 62:338–343
8. Sevin et al (1988)
9. Kurbacher CM, Cree IA, Brenne U, Bruckner HW, Kurbacher JA, Mallmann P, Andreotti PE, Krebs D (1996) Heterogeneity of in vitro chemosensitivity in perioperative breast cancer cells to mitoxantrone versus doxorubicin evaluated by a microplate ATP bioluminescence assay. Breast Cancer Res Treat 41:161–170
10. Untch M, Sevin BU, Perras JP, Angioli R, Untch A, Hightower RD, Köchli OR, Averette HE (1994) Evaluation of Paclitaxel (Taxol), Cisplatin, and the Combination Paclitaxel-Cisplatin in Ovarian Cancer in vitro with the ATP Cell Viability Assay. Gynecol Oncol 54:44–49
11. Andreotti PE, Cree IA, Kurbacher CM et al. (1995) Chemosensitivity testing of human tumors using a microplate adenosine triphosphate luminescence assay: clinical correlation for cisplatin resistance of ovarian carcinoma. Cancer Res 55:5276–5282
12. Ackermann T, Kurbacher CM, Mallmann P et al. (1996) Wachstumscharakteristika von Normalzellen im ATP-Tumor-Chemosensitivitäts-Assay. Arch Gynecol Obstet 258 (suppl 1):86
13. Cree IA, Kurbacher CM, Untch M et al. (1996) Correlation of the clinical response to chemotherapy in breast cancer with ex vivo chemosensitivity. Anti-Cancer Drugs 7:630–635
14. Andreotti PE, Cree IA, Kurbacher CM, Hartmann DM, Linder D, Harel G, Gleiberman I, Caruso PA, Ricks SH, Untch M, et al. (1995) Chemosensitivity testing of human tumors using a microplate adenosine triphosphate luminescence assay: clinical correlation for cisplatin resistance of ovarian carcinoma. Cancer Res 55:5276–5282
15. Gerhardt RT, Perras JP, Sevin BU, Petru E, Ramos R, Guerra L, Averette HE (1991) Characterization of in vitro chemosensitivity of perioperative human ovarian malignancies by adenosine triphosphate assay. Am J Obstet Gynecol 165:245–255
16. Konecny G, Crohns C, Pegram M, Felber M, Lude S, Kurbacher C, Cree IA, Hepp H, Untch M (2000) Correlation of drug response with the ATP tumorchemosensitivity assay in primary FIGO stage III ovarian cancer. Gynecol Oncol 77(2):258–63
17. McGuire WP, Hoskins WJ, Brady MF, Kucera PR, Partridge EE, Look KY, Clarke-Pearson DL, Davidson M (1996) Cyclophosphamide and cisplatin compared with paclitaxel and cisplatin in patients with stage III and IV ovarian cancer. New Engl J Med 334:1–6
18. Untch M, Sevin BU, Perras JP, Angioli R, Untch A, Hightower RD, Koechli O, Averette HE (1994) Evaluation of paclitaxel (Taxol), cisplatin, and the combination paclitaxel-cisplatin in ovarian cancer in vitro with the ATP cell viability assay. Gynecol Oncol 53:44–49
19. Kurbacher CM, Bruckner HW, Cree IA, Kurbacher JA, Wilhelm L, Poch G, Indefrei D, Mallmann P, Andreotti PE (1997) Mitoxantrone combined with paclitaxel as salvage therapy for platinum-refractory ovarian cancer: laboratory study and clinical pilot trial. Clin Cancer Res 3:1527–1533
20. Kurbacher CM, Bruckner HW, Cree IA et al. (1999) A prospective clinical trial on individualized chemotherapy directed by a tumor chemosensitivity assay versus physiciańs choice in patients with platinum-resistant ovarian adenocarcinoma.
21. Hunter EM, Sutherland LA, Cree IA et al. (1993) Heterogeneity of chemosensitivity in human breast carcinoma: use of an adenosine triphosphate (ATP) chemiluminescence assay. Eur J Surg Oncol 19:242–249
22. Kurbacher CM, Brenne U, Kurbacher JA, Mallmann P, Krebs D. (1996) Vergleich der zytostatischen Wirkung von Epirubicin und Mitoxantron auf native Mammakarzinomzellen mit Hilfe des ATP-Tumor-Chemosensitivitäts-Assays. Zentbl Gynäkol 118:271–278

23. Cree IA, Kurbacher CM, Untch M, Sutherland LA, Hunter EM, Subedi AM, James EA, Dewar JA, Preece PE, Andreotti PE, Bruckner HW. (1996) Correlation of the clinical response to chemotherapy in breast cancer with ex vivo chemosensitivity. Anti-Cancer Drugs 7:630–635
24. Kurbacher CM, Bruckner HW, Goor A et al. (1998) Influence of p53 and bcl-2 on the ex vivo chemosensitivity of clinical ovarian carcinomas. Proc Am Assoc Cancer 39:236
25. Janát M-M, Kurbacher CM, Goor A et al. (1998) Lack of correlation between p53/bcl-2 expression and breast chemosensitivity ex vivo. J Cancer Res Clin Oncol 124:R154
26. Rein DT, Schondorf T, Breidenbach M, Janat MM, Weikelt A, Gohring UJ, Becker M, Mallmann P, Kurbacher CM (2000) Lack of correlation p53 expression, bcl-2 expression, apoptosis and ex vivo chemosensitivity in advanced human breast cancer. Anticancer Res 20 (6D):5069–5072
27. Petty R, Evans A, Duncan I, Kurbacher C, Cree I (1998) Drug resistance in ovarian cancer – the role of p53. Path Oncol Res 4:97–102
28. Muss HB, Thor AD, Berry DA, Kute T, Liu ET, Koerner F, Cirrincione CT, Budman DR, Wood WC, Barcos M, et al. (1994) C-erbB-2 expression and response to adjuvant therapy in women with node-positive early breast cancer. New Engl J Med 330:1260–1266
29. Untch M, Konecny G, Lebeau A et al. (1998) Dose intensification (DI) of anthracycline in the adjuvant treatment of high risk breast cancer (HRBC) and c-erbB-2 overexpression. Proc ASCO 17:103a
30. Kurbacher CM, Brenne U, Göhring UJ et al. (1999) HER2 status of primary breast carcinomas and ex vivo chemosensitivity against anthracyclines and taxanes. 1st HER2 State-of-the-Art Conference, San Antonio Breast Cancer Meeting 12/2000
31. Isola J, Järunen T, Tanner M et al. (1999) Topoisomerase-IIα aberrations may explain altered chemosensitivity of HER2-amplified breast cancers. 1st HER2 State-of-the-Art Conference, San Antonio Breast Cancer Meeting 12/2000
32. Crohns C, Untch M, Konecny G (2001) Different Bisphosphonates have direct cytotoxic effects on three breast cancer lines and fresh breast cancer tumor tissue. 37th Annual Meeting ASCO 2001
33. Kurbacher CM (2000) DGGG 2000
34. Powles et al. Breast Cancer Research Treatment.

Treosulfan in the Treatment of Metastatic Melanoma: From Chemosensitivity Testing to Clinical Trials

Karsten Neuber

Department of Dermatology, University Hospital Hamburg,
Martinistraße 52, 20246 Hamburg, Germany
e-mail: neuber@uke.uni-hamburg.de

Abstract

The therapy of metastatic malignant melanoma is limited by poor responses and short overall survival. Thus it remains important to identify and test potential new drugs in this disease. To examine the effects of the bifunctional alkylating cytostatic treosulfan, an in vitro microplate ATP bioluminescence assay (ATP-TCA) was used. Five highly chemoresistant melanoma cell lines and melanoma cells freshly isolated from metastases surgically resected from stage IV melanoma patients (n=10) were incubated with treosulfan. Three cell lines and eight of ten tested tumor cells isolated from melanoma metastases showed tumor growth inhibition after incubation with treosulfan. Therefore, 14 patients with rapidly progressing stage IV malignant melanoma who were pretreated with at least one standard chemotherapy regimen received treosulfan. In this population of patients with highly refractory advanced melanoma one complete remission (7.1%), two partial remissions (14.3%), and three cases of stable disease (21.4%) were observed. Median time to progression and median overall survival for all patients measured from the beginning of treosulfan treatment were 5 months [95% confidence interval (CI) 1.98–2.57 months] and 9 months (95% CI 3.92–8.69 months), respectively. On the basis of these data a multicenter phase II trial was initiated. A total of 31 patients with stage IV melanoma were included and treated second-line with 8 g/m^2 i.v. treosulfan. From this group 26 patients were evaluable. No objective remission (CR, PR) was observed, 5 of 26 patients (19%) had stable disease, and 21 patients had progressive disease. Median overall survival was 6.5 months (95% CI 3.1–10 months). Toxicity of treosulfan was moderate. Patients with treosulfan-sensitive melanoma metastases showed better response rates and prolonged survival compared with patients who were not tested before treosulfan treatment. We therefore suggest further studies with first-line treosulfane alone or in combination with gemcitabine or cytosine arabinoside together with prether-

Recent Results in Cancer Research, Vol. 161

apeutic chemosensitivity testing that may help to select patients who might benefit from specific chemotherapy.

Introduction

Biochemotherapy of Metastatic Malignant Melanoma

The incidence of melanoma is increasing at a rate higher than that of any other type of cancer (Rigel et al. 1996) For patients with metastatic melanoma that is not amenable to surgical extirpation, dacarbazine (DTIC) is the most efficacious single chemotherapeutic agent, with an overall response rate of about 10–20% (Lee et al. 1995; Stadelmann et al. 1998). Besides DTIC, other single agents including cisplatin, carmustine (BCNU), paclitaxel, and the vinca alkaloids vindesine and vinblastine produce consistent responses that typically range from 15 to 20% (Flaherty 2000). Combination chemotherapy regimens result in objective response rates up to 55% (Del Prete et al. 1984; McClay et al. 1987, 1992; Legha et al. 1989), but the duration of response is generally quite poor, ranging from 6 to 9 months (Margolin et al. 1998; Fletcher et al. 1993). Prospective phase III trials failed to demonstrate a superiority of many of these regimens over dacarbazine alone (Luikart et al. 1984; Chapman et al. 1999).

A further increase in the rate of objective responses may be achieved by introducing cytokines into therapeutic regimens, with interleukin-2 and interferon-αα",4> being the most widely acclaimed. However, in a small proportion of patients, long-lasting remissions can be achieved (Atzpodien et al. 1995; Legha et al. 1998; Hoffmann et al. 1998). In contrast, other clinical trials on biochemotherapy did not confirm these results (Jonston et al. 1998, Rosenberg et al. 1999).

Therefore, it remains important to identify and test potential new drugs in malignant melanoma.

Treosulfan

Treosulfan (L-threitol-1,4-bis-methanesulfonate, Ovastat) is a prodrug of a bifunctional alkylating cytostatic. Its mechanism of action is based on a nonenzymatic, pH- and temperature-dependent formation of mono- and diepoxybutane derivatives (Fig. 1). These derivatives are responsible for a DNA alkylation and DNA-interstrand crosslinking, followed by DNA fragmentation and cell death (Feit et al. 1970).

In several European countries treosulfan (Ovastat) is registered as an oral and intravenous treatment for patients with advanced ovarian cancer (Breitbach et al. 1994). The combination of cisplatin (70 mg/m^2 i.v., day 1) and treosulfan (5,000 mg/m^2 i.v., day 1) repeated every 3–4 weeks is an established, active, and well-tolerated first-line chemotherapy for patients with ovarian car-

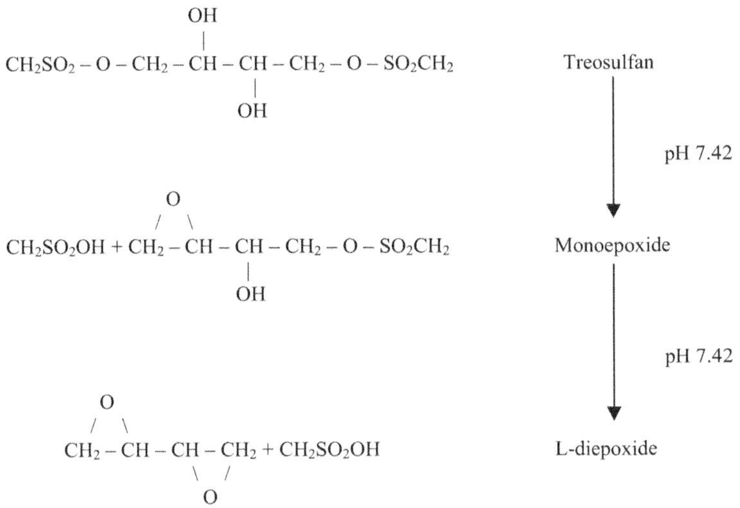

Fig. 1. Formation of treosulfan mono- and diepoxybutane-derivatives responsible for DNA alkylation and DNA-interstrand crosslinking

cinoma (Duncan 1985). Second-line therapy and palliation is recommended with intravenous administration of 7–8 g/m^2 treosulfan every 4 weeks or with a daily oral treatment using treosulfan capsules (Masding et al. 1990). Moreover, significant antitumor activity of treosulfan has been demonstrated in human breast (Köpf-Maier and Sass 1992), small-cell lung, and non-small-cell lung carcinoma (Köpf-Maier and Sass 1996).

Chemosensitivity Testing

Measurement of ATP bioluminescence utilizing the luciferin-luciferase reaction has been proven to be a sensitive and valid method to assess the cytotoxicity of anticancer agents in human tumor cells in vitro (Andreotti et al. 1995). The ATP tumor chemosensitivity assay (TCA) seems to be a valuable method to test the chemosensitivity of both tumor cell lines and clinical tumors (Kurbacher et al. 1995) and is thus regarded as a suitable method to evaluate the cytotoxicity of treosulfan in human melanoma.

Aim of the Study

The anticancer activity of treosulfan in established melanoma cell lines as well as in freshly isolated melanoma cells obtained from surgically resected metastases was investigated. Moreover, we report on response rates, time to progression, and overall survival after second-line treosulfan treatment in patients with DTIC-resistant stage IV melanoma.

Patients, Materials, and Methods

Melanoma Cell Lines

Five different human melanoma cell lines highly resistant to different chemotherapeutic agents were studied. Cell lines IGR-39, IPC-298, RVH-421, COLO-800, and COLO-792 were purchased from the German Collection of Microorganisms and Cell Cultures (DSMZ, Dept. of Human and Animal Cell Cultures). Cell lines were maintained as monolayer cultures in RPMI-1640 medium (GIBCO, Paisley, UK) supplemented with 10% fetal bovine serum (FBS), 100 U/ml penicillin, and 100 mg/ml streptomycin at 37°C, in a humidified 95% air-5% CO_2 atmosphere.

Drugs for In Vitro Experiments

Commercial formulations of treosulfan (Ovastat; kindly supplied by medac GmbH, Hamburg, Germany), paclitaxel, cisplatin, BCNU, fotemustine, and vincristine were used for this study. Temozolamide (similar to DTIC) was a kind gift from Schering-Plough (New Jersey, USA). Treosulfan and the other drugs were dissolved freshly for each assay with an appropriate amount of complete assay medium (CAM) or RPMI-1640.

Specimen Preparation

Surgical biopsy specimens of melanoma metastases from 10 different patients were transported in DMEM (GIBCO) containing 300 U/ml penicillin and 300 μg/ml streptomycin. Specimens were obtained according to protocols approved by the hospital Institutional Review Board after patient informed consent was obtained. Specimens were tested only after selection of appropriate tissue for histological and other clinical diagnostic evaluation.

The tumors were minced into 0.5- to 2.0-mm^3 fragments under sterile conditions after excess fat and normal tissue were excised. Fragments were then dissociated into a cell suspension of single cells and small aggregates by incubation in 5–10 ml of sterile tumor dissociation enzyme reagent (from DCS Innovative Diagnostik Systeme, Hamburg, Germany) for 4–18 h at 37°C. Cells were washed twice and resuspended for assay in CAM (DCS Innovative Diagnostik Systeme, Hamburg, Germany) at $1.0–2.0 \times 10^5$ cells/ml.

Tumor cells from subconfluent monolayers were harvested by trypsinization (0.02% NaEDTA in 0.05% trypsin; Boehringer, Mannheim, Germany). After washing in Hanks' balanced salt solution (HBSS; GIBCO) and centrifugation (5 min at 100 $\times g$) cells were resuspended in RPMI-1640 + 10% FBS and aspirated several times to disperse cell aggregates. Viability of the resultant single-cell suspensions were determined by trypan blue dye exclusion (0.2%;

Table 1. Drug concentrations used in the assay and their clinically relevant doses

Drug name	TDC (µg/ml)	Drug dose correlation
Paclitaxel	13.6	i.v. 275 mg/m^2
Cisplatin	3.8	i.v. 100 mg/m^2
BCNU	8	i.v. 150 mg/m^2
Vincristine	0.4	i.v. 1,5 mg/m^2
Fotemustine	8	i.v. 100 mg/m^2
Treosulfan	20	oral 1 g/m^2
Temozolamide	10	i.v. 150 mg/m^2

Merck, Darmstadt, Germany). Suspensions then were adjusted to a final concentration of 1×10^4 viable cells/ml.

Chemosensitivity Assay

TCA-100 reagents were obtained from DCS Innovative Diagnostik Systeme (Hamburg, Germany). Treosulfan as well as other cytotoxic agents (paclitaxel, cisplatin, BCNU, vincristine, fotemustine, temozolamide) were tested at six dilutions corresponding to 200%, 100%, 50%, 25%, 12.5%, and 6.25% of a standard tumor drug concentration (TDC). TDCs are based on pharmacokinetic data adjusted to provide good discrimination between tumors (Table 1). Cultures of 10,000–20,000 cells/well were tested in 96-well round-bottom polypropylene microplates (Costar 3790; for melanoma cells obtained freshly from metastases) or in 96-well flat-bottom polystyrene plates (Falcon; Becton-Dickinson, Heidelberg, Germany; for melanoma cell lines). Each drug was tested at six concentrations in triplicate as described elsewhere. Microplates contained 12 M0 control wells (0.1 ml cell suspension + 0.1 ml CAM) and 12 MI control wells (0.1 ml cell suspension + 0.1 ml maximum ATP inhibitor). Test drug dilutions were set up in culture microplates by doubling dilutions of fresh 800% TDC solutions in 0.1 ml CAM/well before adding 0.1 ml cells/well.

ATP Extraction and Luminometry

After incubation of the cultures for 2–4 days (cell lines) or 6 days (melanoma cells from metastases) at 37°C in a <98% humidified, 95% air-5% CO_2 atmosphere, cellular ATP was extracted and stabilized by mixing 0.05 ml of tumor cell extraction reagent (DCS Innovative Diagnostik Systeme, Hamburg, Germany) into each well. ATP was measured in a Berthold LB-953 luminometer using 0.05 ml of culture extract injected with 0.05 ml of luciferin-luciferase counting reagent. A 10-s count integration time with a 4-s delay was used. Light output expressed as relative light units (RLU) was used to determine the mean percent inhibition of cell growth/survival in triplicate wells at each drug concentration according to the following equation: 1–[(Test–MI)/M0–MI)]×100.

An ATP standard curve was performed for all studies with 0.05-ml aliquots of a 250 ng/ml ATP standard serially diluted 1:3 in dilution buffer. Microplates were stored at –20°C for repeat measurements if required.

Patients and Study Design

Metastases were surgically removed from 10 different stage IV melanoma patients to obtain cells for chemosensitivity testing. Moreover, between June 1996 and April 1998 14 patients (age: 28–82 years, median: 67.5 years) with histologically confirmed metastatic malignant melanoma, ECOG performance grade of ≤2, and life expectancy ≥3 months were treated with treosulfan (study 1). Informed consent was obtained from each patient before surgery (chemosensitivity testing) or administration of any medication.

Additionally, 31 patients (age: 44–83 years, median: 64 years) with progressive metastatic malignant melanoma after first-line chemotherapy with a DTIC-containing regimen with or without immunotherapy were included in a multicenter phase II protocol. All patients had a good performance status (WHO Performance Index: 0–2) and a life expectancy of more than 3 months. Patients with cerebral metastases were excluded. End points of the study were (1) efficacy (tumor response, median time to progression, median survival time) and (2) toxicity of treosulfan treatment (study 2).

Study Medication

Treatment consisted of up to 5 cycles of treosulfan (Ovastat capsules 3×500 mg/d oral, days 1–7, every 28 days or i.v. treosulfan 8 g/m^2, day 1, every 4 weeks up to a maximum of 6 cycles). Each patient receiving treosulfan had progressive disease after treatment with at least one standard monochemotherapy protocol with either DTIC or fotemustine. Reevaluation of patients was performed according to WHO criteria. Survival and response duration were measured from the initiation of therapy.

Response Evaluation

All patients received two cycles of treatment, unless they had obvious clinical evidence of progressive disease. Tumor response was recorded by standard WHO criteria in measurable and assessable lesions only. Measurable lesions included those with bidimensionable measurements, and assessable disease included disease that was measurable in only one dimension. Only lytic bone lesions were considered assessable. Complete clinical response was defined as disappearance of all tumor on at least two observations, 4 weeks apart. Partial response was defined as 50% or more reduction in the sum of the products of all measurable lesions without any evidence of progression or appearance of new lesions. Stable disease was defined as no change (i.e., <50% decrease or <25% increase) in measurable or assessable disease for at least 8 weeks, whereas progressive disease was defined as more than 25% increase of such disease or the appearance of new lesions.

Patients who showed a response or stable disease in measurable or assessable lesions after the first two cycles received two further cycles.

Dose Modification

Grade III/IV myelosuppression resulted in dose reduction of treosulfan from 8 g/m^2 to 5 g/m^2. Treatment was delayed for up to 2 weeks if the absolute neutrophil count was less than 1,500 μl^{-1} or platelet count was less than 100,000 μl^{-1}. In the case of persistent myelosuppression (>2 weeks), treatment was stopped.

Analysis of Results

Chemosensitivity Testing

For comparison of responses, a simple index was derived by summing the percent inhibition at each level of TDC tested as Index=700–Sum [$Inhibition_{3,13,...200}$]. An arbitrary level of 50% inhibition (Index below 350) was used to assess relative ex vivo sensitivity or resistance.

Clinical Studies

Nominal and ordinal parameters were analyzed via absolute and relative frequencies. Time to progression and overall survival time were calculated from the start date of treatment to the documented date of progressive disease or death, respectively. Patients who had not progressed or who were still alive at the last follow-up were considered censored at this time point. Kaplan-Meier methods were applied for "time to failure" variables. Median progression free survival and median overall survival times were presented with their 95% confidence intervals. In addition, 1-year survival rates were calculated. For differences between study 1 and study 2 the log-rank test and chi-square test were used. The prognostic impact of tumor response on survival was further investigated with the landmark method that eliminates length-biased sampling (Buyse 1996). This method ignores all deaths that occur before a specific landmark time and all progressive diseases documented thereafter. Thus it compares living patients showing a stable disease before the specific landmark time with those living patients having a progressive disease before this time.

Because of the short median time to progression, landmark times of 1 and 2 months were chosen for this exploratory analysis.

Toxicity was analyzed on a per-patient basis by calculating the cumulative toxicity, which was defined as the worst toxicity grade observed during therapy.

Results

Sensitivity of Melanoma Cell Lines to Treosulfan

Data collected with the TCA index is shown in Table 2 for all seven agents and three combinations tested. It is readily apparent that all cell lines are not sensitive or at most weakly sensitive to all alkylating agents except treosulfan. Treosulfan induced more than 50% tumor growth inhibition (Index below 350) in melanoma cell lines IGR-39, IPC-298, and COLO800. Neither one of the combinations nor one of the nonalkylating agents except paclitaxel showed a tumor growth inhibition greater than 50% (Table 2). Paclitaxel inhibited the growth of cell line COLO-800 up to 100% at test drug concentrations of 200% to 50%. At low test drug concentrations (12.5%–6.25%) treosulfan showed stronger growth inhibition of COLO-800 cells than paclitaxel (Fig. 2).

Sensitivity of Freshly Isolated Melanoma Cells to Treosulfan

Chemosensitivity testing of freshly isolated melanoma cells showed significant tumor growth inhibition (>50%) by treosulfan in 8 of 10 cases (Table 3).

Table 2. Sensitivity of five melanoma cell lines to cytotoxic agents frequently used in metastatic melanoma. Results of testing for each melanoma cell line expressed as a simple summary index of inhibition across the range of concentrations tested for single agents as well as for combinations [low values (below 350) indicate considerable inhibition, whereas higher values indicate resistance]

Cell line	Paclitaxel	Cisplatin	BCNU	Vincristine	Fotemustine	Treosulfan	Temozolamide	Cisplatin-paclitaxel	Temozolomide-BCNU-cisplatin	Temozolomide-vincristine-cisplatin
IGR39[a]	540	660	608	529	624	**293**	700	639	450	582
RVH421[b]	626	700	700	378	668	654	650	600	668	419
IPC298[a]	632	670	627	541	447	**299**	575	675	390	480
COLO792[b]	522	700	700	688	700	700	700	516	679	700
COLO800[c]	**216**	608	700	700	424	**295**	700	574	418	608

[a]Cell line derived from primary melanoma.
[b]Cell line derived from brain metastases of malignant melanoma.
[c]Cell line derived from a skin metastasis of malignant melanoma.

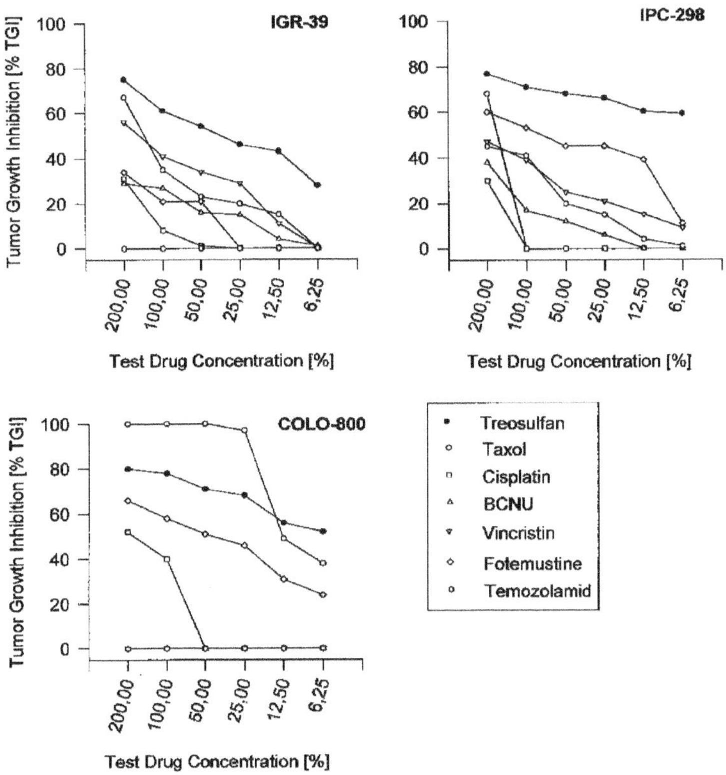

Fig. 2. Growth inhibition of melanoma cell lines IGR-39, IPC-298, and COLO-800 exposed to increasing concentrations of treosulfan, paclitaxel, cisplatin, BCNU, vincristine, fotemustine, and temozolamide. Concentrations are expressed as percent tumor drug concentration

Table 3. Growth inhibition of melanoma cells freshly isolated from metastases of patients (n=10) with stage IV melanoma exposed for 6 days to increasing concentrations of treosulfan

Patient	Loc. of melanoma metastases	Sensitivity in ATP-TCA
1	Skin	255
2	Skin	174
3	Lung	158
4	Skin	402
5	Lymph node	292
6	Skin	166
7	Skin	160
8	Skin	269
9	Skin	305
10	Skin	613

Table 4. Patient characteristics of the two treosulfan trials

	Study 1 (%)	Study 2 (%)
No. of patients	14	31
No. of eligible patients	14	26
Median age (years)	67.5	64
(Range)	(28–82)	(44–83)
Sex		
Male	6 (43)	14 (54)
Female	8 (57)	12 (46)
WHO performance index		
0	9	18 (73)
1	5	6 (23)
2	0	1 (4)
Prior chemotherapy	14	26
No. of disease sites		
1	5 (37)	7 (27)
2	3 (21)	10 (38)
3	3 (21)	7 (27)
≥4	3 (21)	2 (8)
Distribution of disease sites		
Nodes	6 (43)	14 (54)
Skin	5 (36)	3 (12)
Lung	6 (43)	15 (58)
Liver	8 (57)	9 (35)
Spleen	1 (7)	3 (12)
Kidney/Adrenal	1 (7)	5 (19)
Bone	5 (36)	2 (8)
Others	2 (14)	4 (16)

Study Population

Between June 1996 and April 1998, 14 patients with metastatic melanoma resistant to DTIC were treated second-line with treosulfan in a single-center pilot study (study 1). Because of the results of this first study, a multicenter phase II study was initiated (study 2). Between August 1998 and September 1999 a total of 31 patients with the histologically confirmed diagnosis of melanoma and measurable metastatic disease were registered and 28 remained eligible after review of the on-study data. Additionally, two patients were ineligible because of insufficient documentation. All 26 eligible patients were assessable for response and toxicity. The clinical characteristics of all patients from both studies are listed in Table 4. No patient was removed from therapy because of toxicity.

Table 5. Response rate (WHO) after second-line treosulfan treatment in the pilot study and in the phase II trial

	Study 1 (%)	Study 2 (%)
CR	1 (7)	0
PR	2 (14)	0
NC	3 (21)	5 (19)
PD	8 (58)	21 (81)

Tumor Responses

Study 1

One patient had a complete remission, two experienced a partial remission, and stabilization of disease occurred in three patients. Eight patients continued to progress despite therapy (Table 5).

Study 2

No overall objective response (CR or PR) was observed. There were five patients with stable disease (19%). Twenty-one patients (81%) had PD (Table 5). Four patients with PD had a minor or mixed response.

Time to Progression and Survival Analysis

Study 1

The median time to progression in this study (Fig. 3) was 2 months (95% CI, 0.5–9.5 months). Median overall survival (Fig. 4) from the beginning of treosulfan treatment was 9 months (95% CI, 7.9–10.1 months). The median overall survival measured from the initiation of any chemotherapy regimen was 17 months with a range from 5 to 34 months.

Study 2

The median follow-up was 14.3 months (range of those surviving 7.7–25 months). Twenty-five of twenty-six patients (96%) had tumor progression during follow-up. The patient without progression was censored after 14.3 months. The median time to progression (Fig. 3) was 1.8 months (95% CI, 1.6–2.1 months). Twenty patients (77%) died during follow-up. The median overall survival (Fig. 4) for all patients was 6.5 months (95% CI, 3.1–10 months). The 1-year survival rate was calculated as 33.9% (95% CI, 15.4% to 52.3%).

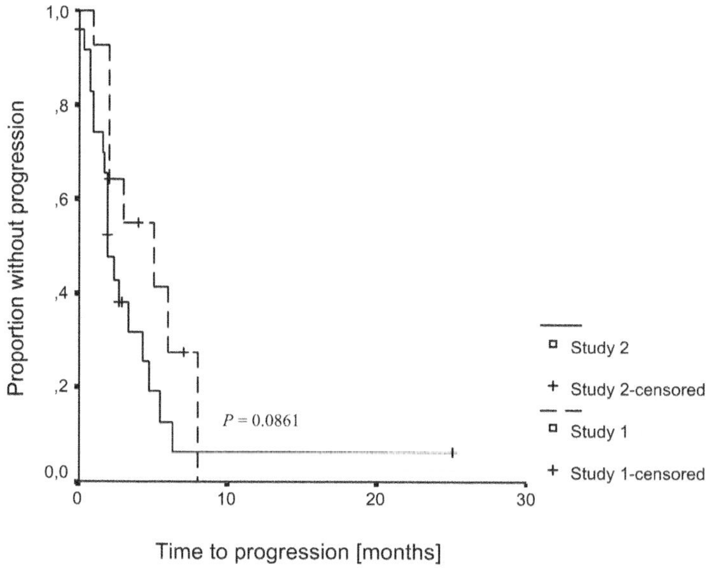

Fig. 3. Time to progression comparing patients treated with treosulfan: study 1 (—) vs. study 2 (—)

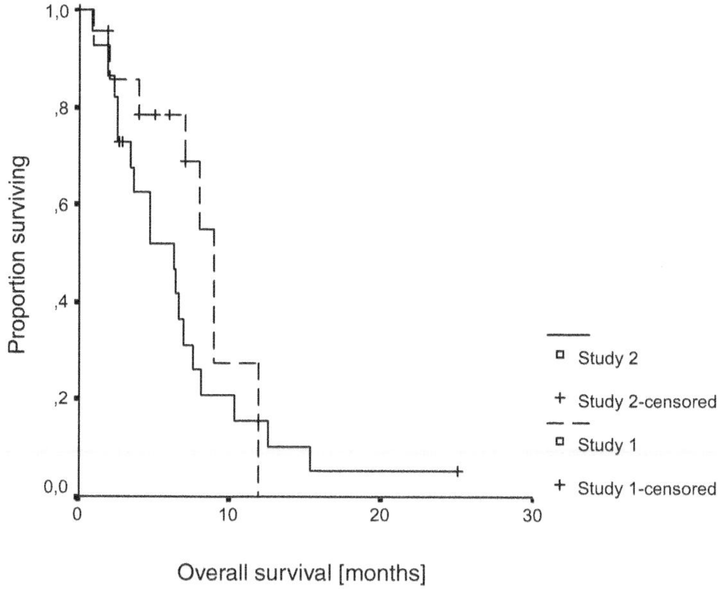

Fig. 4. Overall survival comparing patients treated with treosulfan: study 1 (—) vs. study 2 (—)

With a landmark time of 1 month a statistically significant difference in overall survival was found between the 4 SD and 21 PD patients (log rank, P=0.03), resulting in a median survival time of 7 and 2 months, respectively.

With a landmark time of 2 months, 23 living patients could be analyzed, leading to a median survival of 8 months compared with 5 months, respectively (log rank, P=0.20).

Study 1 Versus Study 2

Comparing the results of the first clinical trial and the phase II trial, the differences in response rate, time to progression, and overall survival were not significant (Figs. 3, 4). However, when the subgroup of patients with in vitro chemosensitivity to treosulfan was compared with the patients without chemosensitivity testing significant differences can be seen. Chi-square analysis of response rates showed significantly (P=0.001) better responses in the group of those patients showing chemosensitivity to treosulfan in the ATP-TCA. Additionally, time to progression [treosulfan sensitive, 6 months (95% CI, 2.8–9.2 months) vs. not tested, 2 months (95% CI, 1.8–2.2 months), P=0.03] and overall survival [treosulfan sensitive, 9 months (95% CI, 7.9–10.1 months) vs. not tested, 4.7 months (95% CI, 1.4–8 months), P=0.049] was significantly prolonged in this subgroup (Figs. 5, 6).

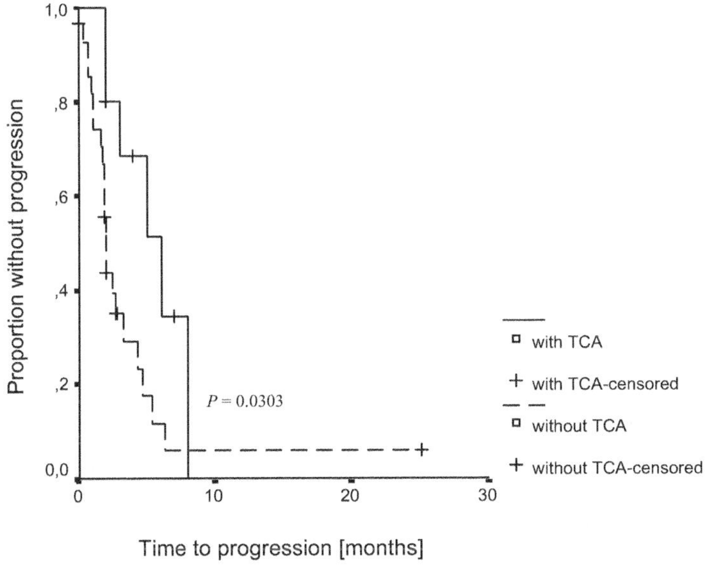

Fig. 5. Time to progression comparing patients treated with treosulfan: without (—) chemosensitivity testing (TCA–) vs. with (—) chemosensitivity testing (TCA+)

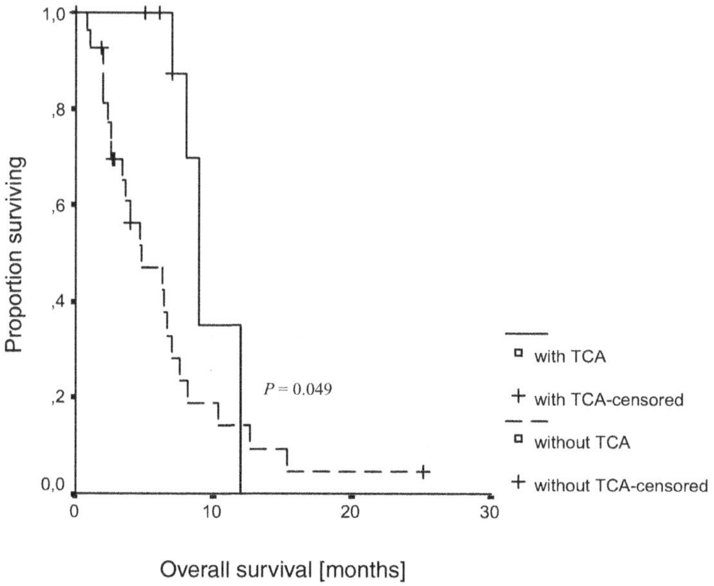

Fig. 6. Overall survival comparing patients treated with treosulfan: without (—) chemosensitivity testing (TCA–) vs. with (—) chemosensitivity testing (TCA+)

Toxicity

All 40 patients treated with treosulfan were assessable for toxicity (Table 6). The major toxicities were hematologic and consisted of lymphocytopenia (grade 3 in 18% and grade 4 in 8% of patients), thrombocytopenia (grade 3 in 5%), and leukocytopenia (grade 3 in 15%). Neither high-grade nonhematological toxicity nor treatment-related death was observed.

Discussion

Chemosensitivity Testing of Treosulfan

In this study, the in vitro activity of treosulfan in five melanoma cell lines as well as in freshly isolated melanoma cells derived from 10 patients has been demonstrated with a microtiter plate ATP bioluminescence assay.

Because the treatment of metastatic melanoma is limited by the lack of effective systemic therapy and the median survival with metastatic disease is less than 1 year, it remains important to identify and test potential new drugs in this disease.

Treosulfan represents a prodrug of a bifunctional alkylating cytostatic. Spontaneous (enzyme independent) activation to the corresponding monoepoxide and diepoxide structures is responsible for the DNA alkylation in gua-

Table 6. Toxicity of treosulfan treatment in both clinical studies (n=40)

	Grade 0	Grade 1	Grade 2	Grade 3	Grade 4
Hematological					
Anemia	30 (75)	4 (10)	6 (15)	0	0
Leukopenia	20 (50)	10 (25)	5 (13)	6 (15)	0
Lymphopenia	29 (73)	0	1 (3)	7 (18)	3 (8)
Neutropenia	39 (98)	0	1 (3)	0	0
Thrombocytopenia	27 (68)	4 (10)	7 (18)	2 (5)	0
Gastrointestinal					
Nausea	35 (88)	4 (10)	1 (3)	0	0
Vomiting	39 (98)	1 (3)	0	0	0
Diarrhea	39 (98)	1 (3)	0	0	0
Constipation	39 (98)	0	1 (3)	0	0
Hepatic disturbance					
γGT	32 (80)	4 (10)	4 (10)	0	0
GOT	38 (95)	1 (3)	1 (3)	0	0
GPT	38 (95)	1 (3)	1 (3)	0	0
AP	37 (93)	3 (8)	0	0	0
LDH	37 (93)	3 (8)	0	0	0
Bilirubin	39 (98)	0	1 (3)	0	0
Fatigue	38 (95)	1 (3)	1 (3)	0	0
Dyspnea	39 (98)	0	0	0	1 (3)
Weight loss	38 (95)	1 (3)	1 (3)	0	0

nine-N^7 position with preference for contiguous runs of guanines and for formation of DNA cross-links (Hartley et al. 1999). The pattern of DNA damage was different from cisplatin and BCNU, which primarily produce blocks at GG or GA sites and O^6 alkylations of guanine, respectively. In vitro cytotoxicity tests, therefore, showed a lack of cross-resistance between treosulfan, cisplatin, or BCNU. This is confirmed by our in vitro tests showing a growth inhibition of melanoma cell lines by treosulfan but not by cisplatin and BCNU either alone or in combination.

DTIC, on the other hand, is enzymatically activated to alkylating metabolites. In consequence, DNA methylation in position N^7, O^6, or O^4 of guanine has been demonstrated, whereas DTIC is not able to induce DNA cross-links. Temozolamide is a derivative of DTIC that is active in vitro. The present data showing a high resistance of the tested cell lines to temozolamide indicate that there is no cross-resistance between temozolamide and treosulfan.

Treosulfan is a clinically well-tolerated prodrug of a bifunctional alkylating cytostatic indicated for the treatment of patients with ovarian carcinoma (Breitbach, et al. 1994; Masding, et al. 1990; Gropp et al. 1998). Although this drug has been used in clinical practice as an oral as well as intravenous formulation for decades, until now activity in malignant melanoma and other human malignancies other than ovarian carcinoma has been scarcely investigated. Recently, preclinical testing of treosulfan showed a broad spectrum of antitumor activity against other carcinomas (Cree et al. 1999; Hunter et al. 1993; Myatt et al. 1997; Neale et al. 1999; Neuber et al. 1999).

With the ATP bioluminescence assay we observed that treosulfan inhibits the growth of melanoma cells in vitro. In established melanoma cell lines as well as in melanoma cells isolated from resected metastases antitumor activity of treosulfan was superior to the other drugs tested, which are known to be effective in malignant melanoma.

Instead of DTIC, which is not metabolized into the active metabolite in vitro, temozolamide has been used. Because it can be assumed that temozolamide and DTIC are similarly effective against malignant melanoma, it is remarkable that melanoma cell growth was more strongly inhibited by treosulfan than by temozolamide.

Clinical Trials

DTIC remains the most efficacious single chemotherapeutic agent, with an overall response rate of about 10%–20% (Stadelmann et al. 1998). Combination chemotherapy regimens resulted in objective response rates up to 55%, but the duration of response was generally quite poor (Chapman et al. 1999). A further increase in the rate of objective responses may be achieved by introducing cytokines into the therapeutic regimens, with interleukin-2 and interferon-γ being the most widely acclaimed (Atzpodien, et al. 1995; Legha et al. 1997, 1998; Hoffmann et al. 1998). However, only in a small proportion of patients can long-lasting remissions be achieved. New chemotherapeutic approaches should, therefore, focus on new drugs with potentially improved efficacy.

Study 1

For ovarian cancer as well as for breast cancer it has been shown that the results of in vitro chemosensitivity testing with the ATP bioluminescence assay correlates with clinical response (Kurbacher et al. 1996; Cree et al. 1996).

Therefore, 14 patients with rapidly progressing stage IV malignant melanoma that were pretreated with at least one standard chemotherapy regimen were treated with treosulfan. In this population of patients with advanced refractory malignant melanoma one complete remission was observed. Partial remission induced by treosulfan was observed in two cases; one patient had stable disease for 8 months. Moreover, survival of these three patients was prolonged to 8 and 12 months, respectively.

Although only a small population of melanoma patients were included in this pilot study, the data indicated that treosulfan might be a promising alkylating cytostatic for the treatment of metastatic malignant melanoma. Thus a multicenter phase II clinical trial was initiated to reconsider the antitumor effectiveness of treosulfan in malignant melanoma.

Study 2

In contrast to the first clinical trial with treosulfan showing complete and partial remissions of advanced metastatic malignant melanoma, in this study no objective responses could be achieved in 26 stage IV melanoma patients. However, in five patients disease progress was stabilized during treosulfan treatment and statistical analysis by the landmark method (Buyse 1996) suggested that patients in whom a stable disease was achieved derived a survival benefit from treosulfan treatment (median overall survival: 7 months). The median survival time for all 26 patients was 6.5 months, and a 1-year survival rate of 33.9% was observed.

The poor response rates in study 2 compared with the results of study 1 (Neuber et al. 1999) may be due to the following reasons: (1) the patients were not preselected by chemosensitivity testing, (2) the proportion of patients with metastases confined to soft tissue sites (skin, lymph nodes, or lung) was higher in the pilot study, and (3) the different pharmacology of oral versus intravenous treosulfan administration.

For ovarian as well as for breast cancer it has been shown that the results of in vitro chemosensitivity testing with an ATP bioluminescence assay correlate with clinical response (Cree et al. 1996; Kurbacher et al. 1996). In vitro sensitivity to treosulfan has been also demonstrated in 8 of 14 melanoma patients and objective responses in vivo after treosulfan treatment were observed in 3 of 10 patients. One possible explanation for the different response rates observed in study 2 is the heterogeneity of tumor chemosensitivity that was not pretested in this study. Indeed, when comparing the subgroup of patients who were sensitive to treosulfan in vitro with the patients that were not tested for chemosensitivity significantly higher response rate and prolonged time to progression as well as prolonged overall survival were observed.

Patients with metastases confined to soft tissue (skin, lymph nodes, or lung) are more likely to respond to chemotherapy and, in many databases, have a better prognosis than patients with metastases to other sites. Of the patients assessable for tumor response in study 2, 77% had metastases confined to soft tissue sites, in contrast to 64% in study 1, so that poor response rates in the phase II trial seems not to be due to the number of soft tissue sites.

The plasma concentrations of treosulfan after intravenous administration (day 1) are different compared with oral treosulfan therapy (days 1–5). The intravenous protocol used in the phase II trial results in a short-lasting peak of treosulfan metabolites in plasma, whereas daily repeated oral application for 1 week results in a plateau of cytostatic mono- and diepoxides (Hilger et al. 2000). One may hypothesize that long lasting plasma levels of treosulfan metabolites after oral administration may have superior antitumor activity. Comparing response rates and survival time of patients with oral versus intravenous treosulfan, no differences were observed (data not shown) However, no clinical trial has been performed that addresses this question.

Toxicity

The treatment protocol used in this study did not require hospitalization. The majority of grade 3 or 4 toxicities were leukocytopenia (15%), lymphocytopenia (39%), and thrombocytopenia (8%). Grade 4 dyspnea in one patient was not related to treosulfan treatment. The toxicities observed in this study are quite similar to those described in previous phase I and II studies with treosulfan alone or in combination regimens (Gropp et al. 1998; Merkle et al. 2000). The intravenous treosulfan regimen used in this study was well tolerated.

Second-Line Chemotherapy in Metastatic Melanoma

There are very few phase II studies of patients with metastatic melanoma previously treated with DTIC receiving second-line chemotherapy with conventional cytotoxic agents (Porcile et al. 1979; Bajetta et al. 1995; Propper et al. 2000; Guven et al. 2001). The objective response rates in these trials using toxic multidrug regimens ranged from 5.7% (DTIC + BCNU + cisplatin + tamoxifen; Propper et al. 2000) to 19% (carboplatin + cytosine arabinoside; Bajetta et al. 1995) and to 26.4% (cisplatin + carboplatin; Guven et al. 2001). The median overall survival time ranged from 4.2 months to 12.5 months. Another phase II study with interleukin-2 and interferon-α2a in patients with progressive metastatic melanoma after chemotherapy revealed no objective responses (Eton et al. 2000). Median time to progression and median survival in this study were 2 months and 6 months, respectively.

The results of the two second-line studies with treosulfan revealed objective responses and survival time that are similar to those in trials performed with much more toxic regimens.

Conclusion

In DTIC-resistant metastatic melanoma, there appears to be no advantage in changing to either single-agent or multi-drug chemotherapy. If patients are to be considered for second-line treatment, identifying patterns of in vitro cross-resistance with newly developed cellular chemosensitivity assays (Cree and Kurbacher 1997) may suggest other therapeutic possibilities. We therefore suggest further studies with first-line treosulfane alone or in combinations with gemcitabine or cytosine arabinoside together with pretherapeutic chemosensitivity testing that may help to select patients who might benefit from specific chemotherapy.

References

Andreotti PE, Cree IA, Kurbacher CM, Hartmann DM, Linder D, Harel G, Gleiberman I, Caruso PA, Ricks SH, Untch M, Sartori C, Bruckner HW (1995) Chemosensitivity testing of human tumors using a microplate adenosine triphosphate luminescence assay: clinical correlation for cisplatin resistance of ovarian carcinoma. Cancer Res 55:5276–5282

Atzpodien J, Lopez-Hänninen E, Kirchner H, Franzke A, Körfer A, Volkenandt M, Duensing S, Schomburg A, Chaitik S, Poliwoda H (1995) Chemoimmunotherapy of advanced malignant melanoma: sequential administration of subcutaneous interleukin-2 and interferon-alpha after intravenous dacarbazine and carboplatin or intravenous dacarbacine, cisplatin, carmustine, and tamoxifene. Eur J Cancer 31:876–881

Bajetta E, Buzzoni R, Vicario G (1995) Combined carboplatin and cytosine arabinoside in metastatic melanoma refractory to dacarbazine. Tumori 81:238–240

Breitbach GP, Villena C, Schwickerath J, Kunz T, Hurst U, Schmidt-Rhode P, Friedrich EJ, Artmeyer E, Schröder M, Eberl M, Franck J, Meinen K, Schiller S, Wernicke K, Sass G, Schmidt H, Bastert G (1994) Treosulfan bei fortgeschrittenem Ovarialkarzinom: eine Phase-III-Studie. Arch Gynecol Obstet 225 [Suppl 1]:80

Buyse M (1996) On the relationship between response to treatment and survival time. Stat Med 15:2797–2812

Chapman PB, Einhorn LH, Meyers ML, Saxman S, Destro AN, Panageas KS, Begg CB, Agarwala SS, Schuchter LM, Ernstoff MS, Houghton AN, Kirkwood JM (1999) Phase III multicenter randomized trial of the Dartmouth regimen versus dacarbazine in patients with metastatic melanoma. J Clin Oncol 17:2745–2751

Cree IA, Kurbacher CM (1997) Individualizing chemotherapy for solid tumors: is there any alternative? Anti-Cancer Drugs 8:541–548

Cree IA, Kurbacher CM, Untch M, Sutherland LA, Hunter EMM, Subedi AMC, James EA, Dewar JA, Preece PE, Andreotti PE, Bruckner HW (1996) Correlation of the clinical response to chemotherapy in breast cancer with ex vivo chemosensitivity. Anti-Cancer Drugs 7:630–635

Cree IA, Neale MH, Myatt NE, de Takats PG, Hall P, Grant J, Kurbacher CM, Reinhold U, Neuber K, MacKie RM, Chana J, Weaver PC, Khoury GG, Sartori C, Andreotti PE (1999) Heterogeneity of chemosensitivity of metastatic cutaneous melanoma. Anti-Cancer Drugs 10:437–444

DelPrete SA, Maurer LH, O'Donnell (1984) Combination chemotherapy with cisplatin, carmustine, dacarbazine, and tamoxifene in metastatic malignant melanoma. Cancer Treat Rep 68:1403–1405

Duncan I (1985) Combination chemotherapy of ovarian carcinoma with cisplatinum and treosulfan – a phase II study. Br J Obstet Gynaecol 92:762–767

Eton O, Buzaid AC, Bedikian AY, Smith TM, Papadopoulos NE, Ellerhorst JA, Hibberts JL, Legha SS, Benjamin RS (2000) A phase II study of "decrescendo" interleukin-2 plus interferon-α-2a in patients with progressive metastatic melanoma after chemotherapy. Cancer 88:1703–1709

Feit PW, Rastrup-Anderson N, Matagne R (1970) Studies in epoxide formation from (2S,3S)-threitol-1,4-bismethanesulfonate. The preparation and biological activity of (2S,3S)9-1,2-epoxy-3,4-butanediol-4-methanesulfonate. J Med Chem 13:1173–1175

Flaherty LE (2000) Rationale for intergroup trial E-3695 comparing concurrent biochemotherapy with cisplatin, vinblastine, and DTIC alone in patients with metastatic melanoma. Cancer J Sci Am 6 [Suppl 1]:S15–20

Fletcher WS, Daniels DS, Sondak VK (1993) Evaluation of cisplatin and DTIC in inoperable stage III and IV melanoma. A Southwest Oncology Group study. Am J Clin Oncol 16:359–362

Gropp M, Meier W, Hepp H (1998) Treosulfan as an effective second-line therapy in ovarian cancer. Gynecol Oncol 71:94–98

Guven K, Kittler H, Wolff K, Pehamberger H (2001) Cisplatin and carboplatin combination as second-line chemotherapy in dacarbazine-resistant melanoma patients. Melanoma Res 11:411–415

Hartley JA, O'Hare CC, Baumgart J (1999) DNA alkylation and interstrand cross-linking by treosulfan. Br J Cancer 79:264–266

Hilger RA, Jacek G, Oberhoff C, Kredtke S, Baumgart J, Seeber S, Scheulen ME (2000) Investigation of bioavailability and pharmacokinetics of treosulfan capsules in patients with relapsed ovarian cancer. Cancer Chemother Pharmacol 45:483–488

Hoffmann R, Müller I, Neuber K, Lassmann S, Probst M, Oevermann K, Franzke A, Kirchner H, Ganser A, Atzpodien J (1998) Risk and outcome in metastatic malignant melanoma patients receiving DTIC, cisplatin, BCNU, and tamoxifen followed by immunotherapy with interleukin-2 and interferon alpha-2a. Br J Cancer 78:1076–1080

Hunter EM, Sutherland LA, Cree IA, Dewar JA, Preece PE, Wood RAB, Linder D, Andreotti PE (1993) Heterogeneity of chemosensitivity in human breast carcinoma: use of an adenosine triphosphate (ATP) chemiluminescence assay. Eur J Surg Oncol 19:242–249

Johnston SRD, Constenia DO, Moore J, Atkinson H, A'Hern RP, Dadian G, Riches PG, Gore ME (1998) Randomized phase II trial of BCDT [carmustine (BCNU), cisplatin, dacarbazine (DTIC) and tamoxifen] with or without interferon alpha (IFN-α) and interleukin (IL-2) in patients with metastatic melanoma. Br J Cancer 77:1280–1286

Köpf-Maier P, Sass G (1992) Antitumor activity of treosulfan against human breast carcinomas. Cancer Chemother Pharmacol 31:103–110

Köpf-Maier P, Sass G (1996) Antitumor activity of treosulfan in human lung carcinomas. Cancer Chemother Pharmacol 37:211–221

Kurbacher CM, Bruckner HW, Andreotti PE, Kurbacher JA, Saß G, Krebs D (1995) In vitro activity of titanocenedichloride versus cisplatin in four ovarian carcinoma cell lines evaluated by a microtiter plate ATP bioluminescence assay. Anti-Cancer Drugs 6:697–704

Kurbacher CM, Mallmann P, Kurbacher JA, Hübner H, Krebs D (1996) Chemosensitivity testing in gynaecological oncology: experiences with an ATP-bioluminescence assay. Geburtsh Frauenheilk 56:70–78

Lee SM, Betticher DC, Thatcher N (1995) Melanoma: chemotherapy. Br Med Bull 51:609–630

Legha SS, Ring S, Papadopoulos N, Plager C, Chawla S, Benjamin R (1989) A prospective evaluation of a triple-drug regimen containing cisplatin, vinblastine, and dacarbazine (CVD) for metastatic melanoma. Cancer 64:2024–2029

Legha SS, Ring S, Eton O, Bedikian A, Plager C, Papadopoulos N (1997) Development and results of biochemotherapy in metastatic melanoma: The University of Texas M.D. Anderson Cancer Center experience. Cancer J Sci Am 3 [Suppl 1]:S9–S15

Legha SS, Ring S, Eton O, Bedikian A, Buzaid AC, Plager C, Papadopoulos N (1998) Development of a biochemotherapy regimen with concurrent administration of cisplatin, vinblastine, dacarbazine, interferon alpha, and interleukin-2 for patients with metastatic melanoma. J Clin Oncol 16:1752–1759

Luikart SD, Kennealey GT, Kirkwood JM (1984) Randomized phase III trial of vinblastine, bleomycin, and cis-dichlorodiammine-platinum versus dacarbazine in malignant melanoma. J Clin Oncol 2:164–168

Margolin KA, Liu PY, Flaherty LE, Sosman JA, Walker MJ, Smith JW 3rd, Fletcher WS, Weiss GR, Unger JM, Sondak VK (1998) Phase II study of carmustine, dacarbazine, cisplatin, and tamoxifen in advanced melanoma: a Southwest Oncology Group study. J Clin Oncol 16:664–669

Masding J, Sarkar TK, White WF, Barley VL, Chawla SL, Boesen E, Rostom AY, Menday AP (1990) Intravenous treosulfan versus intravenous treosulfan plus cisplatinum in advanced ovarian carcinoma. Br J Obstet Gynecol 97:342–351

McClay EF, Mastrangelo MJ, Bellet RE, Berd D (1987) Combination chemotherapy and hormonal therapy in the treatment of malignant melanoma. Cancer Treat Rep 71:465–469

McClay EF, Mastrangelo MJ, Berd D, Bellet RE (1992) Effective combination chemo/hormonal therapy for malignant melanoma: experience with three consecutive trials. Int J Cancer 50:553–556

McClay EF, McClay ME (1996) Systemic chemotherapy for the treatment of metastatic malignant melanoma. Sem Oncol 23:744–753

Merkle E, Ackermann S, Beck EP, Jäger W, Lang N (2000) High-dose versus low-dose cisplatin chemotherapy plus treosulfan in epithelial ovarian carcinoma FIGO II–IV: Results of a prospective randomized trial. Onkologie 23:232–238

Myatt N, Cree IA, Kurbacher CM, Fross AJE, Hungerford JL, Plowman PN (1997) The ex vivo chemosensitivity profile of choroidal melanoma. Anti-Cancer Drugs 8:756–762

Neale MH, Myatt N, Cree IA, Kurbacher CM, Foss AJE, Hungerford JL, Plowman PN (1999) Combination chemotherapy for choroidal melanoma: ex vivo sensitivity to treosulfan with gemcitabine or cytosine arabinoside. Br J Cancer 79:1487–1493

Neuber K, tom Dieck A, Blödorn-Schlicht N, Itschert G, Karnbach C (1999) Treosulfan is an effective alkylating cytostatic for malignant melanoma in vitro and in vivo. Melanoma Res 9:125–132

Porcile G, Musso M, Boccardo F, Rosso R, Santi L (1979) Combination chemotherapy with vinblastine, bleomycin and methotrexate in DTIC-resistant metastatic melanoma. Tumori 30:237–240

Propper DJ, Braybrooke JP, Levitt NC, O'Byrne K, Christodoulos K, Han C, Talbot DC, Ganesan TS, Harris AL (2000) Phase II study of second-line therapy with DTIC, BCNU, cisplatin and tamoxifen (Dartmouth regimen) chemotherapy in patients with malignant melanoma previously treated with dacarbazine. Br J Cancer 82:1759–1763

Rigel DS, Friedman RJ, Kopf AW (1996) The incidence of malignant melanoma in the United States: issues as we approach the 21st century. J Am Acad Dermatol 34:839–847

Rosenberg SA, Yang JC, Schwartzentruber DJ, Hwu P, Marincola FM, Topalian SL, Seipp CA, Einhorn JH, White DE, Steinberg SM (1999) Prospective randomized trial of the treatment of patients with metastatic melanoma using chemotherapy with cisplatin, dacarbazine, and tamoxifen alone or in combination with interleukin-2 and interferon alfa-2b. J Clin Oncol 17:968–975

Stadelmann WK, Rapaport DP, Soong SJ, Reintgen DS, Buzaid AC, Balch CM (1998) Prognostic clinical and pathological features. In: Balch CM, Houghton AN, Sober AJ, Soong SJ (eds) Cutaneous melanoma, 3rd edn. Quality Medical Publishing, St. Louis, pp 11–36

Chemosensitivity Testing and Test-Directed Chemotherapy in Human Pancreatic Cancer

Marko Kornmann, Hans G. Beger, Karl H. Link

M. Kornmann (✉)
Department of General Surgery, University of Ulm, Steinhövelstraße 9, 89075 Ulm, Germany
e-mail: marko.kornmann@medizin.uni-ulm.de

Abstract

Human pancreatic cancer is a devastating disease with poor prognosis. In many cases it is diagnosed at stages in which a complete resection is not possible. However, even after complete resection most tumors recur. Therefore, several chemotherapeutic strategies have been developed, so far, with little impact on the clinical outcome. Because one of the hallmarks of human pancreatic cancer is its general resistance to chemotherapeutic agents, it seems important to develop strategies to individualize chemotherapy and to render cells more sensitive to chemotherapeutic agents. In this summary we describe our methods of in vitro chemosensitivity testing using the human tumor colony-forming assay for pancreatic cancer in comparison with other solid tumors and describe how the in vitro results influence chemotherapy. Furthermore, we point out new developments of mRNA quantitation of chemoresistance target enzymes based on real-time PCR, which may help in the future to individualize chemotherapy of pancreatic cancer. Finally, we present results of studies of cyclin D1 inhibition. Suppression of cyclin D1 by cyclin D1 antisense mRNA expression was associated with growth inhibition and an increase in chemosensitivity to fluoropyrimidines and platinum compounds. Because human pancreatic cancers are relatively chemoresistant and material for chemosensitivity testing with the human tumor colony-forming assay (HTCA) is in most cases difficult to obtain, future investigations should aim at the development of methods requiring only very small samples to analyze markers of chemosensitivity. Our results further suggest that chemotherapy in combination with strategies to increase chemosensitivity may be a reasonable regimen for the treatment of human pancreatic cancer in the future.

Recent Results in Cancer Research, Vol. 161

Introduction

Pancreatic Cancer

Human pancreatic cancer is a devastating disease with poor prognosis (Link et al. 1999b). Because of difficulties in diagnosis, its fast and aggressive growth, and its propensity to metastasize it is frequently diagnosed at an advanced stage, precluding complete operative removal. Because of its resistance to chemotherapeutic agents including fluoropyrimidines and platinum compounds and the lack of other effective systemic therapies, only 1%–5% of patients with ductal adenocarcinoma of the pancreas will be alive 5 years after diagnosis (Link et al. 1999b). Although the reasons for the aggressiveness of this disorder are not known, a number of observations have pointed to the important role of oncogenes, tumor suppressor genes, and growth factors in its pathobiology. Thus many of these cancers harbor K-*ras* oncogene (Bos 1989) and *p53* (Casey et al. 1993) and *DPC4* (Hahn et al. 1996) tumor suppressor gene mutations and frequently overexpress multiple growth factors and their receptors (Korc 1998), which are involved in cell cycle regulation and cell proliferation (Aaronson 1991).

Chemotherapy of Human Pancreatic Cancer

Many drugs have been evaluated in pancreatic cancer with disappointing results. Systemic treatment of advanced pancreatic cancer has been generally carried out with 5-FU alone or in combination with other agents or radiotherapy, with median survival times of approximately 4–12 months (Link et al. 1999b). However, recent studies have demonstrated statistically significant higher response rates, improved symptom control, and prolonged survival with gemcitabine (Carmichael 1997). Despite these improvements, the outcome of systemic treatment in these patients remains extremely poor. In our institution, palliative chemotherapy of pancreatic cancer is also attempted with regional chemotherapy via the celiac arterial axis using mitoxantrone, 5-FU/folinic acid, and cisplatinum as a triple combination (Link et al. 1999b). This protocol has shown favorable local and distant disease control, however, without impact on overall survival (Beger et al. 1999).

In Vitro Chemosensitivity Testing Using a Soft Agar Assay

Human Tumor Colony-Forming Assay

Based on the double-layer soft agar system described by Hamburger and Salmon (Hamburger and Salmon 1977), we established an in vitro procedure of chemosensitivity testing using cultured tumor cell lines and vital tumor cells derived from patients. Patient-derived tumor samples are minced into small pieces immediately after surgical tumor removal and digested to obtain a single-cell suspension. After cell counting, the tumor cells are incubated in the presence of absence of various drugs for certain periods of time. After removal of the drugs cells are seeded onto an agar base layer and fed every 5–7 days. Colony formation is counted after 2–3 weeks, and inhibition of colony formation by each drug for a certain incubation time is determined in relation to untreated controls (Link et al. 1996; Kornmann et al. 2000a; Kornmann et al. 2000b).

We are presently using this assay for two major purposes: first, to estimate the potential efficacy of drugs for regional chemotherapy of gastrointestinal malignancies and, second, to select potential active drugs for regional chemotherapy of various gastrointestinal tumors.

Preclinical Evaluation of Drug Activity for Regional Chemotherapy

In recent years, systemic treatment with agents other than 5-FU, e.g., gemcitabine and oxaliplatin, has demonstrated significant antitumor activity in various gastrointestinal malignancies (Carmichael 1998; Raymond et al. 1998). In comparison to systemic chemotherapy the advantage of regional chemotherapy is the high local drug concentration in association with a lower systemic concentration, resulting in less frequent systemic toxicity (Link et al. 1998). To be eligible for regional administration the drugs must show a clear dose-dependent inhibition of colony formation at a certain incubation time (Link et al. 1998). In Figs. 1 and 2, the dose-response curves of gemcitabine and oxaliplatin, respectively, are shown for MIA PaCa-2 and PMH 2/89 human pancreatic cancer cells. To further find out the optimal infusion time, time-dependent inhibition of colony-formation is also determined as shown in Figs. 1 and 2. In general, the pancreatic cancer cell lines tended to higher chemoresistance than colon cancer cells when comparing the concentration and time products to achieve an inhibition of colony formation (IC_{50}) of at least 50% (Table 1).

After establishing the assay conditions with cultured cell lines, we performed human tumor colony-forming assays (HTCAs) with tumor cells isolated from pancreatic and colorectal liver metastases (Kornmann et al. 2000a,b). Despite the fact that half of the patients with colorectal liver metastases had been pretreated with various chemotherapeutic agents, the concentrations of oxaliplatin and gemcitabine required to achieve an inhibition of colony formation of at least 50% were relatively high for the pancreatic sample (Table 2), supporting the hypothesis that pancreatic cancers are more chemoresistant to platinum compounds and antimetabolites in comparison with other GI cancers. On the basis of theoretical considerations of drug concentrations during hepatic arterial infusion assuming a hepatic arterial blood flow of 250 ml/min (Link et al. 1998), the concentration achievable during the infusion time in a standard patient with 1.9-m^2 body surface area may be determined for clinical

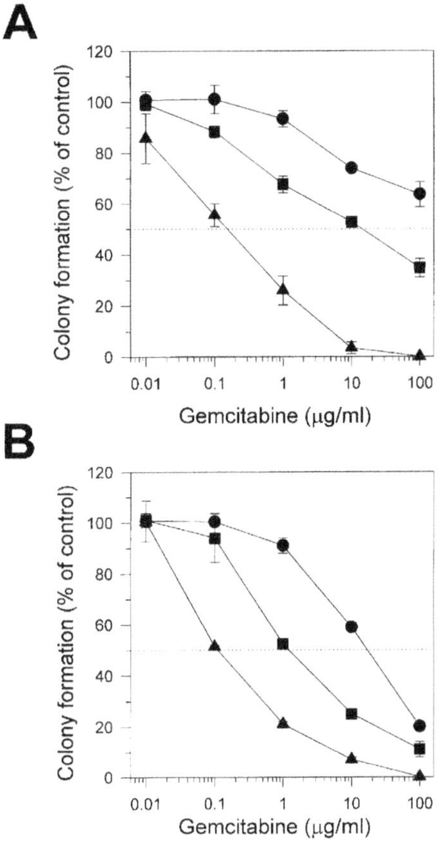

Fig. 1. Antiproliferative effects of gemcitabine in MIA PaCa-2 (**A**) and PMH2/89 (**B**) human pancreatic cancer cells in the human tumor colony-forming assay. Cells were incubated for 2 (●), 4 (■),and 24 h (▲) with increasing concentrations of gemcitabine and then plated in a soft-agar double layer system. Colony formation was evaluated after 2–4 weeks. Results are means (±SD) of triplicate determinations of each test point and are shown as percentage of untreated control. (Adapted from Kornmann et al. 2000a)

protocols. Oxaliplatin may be used at a concentration of 130 mg/m^2 body surface area and an infusion time of 120 min for systemic treatment (Raymond et al. 1998). The in vitro results of oxaliplatin in the cell lines showing lowest

Table 1. IC$_{50}$ values and concentration × time products of gemcitabine and oxaliplatin in relation to exposure time in MIA PaCa-2 and PMH2/89 pancreatic and HT29 and NMG64/84 colon cancer cells

	IC$_{50}$ (μg/ml)/concentration × time products (μg/ml/h)					
	Gemcitabine			Oxaliplatin		
Cell lines	2-h incubation	4-h incubation	24-h incubation	1-h incubation	2-h incubation	24-h incubation
MIA PaCa-2	>100/>200	15/60	0.2/4.8	>100/>100	7.0/14	1.7/41
PMH2/89	18/36	1.2/4.8	0.1/2.4	10/10	6.0/12	0.4/9.6
HT29	100/200	45/180	1.8/43	6.0/6.0	2.5/5.0	0.5/12
NMG64/84	2.5/5.0	0.5/2.0	0.1/2.4	5.0/5.0	1.6/3.2	1.0/24

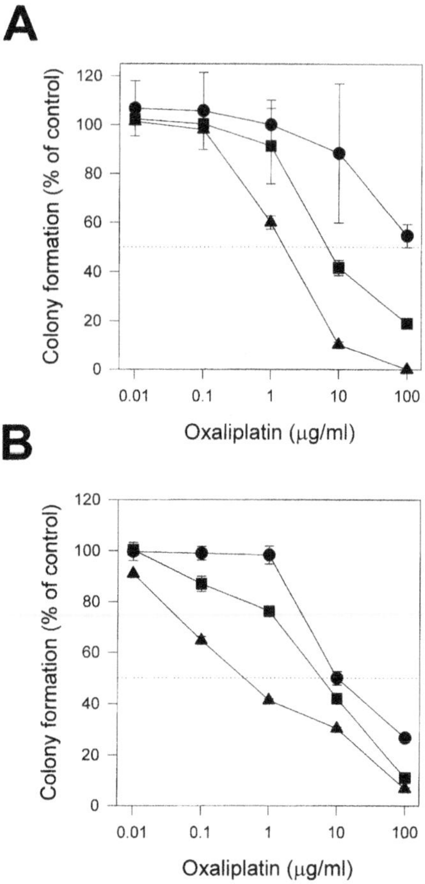

Fig. 2. Antiproliferative effects of oxaliplatin in MIA PaCa-2 (**A**) and PMH2/89 (**B**) human pancreatic cancer cells in the human tumor colony-forming assay (Kornmann et al. 2000b). Cells were incubated for 1 (●), 2 (■), and 24 h (▲)h with increasing concentrations of oxaliplatin. The assay was carried out as described in Fig. 1. Results are means (±SD) of triplicate determinations of each test point and are shown as percentage of untreated control. (Adapted from Kornmann et al. 2000b)

Table 2. IC_{50} values for liver metastases of patients receiving hepatic resection determined by HTCA after a 2-h incubation with gemcitabine or oxaliplatin

	IC_{50} (μg/ml)		
Primary tumor	Gemcitabine	Oxaliplatin	Prior chemotherapy
Rectum	>100	65	Mitoxantrone, 5-FU, cisplatin
Colon	2.5	1.1	No
Colon	22	0.6	No
Colon	100	6.5	5-FU
Pancreas	>100	4.5	No
Colon	70	1.1	No
Colon	>100	1.3	5-FU, irinotecan
Colon	60	0.6	5-FU
Rectum	75	0.2	Mitoxantrone, 5-FU, mitomycin C
Colon	>100	0.8	No

concentration x time products to obtain an inhibition of colony-formation of at least 50% during the 120-min incubation (Fig. 2, Table 1) also support the clinical use of the 120-min infusion time. Assuming the above-mentioned conditions for hepatic arterial infusion, a theoretical oxaliplatin concentration of 8.2 μg/ml may be achieved during the 120-min infusion (130 $mg/m^2 \times 1.9\ m^2$: 120 min : 250 ml/min) (Kornmann et al. 2000b). Under these conditions in 9 of 10 tumors an inhibition of colony-formation of at least 50% (IC_{50}) was achieved, suggesting that oxaliplatin may be also an in vivo active drug for regional chemotherapy of these tumors including pancreatic cancers (Kornmann et al. 2000b).

The IC_{50} values of gemcitabine were below 100 μg/ml for half of the samples (Table 2). However, to achieve this concentration in vivo gemcitabine must be administered as a 120-min hepatic arterial infusion using 1,500 mg/m^2 body surface area, which has been suggested by several authors for systemic treatment. However, currently gemcitabine is mainly delivered as a 30-min infusion using 1,000 mg/m^2 (Carmichael 1998; Pollera 1997; Vermorken et al. 1997; Mani et al. 1998).

Regional Chemotherapy Directed by Individual Chemosensitivity Testing

Among the major intrinsic parameters of response to regional chemotherapy are tumor vascularity (Daly et al. 1985; Rougier et al. 1992) and chemosensitivity. Chemosensitivity testing might improve the response to regional therapy (Kanematsu et al. 1990). In a prospective correlative trial analyzing the results of individual HTCAs there was a highly significant correlation between in vitro drug sensitivity and clinical response (Link et al. 1986). On the basis of these observations we started treatment of patients with evaluable HTCA according to their individual in vitro test results. Thirty-six consecutive patients with isolated liver metastases including carcinoid (3), islet cell (2), and ductal pancreatic (1) cancers received treatment based on the HTCA with regional infusion chemotherapy (Link et al. 1996). In vitro sensitivity of a drug was defined as an inhibition of colony formation of at least 50% and in vitro resistance as inhibition of less than 50%. In this study, patients receiving at least one in vitro sensitive drug showed an intrahepatic progression rate of 7%, whereas patients who only received in vitro resistant drugs had an intrahepatic progression rate of 57% (Link et al. 1996). These results indicated that the HTCA could identify active drugs for individualized hepatic artery infusion chemotherapy and that patients may profit from the use of in vitro sensitive drugs. In a subsequent study, the HTCA results were combined with thymidylate synthase (TS) mRNA quantitation (Link et al. 2000). TS is a key enzyme of DNA synthesis and is irreversibly blocked by 5-FU after its intracellular metabolism (Heidelberger et al. 1983). The analysis of the test combination in 24 consecutive patients including 2 patients with carcinoid liver metastases revealed that 77% (10 of 13) of the sensitive and only 9% (1 of 11) of the resistant patients responded to regional chemotherapy. Patients grouped as in vitro sensitive also displayed a longer median survival (32 months; range: 5–75 months) than in vitro resistant patients (17 months; range: 3–28 months). This study demonstrated for the first time that patients receiving in vitro sensitive tested drugs via regional chemotherapy may benefit from this strategy when HTCA testing and TS mRNA quantitation are combined.

Limitation of Individual Chemosensitivity Testing with the HTCA

Despite the success of this test procedure, one major disadvantage of individual drug testing with the HTCA is the limited growth rate of solid tumors (Flentje and Schlag 1985; Bertelsen et al. 1984; von Hoff 1990). Our own growth rate has been 58% in more than 300 assays with various solid tumors. Another major drawback, especially for human pancreatic cancer, is the limited availability of tumor tissue. Most ductal pancreatic cancers contain, if at all, 5%–10% tumor cells, which are embedded in a fibrotic stroma containing fibroblasts and pancreatic stellate cells (Kornmann et al. 1998b; Bachem et al. 1998). To perform HTCA testing a certain amount of viable tumor cells is required per test drug. Because of the low number of tumor cells per volume of tumor tissue a large sample is required to test five or six different drugs (Link et al. 1996). However, in most cases of advanced pancreatic disease, a diagnostic laparoscopy with a small biopsy is performed to verify diagnosis rather than a major tumor resection to obtain additional material for HTCA testing. Moreover, in contrast to colorectal cancer, only in selected cases is a partial liver resection to remove liver metastases or resection of single peritoneal implanted nodes going to be carried out (Link et al. 1996, 1999b, 2000). Taking into account that tumor tissue is only available in about 50% of all of our patients with advanced malignant diseases (Link et al. 1996), because the scope of surgery should not be substantially expanded to obtain biopsies, evaluable HTCA results presently may be expected in only 20%–30% of all patients. The number of cases yielding tumor tissue of pancreatic cancer is even more limited. Therefore, to expand the potential benefit of HTCA testing, we developed regional chemotherapy protocols for patients without available individual HTCA results based on in vitro concentration-response studies of solid tumors with various agents demonstrating potent activity in certain tumor types (Link et al. 1998). Thus regional treatment of pancreatic cancer via the celiac axis is carried out with mitoxantrone, 5-FU/folinic acid, and cisplatinum (Link et al. 1999b) and of colorectal liver metastases with mitoxantrone, 5-FU, folinic acid, and mitomycin C (Link et al. 1999a).

Chemosensitivity Testing with Molecular Markers of Response

Thymidylate Synthase mRNA Quantitation

Another way to individually assess chemosensitivity may be the determination of pharmacogenetic markers of tumor cells with molecular biological methods (Kleyn and Vesell 1998). Thymidylate synthase (TS) catalyzes the methylation of deoxyuridine monophosphate with 5,10-methylentetrahydrofolate as a cofactor (Santi et al. 1974). This reaction is crucial for DNA synthesis, because it provides the sole intracellular de novo source of thymidylate, and is irreversibly inhibited by 5-FU (Santi et al. 1974; Heidelberger et al. 1983). Overexpression of TS protein or mRNA has been shown to confer resistance to 5-FU and other fluoropyrimidines in several preclinical and clinical studies including colorectal and gastric malignancies (Lenz et al. 1996; Leichman et al. 1997). We have previously shown that TS mRNA expression is a predictor for response and resistance of patients with isolated nonresectable liver metastases of colorectal and other solid tumors receiving fluoropyrimidine-based regional chemotherapy (Kornmann et al. 1997; Link et al. 2000). Only patients with TS mRNA levels below a certain cut-off had a high probability of responding, whereas no patients with a TS mRNA level above the cut-off responded (Fig.3). A similar TS mRNA cut-off value has been reported for systemic 5-FU-based chemotherapy of advanced colorectal and gastric cancers (Lenz et al. 1996; Leichman et al. 1997). As mentioned above, in a subsequent study the TS results were combined with the HTCA (Link et al. 2000). The analysis of the test combination in 24 consecutive patients including 2 patients with carcinoid liver metastases revealed that 77% (10 of 13) of the sensitive and only 9% (1 of 11) of the resistant patients responded to regional chemotherapy. Patients grouped as in vitro sensitive by the test combination displayed a significantly longer survival than in vitro resistant patients (log-rank test: $P<0.05$). This study demonstrated for the first time that patients receiving in vitro sensitive tested drugs via regional chemotherapy and having low TS levels may benefit from this strategy (Fig. 4).

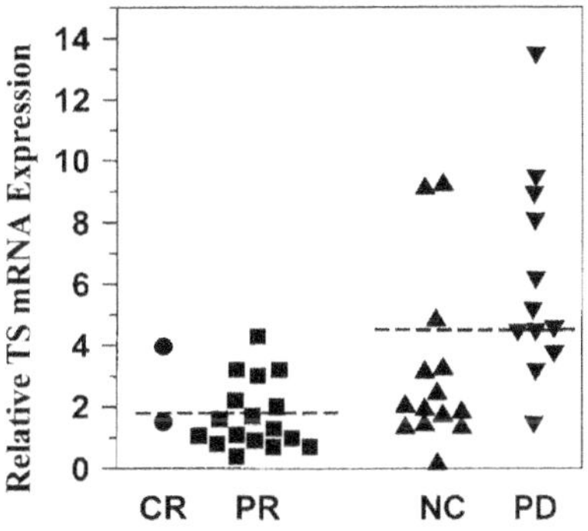

Fig. 3. Association of response to 5-FU-based hepatic arterial infusion chemotherapy and intratumoral thymidylate synthase (TS) mRNA levels in 45 patients with isolated liver metastasis from colorectal (35), carcinoid (2), stomach (2), renal cell (1), c-cell (1), unknown primary (1) carcinoma, and cholangio (2) and hepatocellular (1) carcinoma. The dotted lines show the median TS levels of the 19 responders (1.8×10^{-3}, range: 0.4–4.3×10^{-3}) and 26 nonresponders (4.5×10^{-3}, range: 0.1–13.5×10^{-3}). P=0.0011

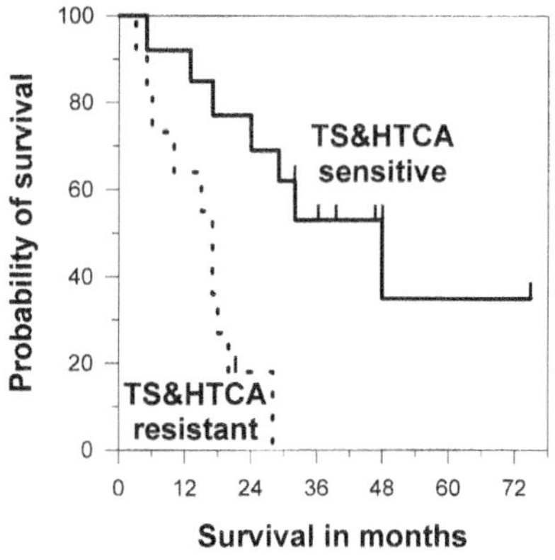

Fig. 4. Association of survival of patients with isolated liver tumors of solid tumors receiving 5-FU-based hepatic arterial infusion chemotherapy with HTCA testing and TS mRNA quantitation (Link et al. 2000). TS and HTCA sensitive patients (n=13, solid line) and TS and HTCA resistant patients (n=11, dotted line). Log-rank test: $P<0.05$

Strategies of mRNA Quantitation in Pancreatic Cancer

However, presently it is not known whether TS mRNA levels also predict for fluoropyrimidine sensitivity in human pancreatic cancer. The reasons for this may be the low percentage of tumor cells in pancreatic cancer specimens. Performing TS mRNA quantitation from pancreatic cancer samples may result in mainly low values because of the low content of tumor cells in the specimens. As mentioned above, most ductal pancreatic cancers contain only 5% tumor cells and are surrounded by a large fibrotic stroma containing fibroblasts and pancreatic stellate cells. Moreover, in the noncancerous pancreas adjacent to pancreatic cancer areas often chronic pancreatitis-like alterations are found (Kornmann et al. 1998a). Altogether this may result in the determination of low TS levels although the cancer cells express high TS levels.

Therefore, new strategies to determine the TS expression of pancreatic cancer cells must be developed. One way to avoid this problem is the determination of TS protein expression with immunohistochemical staining. However, the quantitative comparison with immunohistochemistry is not very subtle (low vs. high staining intensity) and is dependent on the investigator. Another way to quantitatively analyze TS expression is the determination of the relative TS mRNA expression using β-actin as denominator (Horikoshi et al. 1992). Recently, this method has been established with real-time RT-PCR (Kornmann et al. 1999a), a very sensitive PCR method for analysis of small samples (Lockey et al. 1998). In the future, this procedure, in combination with microdissection (Specht et al. 2001), may allow us to accurately determine TS mRNA expression in small pancreatic cancer samples, e.g., biopsy specimens.

Quantitation of Other Possible Target Genes Conferring Chemosensitivity

Another advantage of this PCR procedure is the establishment of a cDNA library of each tumor. Thus, in parallel to TS mRNA quantification, other possible target genes involved in chemosensitivity of various drugs may be investigated. For example, dihydropyrimidine dehydrogenase (DPD) is the key enzyme of fluoropyrimidine inactivation and has been associated with 5-FU resistance (Allegra 1999; Diasio 1999). An enzyme that is responsible for DNA repair, ERCC-1, has been shown to correlate with cisplatinum resistance (Metzger et al. 1998). Using this strategy of characterizing the individual gene expression pattern may help in the future to select potentially active agents for each patient.

Inhibition of Cyclin D1 mRNA Expression

Cyclins are regulatory subunits of a protein kinase family that are involved in cell cycle regulation (Pines 1994). Cyclin D1 controls the G_1 phase, an essential period in which cell differentiation and proliferation are initiated (Pardee 1989; Sherr 1994). Elevated cyclin D1 mRNA levels shorten the G_1 phase and reduce dependence on exogenous mitogens (Jiang et al. 1993; Quelle et al. 1993; Resnitzky et al. 1994). The inhibition of cyclin D1 function by antibody microinjection or suppression of its expression by transfection with a cyclin D1 antisense expression construct (CD1AS) attenuated the growth of colon, esophageal, lung, and pancreatic cancer cells (Zhou et al. 1995; Arber et al. 1997; Schrump et al. 1996; Kornmann et al. 1998a). Elevated cyclin D1 mRNA levels are also associated with decreased survival of patients with cancers of the breast, esophagus, colon, and pancreas (McIntosh et al. 1995; Naitoh et al. 1995; Maeda et al. 1998; Kornmann et al. 1998c).

Decreasing the cyclin D1 mRNA and protein level by expression of the human full-length cyclin D1 antisense cDNA (Zhou et al. 1995) in a stable manner in the human pancreatic cancer cell lines ASPC-1 and COLO-357 resulted in significant in vitro and in vivo growth inhibition (Kornmann et al. 1998a). In parallel to this growth inhibition with accumulation of the cells in the G_0/G_1 phase (Kornmann et al. 1999b), the reduction of cyclin D1 was associated with an increase of chemosensitivity (Kornmann et al. 1998a, 1999a). First, the inhibitory effects of the platinum compounds cisplatinum (Kornmann et al. 1998a) and carboplatinum (Fig. 5) on cell proliferation were markedly enhanced in the antisense-expressing clones. However, the increase in platinum sensitivity was not accompanied by alterations of ERCC-1 (unpublished observation).

The sensitivity of antisense-expressing clones to the fluoropyrimidines 5-FU and 5-FUdR was also significantly enhanced (Kornmann et al. 1999a). In contrast to the platinum compounds, the increased fluoropyrimidine sensitivity was associated with alterations of specific resistance genes (Kornmann et al. 1999a). Thus the TS mRNA levels in cyclin D1 antisense-expressing clones was decreased up to twofold compared with sham-transfected and wild-type cells (Fig. 6).

Cyclin D1 suppression also enhanced the cytotoxic effects of mitoxantrone, an anthracenedione derivative related to the anthracycline antibiotics that inhibit DNA topoisomerase II (Harris and Hochhauser 1992; Thomas and

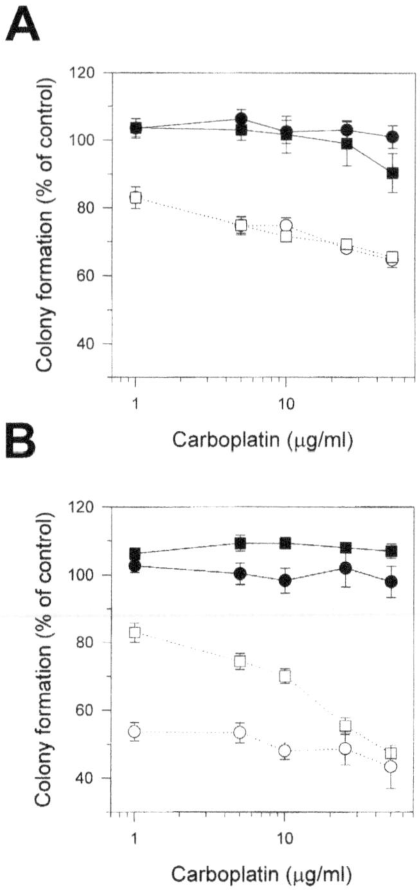

Fig. 5. Antiproliferative effects of carboplatin in PANC-1 (**A**) and COLO-357 (**B**) human pancreatic cancer cells with the MTT assay. Wild-type (●) and sham-transfected (■)cells and corresponding cyclin D1 antisense-transfected cell clones (○, □). Cells were seeded in 96-well plates and incubated for 1 h in the absence or presence of increasing concentrations of carboplatinum. Growth was determined after 48 h by the MTT assay. Results are expressed as growth in % of control and are means (±SE) of quadruplicate determinations of at least three separate experiments

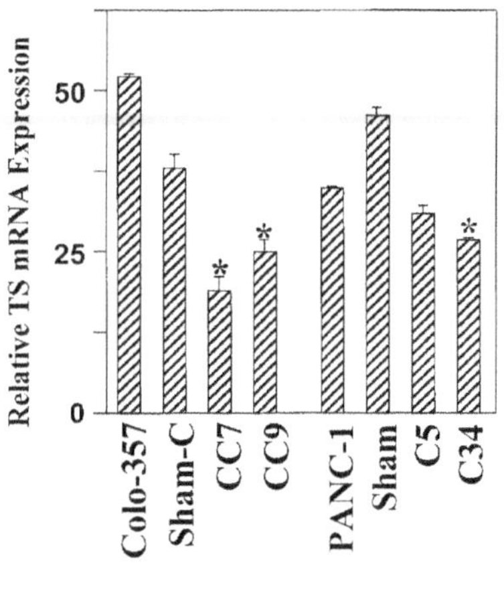

Fig. 6. Quantitation of relative TS mRNA expression with real-time fluorescence PCR in COLO-357 and PANC-1 cells and corresponding sham- and cyclin D1 antisense-transfected clones. Results are means (±SD) from at least three separate determinations. *P<0.05

Archimbaud 1997). Multidrug selection experiments have demonstrated that resistance to mitoxantrone can be associated with MDR1 and/or MRP overexpression (Zhou et al. 1996; Schurr et al. 1989; Schneider et al. 1994). The expression of both transporter genes MDR1 and MRP, which encode for transmembrane drug-transporting efflux pumps, was found to be decreased after cyclin D1 suppression (Kornmann et al. 1999a). More recent findings show that multiple mechanisms may confer drug resistance to mitoxantrone including the expression level of topoisomerase II and other ATP efflux pumps (Hazlehurst et al. 1999).

These findings demonstrate that inhibition of cyclin D1, in addition to suppressing the growth of pancreatic cancer cells, enhances their responsiveness to several chemotherapeutic agents including fluoropyrimidines and platinum compounds.

Concluding Remarks

The present review has summarized in the main part the data on chemosensitivity testing of human pancreatic cancer generated in collaboration with our institution. The data presented here demonstrate that patients can profit from chemosensitivity testing followed by test-directed individual therapy. Therefore, as shown for gemcitabine and oxaliplatin with the human tumor colony-forming assay, it seems important to mimic conditions and drug concentrations in vitro that are also achievable in vivo. Because the in vitro tests using vital tumor cells depend on the availability of large amounts of tissue and are not evaluable in all cases, the molecular analysis of resistance genes, e.g., thymidylate synthase mRNA quantitation, should also become established in human pancreatic cancer. The analysis based on a real-time RT-PCR procedure is very sensitive, allowing the use of tiny samples in contrast to HTCA testing. Recently, a commercially available kit for TS mRNA quantitation using a real-time PCR procedure has become available and may also be used with RNA extracted from paraffin-embedded microdissected tissue specimens.

The data presented here also point out the high chemoresistance of human pancreatic cancer cells to antimetabolites and platinum compounds in comparison with other gastrointestinal malignancies. Therefore, it seems especially important in human pancreatic cancer, besides the individual selection of active drugs, to increase the general chemosensitivity of pancreatic cancer cells. Although the exact molecular mechanisms by which the suppression of cyclin D1 leads to alterations in the expression levels of multiple drug resistance genes are not known, the presented findings suggest that future therapeutic strategies aimed at cyclin D1 inhibition may have the dual advantage of suppressing pancreatic cancer growth and enhancing chemosensitivity.

Acknowledgements. We thank Prof. P.V. Danenberg and K.D. Danenberg from the University of Southern California School of Medicine, Los Angeles, California for their collaboration regarding TS mRNA quantitation and Prof. M. Korc from the University of California, Irvine, California for his collaboration regarding cyclin D1 antisense expression.

References

Aaronson SA (1991) Growth factors and cancer. Science 254:1146–1153
Allegra CJ (1999) Dihydropyrimidine dehydrogenase activity: prognostic partner of 5-fluorouracil? Clin Cancer Res 5:1947–1949
Arber N, Doki Y, Han EK, Sgambato A, Zhou P, Kim NH, Delohery T, Klein MG, Holt PR, Weinstein IB (1997) Antisense to cyclin D1 inhibits the growth and tumorigenicity of human colon cancer cells. Cancer Res 57:1569–1574
Bachem MG, Schneider E, Gross H, Weidenbach H, Schmid RM, Menke A, Siech M, Beger H, Grunert A, Adler G (1998) Identification, culture, and characterization of pancreatic stellate cells in rats and humans. Gastroenterology 115:421–432
Beger HG, Gansauge F, Buchler MW, Link KH (1999) Intraarterial adjuvant chemotherapy after pancreaticoduodenectomy for pancreatic cancer: significant reduction in occurrence of liver metastasis. World J Surg 23:946–949
Bertelsen CA, Sondak VK, Mann BD, Korn EL, Kern DH (1984) Chemosensitivity testing of human solid tumors. A review of 1582 assays with 258 clinical correlations. Cancer 53:1240–1245
Bos JL (1989) ras oncogenes in human cancer: a review. Cancer Res 49:4682–4689
Carmichael J (1997) Clinical response benefit in patients with advanced pancreatic cancer. Role of gemcitabine. Digestion 58:503–507
Carmichael J (1998) The role of gemcitabine in the treatment of other tumours. Br J Cancer 78 [Suppl 3]:21–25
Casey G, Yamanaka Y, Friess H, Kobrin MS, Lopez ME, Buchler M, Beger HG, Korc M (1993) p53 mutations are common in pancreatic cancer and are absent in chronic pancreatitis. Cancer Lett 69:151–160
Daly JM, Butler J, Kemeny N, Yeh SD, Ridge JA, Botet J, Bading JR, DeCosse JJ, Benua RS (1985) Predicting tumor response in patients with colorectal hepatic metastases. Ann Surg 202:384–393
Diasio RB (1999) Clinical implications of dihydropyrimidine dehydrogenase inhibition. Oncology (Huntingt) 13 [7 Suppl 3]:17–21
Flentje D, Schlag P (1985) Is chemosensitivity testing for peri-operative treatment planning in gastro-intestinal cancer by the human tumour colony assay worthwhile? Eur J Surg Oncol 11:227–233
Hahn SA, Schutte M, Hoque AT, Moskaluk CA, da Costa LT, Rozenblum E, Weinstein CL, Fischer A, Yeo CJ, Hruban RH, Kern SE (1996) DPC4, a candidate tumor suppressor gene at human chromosome 18q21.1. Science 271:350–353
Hamburger AW, Salmon SE (1977) Primary bioassay of human tumor stem cells. Science 197:461–463
Harris AL, Hochhauser D (1992) Mechanisms of multidrug resistance in cancer treatment. Acta Oncol 31:205–213
Hazlehurst LA, Foley NE, Gleason-Guzman MC, Hacker MP, Cress AE, Greenberger LW, De Jong MC, Dalton WS (1999) Multiple mechanisms confer drug resistance to mitoxantrone in the human 8226 myeloma cell line. Cancer Res 59:1021–1028
Heidelberger C, Danenberg PV, Moran RG (1983) Fluorinated pyrimidines and their nucleosides. Adv Enzymol Relat Areas Mol Biol 54:58–119
Horikoshi T, Danenberg KD, Stadlbauer TH, Volkenandt M, Shea LC, Aigner K, Gustavsson B, Leichman L, Frosing R, Ray M, Danenberg PV (1992) Quantitation of thymidylate synthase, dihydrofolate reductase, and DT-diaphorase gene expression in human tumors using the polymerase chain reaction. Cancer Res 52:108–116
Jiang W, Kahn SM, Zhou P, Zhang YJ, Cacace AM, Infante AS, Doi S, Santella RM, Weinstein IB (1993) Overexpression of cyclin D1 in rat fibroblasts causes abnormalities in growth control, cell cycle progression and gene expression. Oncogene 8:3447–3457
Kanematsu T, Higashi H, Takenaka K, Matsumata T, Maehara Y, Sugimachi K (1990) Bioenergy status of human liver during and after warm ischemia. Hepatogastroenterology 37 [Suppl 2]:160–162

Kleyn PW, Vesell ES (1998) Genetic variation as a guide to drug development. Science 281:1820–1821

Korc M (1998) Role of growth factors in pancreatic cancer. Surg Oncol Clin N Am 7:25–41

Kornmann M, Arber N, Korc M (1998a) Inhibition of basal and mitogen-stimulated pancreatic cancer cell growth by cyclin D1 antisense is associated with loss of tumorigenicity and potentiation of cytotoxicity to cisplatinum. J Clin Invest 101:344–352

Kornmann M, Beger HG, Korc M (1998b) Role of fibroblast growth factors and their receptors in pancreatic cancer and chronic pancreatitis. Pancreas 17:169–175

Kornmann M, Butzer U, Blatter J, Beger HG, Link KH (2000a) Pre-clinical evaluation of the activity of gemcitabine as a basis for regional chemotherapy of pancreatic and colorectal cancer. Eur J Surg Oncol 26:583–587

Kornmann M, Danenberg KD, Arber N, Beger HG, Danenberg PV, Korc M (1999a) Inhibition of cyclin D1 expression in human pancreatic cancer cells is associated with increased chemosensitivity and decreased expression of multiple chemoresistance genes. Cancer Res 59:3505–3511

Kornmann M, Fakler H, Butzer U, Beger HG, Link KH (2000b) Oxaliplatin exerts potent in vitro cytotoxicity in colorectal and pancreatic cancer cell lines and liver metastases. Anticancer Res 20:3259–3264

Kornmann M, Ishiwata T, Itakura J, Tangvoranuntakul P, Beger HG, Korc M (1998c) Increased cyclin D1 in human pancreatic cancer is associated with decreased postoperative survival. Oncology 55:363–369

Kornmann M, Link KH, Lenz HJ, Pillasch J, Metzger R, Butzer U, Leder GH, Weindel M, Safi F, Danenberg KD, Beger HG, Danenberg PV (1997) Thymidylate synthase is a predictor for response and resistance in hepatic artery infusion chemotherapy. Cancer Lett 118:29–35

Kornmann M, Tangvoranuntakul P, Korc M (1999b) TGF-beta-1 up-regulates cyclin D1 expression in COLO-357 cells, whereas suppression of cyclin D1 levels is associated with down-regulation of the type I TGF-beta receptor. Int J Cancer 83:247–254

Leichman CG, Lenz HJ, Leichman L, Danenberg K, Baranda J, Groshen S, Boswell W, Metzger R, Tan M, Danenberg PV (1997) Quantitation of intratumoral thymidylate synthase expression predicts for disseminated colorectal cancer response and resistance to protracted-infusion fluorouracil and weekly leucovorin. J Clin Oncol 15:3223–3229

Lenz HJ, Leichman CG, Danenberg KD, Danenberg PV, Groshen S, Cohen H, Laine L, Crookes P, Silberman H, Baranda J, Garcia Y, Li J, Leichman L (1996) Thymidylate synthase mRNA level in adenocarcinoma of the stomach: a predictor for primary tumor response and overall survival. J Clin Oncol 14:176–182

Link KH, Aigner KR, Kuehn W, Schwemmle K, Kern DH (1986) Prospective correlative chemosensitivity testing in high-dose intraarterial chemotherapy for liver metastases. Cancer Res 46:4837–4840

Link KH, Kornmann M, Butzer U, Leder G, Sunelaitis E, Pillasch J, Salonga D, Danenberg KD, Danenberg PV, Beger HG (2000) Thymidylate synthase quantitation and in vitro chemosensitivity testing predicts responses and survival of patients with isolated nonresectable liver tumors receiving hepatic arterial infusion chemotherapy. Cancer 89:288–296

Link KH, Kornmann M, Formentini A, Leder G, Sunelaitis E, Schatz M, Pressmar J, Beger HG (1999a) Regional chemotherapy of non-resectable liver metastases from colorectal cancer – literature and institutional review. Langenbecks Arch Surg 1999 384:344–353

Link KH, Leder G, Formentini A, Fortnagel G, Kornmann M, Schatz M, Beger HG (1999b) Surgery and multimodal treatments in pancreatic cancer – a review on the basis of future multimodal treatment concepts. Gan To Kagaku Ryoho 26:10–40

Link KH, Kornmann M, Leder GH, Butzer U, Pillasch J, Staib L, Gansauge F, Beger HG (1996) Regional chemotherapy directed by individual chemosensitivity testing in vitro: a prospective decision-aiding trial. Clin Cancer Res 2:1469–1474

Link KH, Leder G, Pillasch J, Butzer U, Staib L, Kornmann M, Bruckner U, Beger HG (1998) In vitro concentration response studies and in vitro phase II tests as the experimental basis for regional chemotherapeutic protocols. Semin Surg Oncol 14:189–201

Lockey C, Otto E, Long Z (1998) Real-time fluorescence detection of a single DNA molecule. Biotechniques 24:744–746

Maeda K, Chung Y, Kang S, Ogawa M, Onoda N, Nishiguchi Y, Ikehara T, Nakata B, Okuno M, Sowa M (1998) Cyclin D1 overexpression and prognosis in colorectal adenocarcinoma. Oncology 55:145–151

Mani S, Kugler JW, Knost JA, Sciortino DF, Gibbons J, Garcia JC, Ansari RH, Schilsky RL, Vokes EE (1998–99) Phase II trial of 150-minute weekly infusion of gemcitabine in advanced colorectal cancer: minimal activity in colorectal cancer. Invest New Drugs 16:275–278

McIntosh GG, Anderson JJ, Milton I, Steward M, Parr AH, Thomas MD, Henry JA, Angus B, Lennard TW, Horne CH (1995) Determination of the prognostic value of cyclin D1 overexpression in breast cancer. Oncogene 11:885–891

Metzger R, Leichman CG, Danenberg KD, Danenberg PV, Lenz HJ, Hayashi K, Groshen S, Salonga D, Cohen H, Laine L, Crookes P, Silberman H, Baranda J, Konda B, Leichman L (1998) ERCC1 mRNA levels complement thymidylate synthase mRNA levels in predicting response and survival for gastric cancer patients receiving combination cisplatin and fluorouracil chemotherapy. J Clin Oncol 16:309–316

Naitoh H, Shibata J, Kawaguchi A, Kodama M, Hattori T (1995) Overexpression and localization of cyclin D1 mRNA and antigen in esophageal cancer. Am J Pathol 146:1161–1169

Pardee AB (1989) G_1 events and regulation of cell proliferation. Science 246:603–608

Pines J (1994) Protein kinases and cell cycle control. Semin Cell Biol 5:399–408

Pollera CF (1997) More is better but.. how is best: are milligrams over hours better than grams over minutes? The case of gemcitabine. J Clin Oncol 15:2172–2174

Quelle DE, Ashmun RA, Shurtleff SA, Kato JY, Bar-Sagi D, Roussel MF, Sherr CJ (1993) Overexpression of mouse D-type cyclins accelerates G_1 phase in rodent fibroblasts. Genes Dev 7:1559–1571

Raymond E, Chaney SG, Taamma A, Cvitkovic E (1998) Oxaliplatin: a review of preclinical and clinical studies. Ann Oncol 9:1053–1071

Resnitzky D, Gossen M, Bujard H, Reed SI (1994) Acceleration of the G_1/S phase transition by expression of cyclins D1 and E with an inducible system. Mol Cell Biol 14:1669–1679

Rougier P, Laplanche A, Huguier M, Hay JM, Ollivier JM, Escat J, Salmon R, Julien M, Roullet Audy JC, Gallot D, et al (1992) Hepatic arterial infusion of floxuridine in patients with liver metastases from colorectal carcinoma: long-term results of a prospective randomized trial. J Clin Oncol 10:1112-1119

Santi DV, McHenry CS, Sommer H (1974) Mechanism of interaction of thymidylate synthetase with 5-fluorodeoxyuridylate. Biochemistry 13:471–481

Schneider E, Horton JK, Yang CH, Nakagawa M, Cowan KH (1994) Multidrug resistance-associated protein gene overexpression and reduced drug sensitivity of topoisomerase II in a human breast carcinoma MCF7 cell line selected for etoposide resistance. Cancer Res 54:152–158

Schrump DS, Chen A, Consoli U (1996) Inhibition of lung cancer proliferation by antisense cyclin D. Cancer Gene Ther 3:131–135

Schurr E, Raymond M, Bell JC, Gros P (1989) Characterization of the multidrug resistance protein expressed in cell clones stably transfected with the mouse mdr1 cDNA. Cancer Res 49:2729–2733

Sherr CJ (1994) G_1 phase progression: cycling on cue. Cell 79:551–555

Specht K, Richter T, Muller U, Walch A, Werner M, Hofler H (2001) Quantitative gene expression analysis in microdissected archival formalin-fixed and paraffin-embedded tumor tissue. Am J Pathol 158:419–429

Thomas X, Archimbaud E (1997) Mitoxantrone in the treatment of acute myelogenous leukemia: a review. Hematol Cell Ther 39:63–74

Vermorken JB, Guastalla JP, Hatty SR, Seitz DE, Tanis B, McDaniels C, Clavel MD (1997) Phase I study of gemcitabine using a once every 2 weeks schedule. Br J Cancer 76:1489–1493

Von Hoff DD (1990) He's not going to talk about in vitro predictive assays again, is he? J Natl Cancer Inst 82:96–101

Zhou DC, Ramond S, Viguie F, Faussat AM, Zittoun R, Marie JP (1996) Sequential emergence of MRP- and MDR1-gene over-expression as well as MDR1-gene translocation in homoharringtonine-selected K562 human leukemia cell lines. Int J Cancer 65:365–371

Zhou P, Jiang W, Zhang YJ, Kahn SM, Schieren I, Santella RM, Weinstein IB (1995) Antisense to cyclin D1 inhibits growth and reverses the transformed phenotype of human esophageal cancer cells. Oncogene 11:571–580

Clinical Significance of Cellular Drug Resistance in Childhood Leukemia

G.J.L. Kaspers, A.J.P. Veerman

G.J.L. Kaspers (✉)
Department of Pediatric Hematology/Oncology, VU University Medical Center, De Boelelaan 1117, 1081 Amsterdam, The Netherlands
e-mail: gjl.kaspers@vumc.nl

Abstract

Cellular drug resistance is an important determinant of the response to chemotherapy, and its precise measurement may have clinical relevance. Potential applications are: prognostic factor for risk-group stratification, tailored chemotherapy for subgroups or individual patients with a specific cellular drug resistance profile, determination of cross-resistance patterns, study of drug interactions, study of resistance modulation or circumvention, selection of patients for phase II studies and screening for the cytotoxicity of novel compounds. The colorimetric 4-day MTT assay is a frequently used method. However, a distinction between malignant and non-malignant cells cannot be made, which should be taken into account. In the case of a relatively high percentage of contaminating non-malignant cells, the differential staining cytotoxicity (DiSC) assay can be used. The MTT assay's technical success percentage is about 80% for fresh ALL and AML samples. For methotrexate (MTX) a different assay must be used, such as the thymidylate synthase inhibition assay (TSIA). The MTT assay measures the number of living cells that survived drug exposure. Therefore, the effect of many if not most drugs to induce leukemia cell death by apoptosis is also included. This review mainly summarizes the data on cellular drug resistance in childhood leukemia, as obtained by the MTT assay and TSIA, in our laboratory in Amsterdam. These data clearly demonstrate the significant relation between in vitro cellular drug resistance and clinical and cell biological features and short- and long-term clinical outcome in childhood leukemia. In conclusion, cellular drug resistance testing provides clinically relevant information that can be available within 1 week and can be performed successfully in the vast majority of leukemia samples. The data are more and more being used and being considered for use in clinical trials in leukemia.

Recent Results in Cancer Research, Vol. 161

Introduction

Childhood leukemia is one of the most convincing examples that chemotherapy may cure a malignancy. With contemporary protocols, the survival for acute lymphoblastic leukemia (ALL) is up to 80% (Pui and Evans 2000), and for acute myeloid leukemia up to 60% (Creutzig et al. 2001; Stevens et al. 1998). However, treatment failures do occur. In addition to toxic deaths and secondary malignancies, unsuccessful chemotherapy essentially has three causes: pharmacokinetic resistance, cellular drug resistance and regrowth resistance. Pharmacokinetics determine the extent of exposure of the leukemic cells to the drugs, which has been demonstrated to be of clinical significance in childhood ALL (Evans et al. 1998). Regrowth resistance reflects the relapse potential of minimal residual leukemic cells (Preisler and Gopal 1994). These cells have escaped the cytostatic drugs but have also survived in their microenvironment and apparently were not killed by the autoimmune defence system. Cellular drug resistance is another important factor and can be primary (intrinsic, de novo) or acquired. Although the higher response rates in newly diagnosed leukemia than in relapsed disease suggest that drug resistance can be acquired, it is also possible that there is a selection of an intrinsically more drug-resistant subclone which was already present at initial diagnosis. Acquired or secondary drug resistance may be the result of spontaneously occurring cellular changes or may be induced by drug exposure. The latter is frequently used to cause drug resistance in leukemia cell lines in vitro, but it is questionable whether such cell lines and the mechanisms of resistance that have been introduced properly reflect the clinical situation. Therefore, we focus on the use of patient material in our preclinical, translational research program. The first important goal in the research on drug resistance is to find a method that can accurately and reliably determine the extent of drug resistance of malignant cells. In addition, mechanisms of resistance and studies on the modulation and circumvention of drug resistance are important. The cellular drug resistance assay that we have adapted and improved and have been using over the past 15 years is the colorimetric short-term methyl-thiazol-tetrazolium (MTT) assay (Kaspers et al. 1991; Pieters et al. 1988, 1990; Veerman and Pieters 1990a). Because we observed no clear dose-dependent methotrexate-induced cytotoxicity in the MTT assay, we adapted and improved the thymidylate synthase inhibition assay (TSIA) (Rots et al. 1999a). In this review, we will summarize the MTT assay results obtained by us, as well as the results obtained with the TSIA, in our laboratory in Amsterdam. Because of limitations to the length of this paper, the work of others is only referred to in a very limited way. The data clearly demonstrate that cellular drug resistance testing provides clinically relevant information, which partly is useful for rational improvements of current clinical treatment protocols and which may also be used as a prognostic factor and for risk-group stratification and subsequent risk-group adapted treatment. There are a number of other potential applications, as summarized in Table 1 and discussed further later on.

Table 1. Possible applications of cellular drug resistance testing (adapted from Kaspers et al.: Cellular drug resistance in acute myeloid leukemia: Literature review and preliminary analysis of an ongoing collaborative study. Klin Pädiatr 1999, 211: 239–244. Georg Thieme Verlag)

Drug screening
Selection of patients for phase II trials
Study of drug interactions
Study of drug resistance modulation and circumvention
Study of cross-resistance patterns
Tailored therapy for subgroups of patients
Prognostic factor for risk-group stratification and risk-group adapted chemotherapy
Tailored therapy for individual patients (curative or palliative)

Cellular Drug Resistance Assays

MTT Assay

The MTT assay is done as described previously (Pieters et al. 1988, 1990; Kaspers et al. 1991). Briefly, mononuclear cells are isolated from bone marrow or peripheral blood by density gradient centrifugation and washed twice. If necessary, contaminating non-malignant cells are removed by using Dynabeads in a negative cell selection process (Kaspers et al. 1994a). A cell suspension is made, using a RPMI-based culture medium with several supplements, of 1–2×10^6 cells/ml. Eighty microliters of the suspension are added to the wells of 96-well microculture plates, already containing 20 µl of different drug solutions in six different concentrations (or 20 µl of RPMI only for the blanks and control wells). All drug experiments are done in duplicate. Four to six wells contain culture medium only to blank the spectrophotometer. Some drugs affect the optical density (OD) of the medium and require a separate blank (e.g., mercaptopurine). Another six to eight wells contain cells in culture medium but no drugs and serve as control wells to calculate the control cell survival. Culture and drug exposure in the plates takes 96 h in our laboratory. Then 10 µl of 5 mg/ml methyl-thiazol-tetrazolium (MTT, Sigma) is added to each well, and after the plates are shaken for 5 min on a plate shaker (1,500 shakes/min) the plates are incubated for another 6 h. The principle of the assay is that only living cells can convert MTT into colored formazan crystals, which must be dissolved with acidified isopropanol. It is our experience that it is better to acidify the isopropanol well in advance, several weeks before using it. A recent modification of the MTT assay is that the OD of each well is now being measured with a microplate spectrophotometer at dual wavelengths (720 nm subtracted from 562 nm), thereby correcting for "noise signals" such as those caused by debris at the bottom of the wells and by scratches on the bottom of the plates. Within a certain range, OD is linearly related to the number of viable cells, and this must be ascertained for each subgroup of leukemias (and other tissue types) separately (Pieters et al. 1988; Kaspers et al. 1991; Klumper et al. 1995a,b). Leukemic cell survival (LCS) is calculated as: (mean OD treated wells-mean OD blanks)/(mean OD control wells-mean OD blanks)×100. The LC_{50} value, i.e., the drug concentration lethal to 50% of the cells, is calculated from the dose-response curve and used as measure for in vitro drug resistance. We have also calculated area under the dose-response curves (AUC) in the past, but it appeared that these values were strongly (Rho>0.90) and highly significantly correlated with the LC_{50} values (data not shown). Because the AUC has the disadvantage that it becomes impossible to change the drug concentration range, and because the value itself is not very perceptible, we prefer LC_{50} values. The MTT assay data are reliable and representative for leukemic cells if the control OD is 0.050 at least, and if the percentage of leukemic cells in the control wells is 70% at least (Pieters et al. 1990; Kaspers et al. 1994a). The use of either bone marrow or peripheral blood is possible, because the sample source itself does not influence the assay results (Kaspers et al. 1991; Klumper et al. 1995a,b). Similarly, fresh or cryopreserved cells can be used because assay results are similar, although the assay success rate is lower if cryopreserved cells are used (Pieters et al. 1989; Klumper et al. 1995b). The only drug that did not result in dose-response curves was methotrexate, probably because of the salvage effect of nucleosides and bases that are present in the culture medium and that are released by dying cells (Rots et al. 1999a). Therefore, MTX resistance is tested by the TSIA (see below).

Thymidylate Synthase Inhibition Assay

The TSIA measures the methotrexate (MTX)- or other drug-mediated inhibition of the TS-catalyzed conversion of [^{3}H]deoxyuridine monophosphate (dUMP) to dTMP and ^3H_2O. It is an indicator of cellular resistance to MTX (and other antifolates), although it is not a total cell kill assay such as the MTT assay (Rots et al. 1999a,b, 2000, 2001). However, with cell lines the data of the MTT assay and TSIA on methotrexate and other antifolates correlated well (Mauritz et al. 1998). Leukemic cells in suspension (135 µl of 1×10^6 cells/ml) are exposed to five different concentrations of MTX (15 µl drug solution) in duplicates for 21-h continuous exposure or for a 3-h short exposure followed by washing and an additional 18-hs drug-free incubation. 5-[^{3}H]-2'-deoxycytidine at a final concentration of 1 µM (2.5 Ci/mmol) is added 4 h after the start of each experiment as a precursor for [^{3}H]dUMP, the substrate for TS. Blanks in triplicate containing 150 µl of culture medium only and control cell suspensions without MTX (15 µl RPMI instead) in duplicate are included. After the 21 h, cells are put on ice and 150 µl of 35% ice-cold trichloroacetic acid is added together with 750 µl of 10% activated charcoal solution. After vortexing, samples are left on ice for 30 min and centrifuged; 450 µl of the aqueous phase, containing ^3H_2O, is transferred to a scintillation vial and counted for radioactivity. After subtraction of the mean blank counts, the data are expressed as the drug concentration needed to inhibit 50% of the control TS activity, assuming a linear dose-response curve between the two flanking concentration points. The $TSI_{50,cont}$ refers to the continuous exposure condition and the $TSI_{50,short}$ to the short-term exposure.

Determination of In Vitro Cross-Resistance Patterns

Because the MTT assay is semi-automated, it is relatively simple to measure the cytotoxicity of 10–20 drugs or even more in a leukemia sample. The major limitation generally is having enough cells to test all drugs. We have determined cross-resistance patterns in several leukemia subgroups for several major types of drugs. Below, cross-resistance patterns among structurally related drugs are described in greater detail. However, in both newly diagnosed (Kaspers et al. 1998) and relapsed ALL (Klumper et al. 1995a) we also observed significant, weak to moderate cross-resistance between non-related drugs. This suggests the involvement of a common pathway that at least partly contributes to cellular drug resistance. Apoptosis and its regulators are the likely possibility, and indeed we recently found that regulators at different levels (mitochondria, caspase inhibitors) are involved in glucocorticoid resistance (Haarman et al. 2001a).

Anthracyclines

With respect to the anthracyclines and the related anthracenedione mitoxantrone, a strong and statistically significant cross-resistance was found to daunorubicin, doxorubicin, idarubicin and mitoxantrone in both newly diagnosed and relapsed ALL. Spearman's correlation coefficients (Rho) were 0.75. Cross-resistance to aclarubicin was slightly less strong, with Rho values of 0.50–0.57. Therefore, except perhaps for aclarubicin, the structurally related drugs did not appear to be useful to circumvent daunorubicin resistance in childhood ALL (Kaspers et al. 1994b; Klumper et al. 1995c).

Glucocorticoids

With respect to glucocorticoids, predniso(lo)ne is historically the most frequently used drug in the treatment of ALL. A randomized clinical study by the CALGB showed that dexamethasone was superior to predniso(lo)ne in preventing central nervous system relapses in childhood ALL (Jones et al. 1991). A non-randomized clinical study by the Dutch Childhood Leukemia Study Group also suggested that dexamethasone was superior to predniso(lo)ne in childhood ALL (Veerman et al. 1990b, 1996). More recent randomized clinical studies support these findings, although dexamethasone also appears to be more toxic (Gaynon et al. 2000; Hurwitz et al. 2000; Mattano et al. 2000). An explanation may be that dexamethasone is more potent than assumed based on anti-inflammatory and thymolytic activities. We previously found that dexamethasone was median 16-fold more potent in vitro than prednisolone (Kaspers et al. 1996). However, in a more recent analysis we (Haarman et al. unpublished) and others (Ito et al. 1996) found a factor of 7, more in agreement with the generally assumed difference. Despite the possibility of increased potency, leukemic cells were strongly cross-resistant to both glucocorticoids (Kaspers et al. 1996, Haarman et al. 2001c). More recently, cortivazol, which is a novel synthetic analogue, has been tested. It has been reported that the glucocorticoid receptor has two binding sites for cortivazol but only one binding site for the conventional glucocorticoids such as prednisolone and dexamethasone. Although cell line studies showed that cortivazol still had antileukemic activity but dexamethasone did not, our in vitro studies on patient ALL samples suggest that cortivazol may circumvent dexamethasone resistance at best in only a small subgroup of patients with ALL and cannot overcome the glucocorticoid resistance in AML (Haarman et al. 2001b, and unpublished data).

Antifolates

Rots et al. reported that several leukemia subgroups were resistant to methotrexate on short-term exposure. This resistance, as determined using the TSIA, could be overcome in T-cell ALL and in AML by prolonging the exposure to 21 h (Rots et al. 1999a, 2001). However, relapsed ALL remained resistant to MTX, also under the continuous exposure condition (Rots et al. 2000). In testing novel antifolates, it appeared that especially trimetrexate, GW1843U89, raltitrexed and ZD9331 were more potent in inhibiting TS activity than methotrexate itself during continuous exposure (Rots et al. 1999b). Moreover, trimetrexate and GW1843U89 could circumvent the methotrexate of relapsed ALL samples in both the short-term and long-term exposure conditions. The rationale for studying novel antifolates clinically against methotrexate is that some can bypass transport deficiency (trimetrexate), do not require polyglutamylation (trimetrexate, ZD9331), have an increased affinity towards folylpolyglutamate synthetase and reduced folate carrier (GW1843U89, raltitrexed) and target other enzymes than dihydrofolate reductase itself (GW1843U89, ZD9331). From our data, GW1832U89 and trimetrexate seem most interesting to explore further in childhood leukemia (Rots et al. 1999b).

Cellular Drug Resistance in Relation to Clinical and Cell Biological Features

ALL Versus AML Samples Obtained at Initial Diagnosis

A preliminary comparison of 125 ALL and 28 AML samples revealed that AML samples were median more than 75-fold more resistant to glucocorticoids (both to prednisolone and dexamethasone), and 2-fold more resistant to vincristine, than AML samples (Kaspers et al. 1994c). For nine other drugs no statistically significantly different results were found, although l-asparaginase also appeared to be less cytotoxic in AML. Of interest, glucocorticoids induced a significantly higher cell survival than was seen in the controls in about one-third of AML but in only 2% of ALL samples. A similar effect was observed for vincristine and vindesine, but less frequently (11% of AML and 4% of ALL samples). A more recent study by Zwaan et al. (2000b) confirmed these results. However, with much larger numbers (536 ALL and 128 AML samples) differences were now also statistically significant for l-asparaginase (median 7-fold increased resistance in AML), anthracyclines (median 2- to 3-fold), etoposide (5-fold), platinum analogues (2- to 3-fold), 4-HOO-ifosfamide (4-fold) and thiotepa (4-fold). Only for cytarabine and thiopurines (mercaptopurine and thioguanine) did ALL and AML appear equally sensitive with enough samples being tested to draw such a conclusion. For other drugs no statistically significant differences were seen either, but numbers were lower and AML samples were median 1.3- to 5-fold more resistant (busulfan, amsacrine, teniposide and vindesine). A recent analysis of our data on 2-chloro-deoxyadenosine revealed that this is the only drug in our panel with statistically significantly increased cytotoxicity towards AML cells compared with ALL, which was mainly due to increased efficacy in AML FAB type M5 samples (Zwaan et al. 2000a). For methotrexate, the TSIA was used. AML samples were median sixfold more resistant (P=0.001) to methotrexate than ALL samples on short-term 3-h exposure, but this resistance was overcome with continuous 21-h exposure (Rots et al. 1999a, 2001).

Newly Diagnosed Versus Relapsed Disease

The largest study concerned ALL samples, and was reported by Klumper et al. (1995a). Compared with samples from 141 children with initial ALL, those from 137 children with relapsed ALL were statistically significantly more resistant to glucocorticoids (median >24-fold), l-asparaginase (2-fold), anthracyclines (2-fold) and thiopurines (1.5-fold). The time of relapse, early versus late, and whether it concerned a first or multiple (second or higher) relapse provided additional information. It appeared that within the relapsed group, both the early and multiple relapsed samples were significantly more resistant to several drugs than the samples of patients with a late relapse. At multiple relapse, resistance to vincristine (median 3-fold) and teniposide (median 2-fold) had developed. For methotrexate, again the TSIA had to be used (Rots et al. 1999a, 2000). Within only common/pre-B ALL, relapsed samples were median threefold more resistant (P=0.01) to methotrexate than untreated samples in both short- and long-term exposure conditions. AML is more rare, and with improved prognosis, relapsed AML is even more rare. A recently initiated collaboration with several groups will increase the number of successfully tested relapsed AML in the future. So far, only limited data are available. Klumper et al. (1995b) reported that relapsed AML samples (n=16) were median threefold more resistant (P=0.05) to cytarabine in vitro than untreated samples (n=29). This is in agreement with data of Hongo et al. (1993), who also found increased resistance to etoposide. More recently, we confirmed these data, although now relapsed AML samples were only twofold more resistant to cytarabine (Zwaan et al. 2000a). Of potential interest, 2-chloro-deoxyadenosine retained its antileukemic activity in vitro against relapsed AML, especially within the FAB type M5 subgroup. These data support the potential clinical value of 2-chloro-deoxyadenosine in AML FAB type M5, as was also demonstrated by clinical studies performed at the St. Jude Children's Research Hospital (Krance et al. 2001).

Age

Several analyses have confirmed that, at least in part, the prognostic significance of age in childhood ALL may be explained by differences in cellular drug resistance, also taking immunophenotype into account. The largest series included 395 children, of whom 310 had common or pre-B ALL (Pieters et al. 1998). Within the latter subgroup, children aged 10 years or older had ALL cells that were significantly more resistant to glucocorticoids, l-asparaginase, mercaptopurine and idarubicin. In general, children below 1.5 years of age also had more drug resistant ALL cells, but this seemed to be associated with the increased incidence of the immature pro-B ALL phenotype. However, numbers were small in the infant subgroup. Independent of immunophenotype, infants had ALL cells that were relatively resistant to glucocorticoids, l-asparaginase and teniposide but more sensitive to cytarabine.

Immunophenotype in ALL

Several consecutive analyses which included increasing numbers of samples consistently showed that immunophenotypes associated with a worse clinical outcome, the very immature pro-B (B-cell precursor, CD10 and cytoplasmic μ negative) and the T-cell (TdT, CD3 and CD7 positive) phenotypes, had specific drug resistance profiles with increased resistance to several drugs, compared with the common ($CD10^+$, cytoplasmic μ^-) and pre-B ($CD10^{+/-}$, cytoplasmic μ^+) ALL samples. More specifically, T-cell ALL samples showed a strong resistance to glucocorticoids, l-asparaginase and vincristine and a mild but statistically significant resistance to all other drugs except thiopurines and teniposide (Pieters et al. 1998). The pro-B ALL samples were statistically significantly more resistant to all drugs except mitoxantrone, idarubicin, vincristine and teniposide. Most pronounced resistance was seen to glucocorticoids (median >38-fold) and l-asparaginase (8-fold). Of potential interest, pro-B ALL samples were median twofold more sensitive to cytarabine, although it was of borderline statistical significance (P=0.055). Increased sensitivity was not seen in T-cell ALL. As mentioned above, increased methotrexate resistance was seen in T-cell ALL compared with common/pre-B ALL with short-term exposure to methotrexate (median 10-fold, P=0.001), but this resistance could be completely overcome by continuous exposure (Rots et al. 1999a). ALL samples with co-expression of myeloid lineage-associated antigens were significantly more resistant to glucocorticoids in an initial study (Kaspers et al. 1994c), but this could not be confirmed in a subsequent larger study (Den Boer et al. 1999).

FAB Type

In ALL, we did not find different drug resistance profiles in FAB type L1 as compared to L2 samples (Kaspers et al. 1995a). Recently, Zwaan et al. (2000b) of our group reported a detailed analysis of the relation between the morphological FAB type and cellular drug resistance in 128 children with AML. FAB type M1 and M2 samples did not differ in cellular drug resistance and were therefore pooled. FAB type M5 was markedly more sensitive in vitro to cytarabine (3-fold), anthracyclines (2- to 3-fold), mitoxantrone (13-fold) and etoposide (9-fold) compared with FAB type M4 samples and significantly more sensitive to cytarabine (3-fold) and etoposide (5-fold) compared with FAB types M1/M2 as well. Moreover, and of potential clinical relevance, FAB type M5 samples were similarly sensitive as ALL cells to l-asparaginase and vincristine. The l-asparaginase sensitivity may be explained by the lack of or at least low activity of asparagine synthetase in AML M5 samples (Dübbers et al. 2000). In addition, Rots et al. (2001) showed that AML cells are equally sensitive to methotrexate as common/pre-B ALL cells if cells are exposed long enough (21 h). This was especially true for the FAB type M5 samples but, interestingly, could not be explained by increased long-chain polyglutamylation of methotrexate.

DNA Ploidy in ALL

In a relatively small study, Kaspers et al. (1995b) reported that common ALL cells with a hyperdiploid DNA content (DNA-index 1.16–1.35, roughly identical to >51–63 chromosomes) are significantly more sensitive to antimetabolites (thiopurines and cytarabine) and l-asparaginase than non-hyperdiploid ALL cells. This is illustrated in Fig. 1. Recently, Ramakers-Van Woerden et al. (2001) extended this analysis in a larger cohort of children. They confirmed this association and, in addition, found that hyperdiploid ALL cells were also more sensitive to 4-HOO-ifosfamide. Moreover, apart from hyperdiploidy, the gain of specific chromosomes significantly affected the drug resistance profiles.

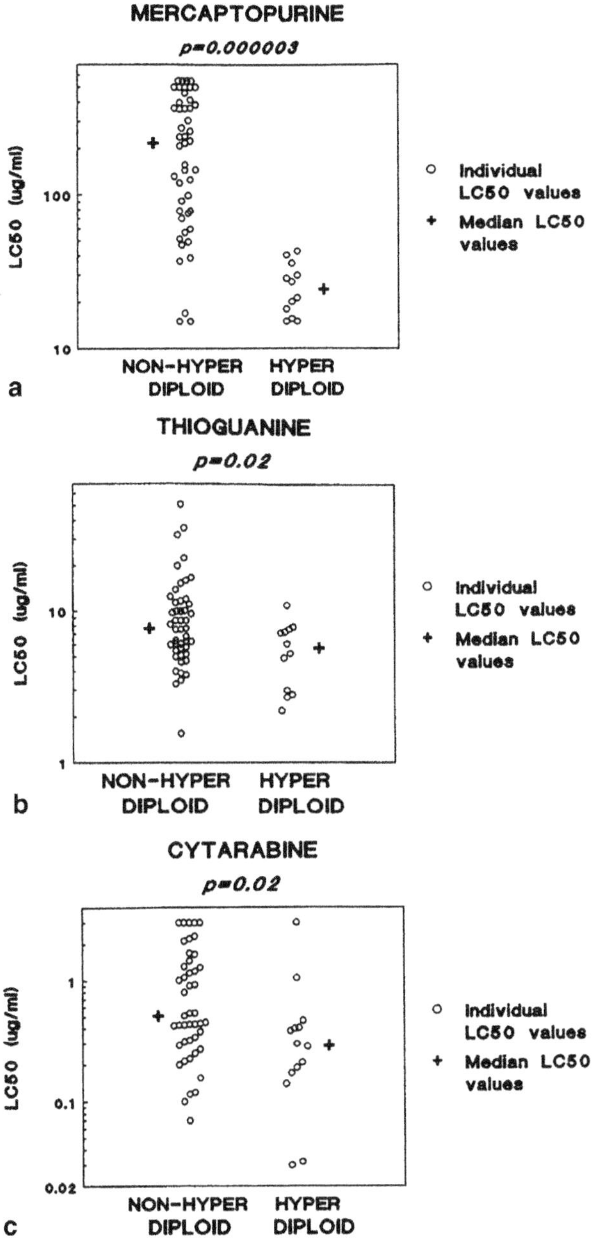

Fig. 1a–d. Significant differences in cellular drug resistance determined by the MTT assay between non-hyperdiploid (DNA-index <1.16 or >1.35) and hyperdiploid (DNA-index 1.16–1.35) common ALL cases. Each open symbol represents the LC_{50} value (drug concentration lethal to 50% of the leukemic cells) for one patient sample; the medians are also indicated. (Reprinted from Kaspers et al.: Favorable prognosis of hyperdiploid common acute lymphoblastic leukemia may be explained by sensitivity to antimetabolites and other drugs: Results of an in vitro study. Blood 1995, 85: 751–756. Copyright American Society of Hematology, used by permission)

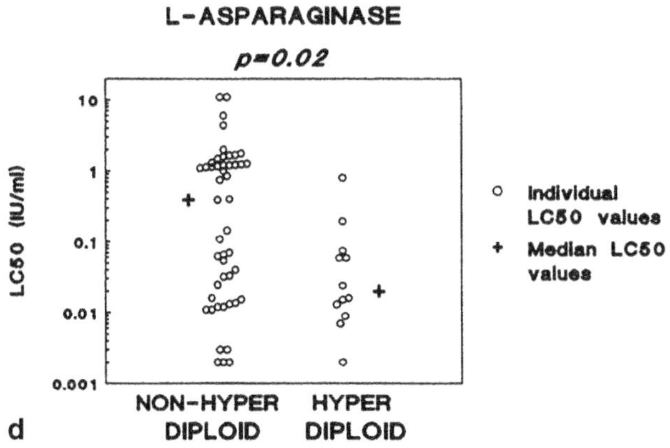

Fig. 1 d

Specific Cytogenetic Abnormalities in ALL and AML

Apart from the above-mentioned studies on DNA ploidy, we also investigated the relation between more specific cytogenetic abnormalities and cellular drug resistance. In ALL, cases with the t(12;21), resulting in the TEL-AML1 gene fusion, had ALL cells that were 11-fold more sensitive to l-asparaginase at a matched comparison (Ramakers-Van Woerden 2000). Within AML, a recent analysis revealed that Down syndrome patients with a constitutive trisomy 21 have AML cells that are markedly more sensitive to most drugs tested, including vincristine (but not l-asparaginase or glucocorticoids), than non-Down syndrome AML cells (Zwaan et al. 2002a). Finally, AML samples with the t(9;11) were markedly more sensitive to several drugs, while samples with chromosome 5 and/or 7 abnormalities were more resistant to cytarabine (Zwaan et al. 2002b).

Cellular Drug Resistance in relation to Short-Term Clinical Outcome

In Vitro Prednisolone Resistance in Newly Diagnosed ALL

Kaspers et al. (1998) reported that the 12 (8%) clinical poor responders after 7 days of prednisone window treatment (systemic monotherapy with prednis(ol)one, but one intrathecal MTX injection as well, according to the Dutch BFM-like protocols DCLSG-ALL-7 and -8) had ALL cells that were median 131-fold more resistant to prednisolone in vitro than 131 good responders (P=0.01). After excluding 17 patients with <1,000 circulating blasts/mm^3 blood before the start of the window treatment (by definition clinical good responders, but obviously not suitable for analysis) resulted in similar results: Poor responders were still 97-fold more resistant to prednisolone (P=0.006), as shown in Fig. 2.

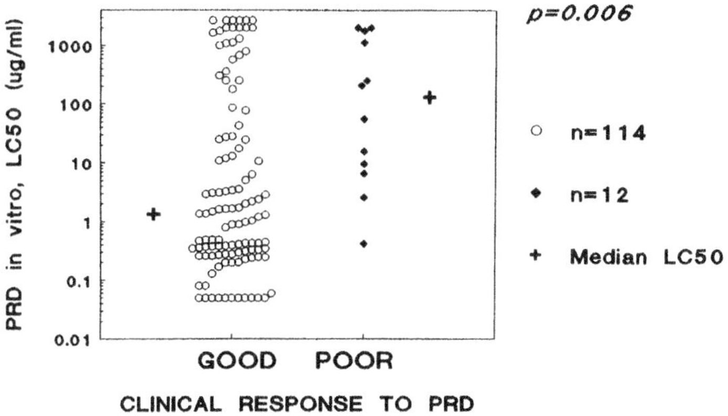

Fig. 2. Significant difference in LC_{50} values for prednisolone (PRD) between ALL patients who responded well (<1,000 leukemic blasts/µl of peripheral blood) and poorly (>1,000 blasts/µl) to a systemic 1-week monotherapy with PRD. Excluded are patients who had less than 1,000 leukemic cells per µl of peripheral blood at initial diagnosis already. (Reprinted from Kaspers et al.: Prednisolone resistance in childhood acute lymphoblastic leukemia: vitro-vivo correlations and cross-resistance to other drugs. Blood 1998, 92: 259–266. Copyright American Society of Hematology, used by permission)

In Vitro l-Asparaginase Resistance in Newly Diagnosed ALL

Asselin et al. (1999) reported that two of five in vitro l-asparaginase-sensitive patients were responders in vivo, whereas seven of eight in vitro resistant patients did not respond clinically to a single-agent l-asparaginase window.

In Vitro Daunorubicin Resistance in Newly Diagnosed ALL

Den Boer (unpublished data) reported on a group of children treated according to the German COALL-92 protocol. It appeared that the 21 clinically poor responders to a systemic monotherapy with daunorubicin were in vitro 1.3-fold more resistant to daunorubicin than 95 good responders (P=0.01). In addition, 15 patients who later appeared to have refractory or relapsed disease had ALL cells at initial diagnosis that were in vitro 1.9-fold more resistant to daunorubicin than ALL cells of 101 patients without a reported event (P=0.004).

In Vitro Drug Resistance in Refractory and Relapsed ALL

Klumper et al. (1995a) reported that all four patients with primary refractory disease were resistant or highly resistant to the induction drugs prednisolone, vincristine, l-asparaginase and daunorubicin. In addition, clinically poor responders to a single-agent idarubicin window treatment (n=17) had ALL cells that were in vitro 3.2-fold more resistant to idarubicin than good responders

(n=10, P=0.04). Finally, 6 of 30 patients with first relapsed ALL failed to achieve a second CR on the ALL-REZ BFM-90 protocol and had ALL cells that were significantly (P<0.05) more resistant to prednisolone (>13.3-fold), dexamethasone (>1.4-fold), daunorubicin (2.7-fold) and doxorubicin (2.9-fold).

In Vitro Drug Resistance in AML

A preliminary analysis of an ongoing study revealed that patients with a relatively poor initial response to combination induction chemotherapy (>5% blasts in the day 15 bone marrow) had AML cells that were more resistant to cytarabine, etoposide, daunorubicin and idarubicin (Kaspers et al. 1999). Previously, we showed (Klumper et al. 1995b) that the group of poor responders (n=14) was threefold more resistant (P=0.05) to cytarabine than the group of 15 good responders to chemotherapy (complete remission already after one course of chemotherapy).

Cellular Drug Resistance in Relation to Long-Term Clinical Outcome

ALL

Our first retrospective study concerned 82 Dutch children with ALL with a median follow-up for patients at risk of 4 years. Forty-four of 82 samples were tested successfully with the MTT assay for resistance to prednisolone, vincristine, l-asparaginase, daunorubicin and/or thioguanine (Pieters et al. 1991). A significantly lower probability of continuous complete remission (CCR) was noted for patients with ALL cells that were in vitro resistant to prednisolone (n=32), daunorubicin (n=22) and thioguanine (n=36), independent from WBC, age, sex and hepatosplenomegaly (but not tested in multivariate analysis). No correlation with outcome was observed for resistance to vincristine (n=38) and l-asparaginase (n=29). In a subsequent prospective study, Kaspers et al. (1997a) reported on samples from 152 children with ALL treated according to the Dutch Childhood Leukemia Study Group protocols ALL-7 and ALL-8, tested with the MTT assay for resistance to 12 drugs. Median follow-up of the patients at risk was 4 years. At risk-group stratified univariate analysis, a significantly (P=0.01) lower probability of disease-free survival (pDFS, including resistant disease and relapse as events) was seen for patients resistant to prednisolone (dexamethasone: P=0.012), vincristine, and l-asparaginase. After multiple regression analysis, a so-called PVA profile emerged with superior prognostic significance compared with single drugs. The pDFS (3 years) for the 20% of patients with a sensitive profile (score 3 or 4) was 100%, for the 40% of patients with an intermediately sensitive profile (score 5 or 6) it was 84%, and for the remaining 40% of patients with a resistant profile (scores 7, 8 or 9) it was 43% (P<0.001; Fig. 3). At multivariate analysis, the PVA profile was the only independent significant (P<0.001) prognostic factor (model also

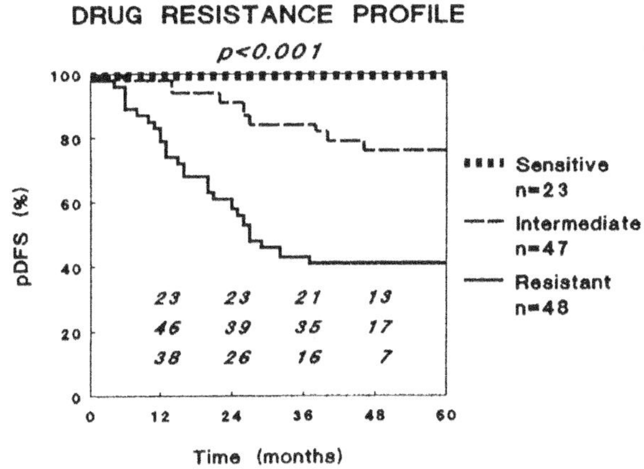

Fig. 3. Significantly different probability of disease-free survival (pDFS) between patients with a sensitive, an intermediately sensitive and a resistant drug resistance profile, combining MTT assay results for prednisolone, vincristine and l-asparaginase. The numbers along the X-axis indicate the patients at risk in the three groups at the different time points. (Reprinted from Kaspers et al.: In vitro cellular drug resistance and prognosis in childhood acute lymphoblastic leukemia. Blood 90: 2723–2729. Copyright American Society of Hematology, used by permission)

including age, WBC, immunophenotype, and DNA ploidy). At risk-group stratified univariate and multivariate analysis, a significantly ($P<0.001$) lower pDFS was observed for patients resistant to prednisolone, also only within the clinical good prednisone responders (see above and Fig. 4). This demonstrates a prognostic value of the in vitro MTT assay additional to that of the clinical response to an initial treatment with prednisone (Kaspers et al. 1998). We have also performed a similar prospective analysis in German children with ALL treated according to the COALL-92 study (Janka-Schaub 1999). The study included samples from 140 patients with a median follow-up of 4 years. Patients with ALL cells with a resistant PVA profile (19% of all patients) had a lower 4-year probability of event-free survival (pEFS) (35%) than intermediately sensitive patients (62% of all patients, pEFS 80%) and in vitro sensitive patients (19% of patients, pEFS 94%). At risk-group stratified multivariate analysis, the PVA profile was the only independent significant ($P<0.001$) prognostic factor (model also including age, WBC, and immunophenotype). The intermediately sensitive group was larger in this study than in the others, because this was defined as a PVA score of 5, 6 or 7 (instead of only 5 or 6). In a larger cohort of retrospectively studied samples from 209 Japanese children with ALL tested with the MTT assay for resistance to 14 drugs, Hongo et al. (1997, 1999) reported similar results. The patients with ALL cells that were sensitive in vitro to two or three drugs (out of 3: prednisolone, vincristine, l-asparaginase), had a significantly better pEFS (3 years) than the patients with relatively resistant ALL cells (sensitivity to no or 1 drug), 0.81 and 0.62, respectively. This was found at both univariate and multivariate analysis. Of interest, in the most recent paper, the presence of a Philadelphia chromosome remained an

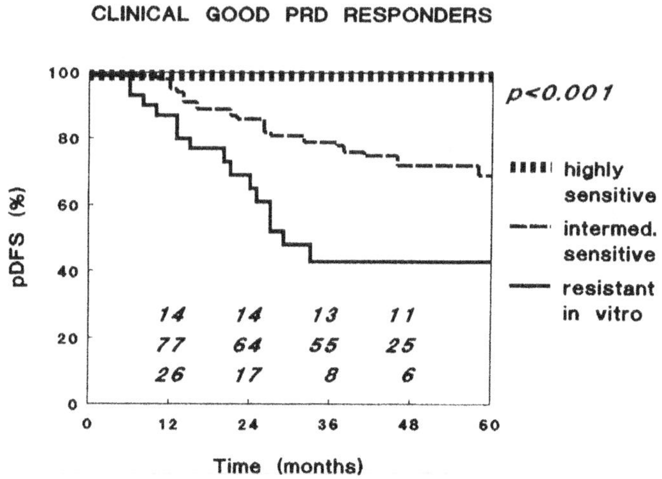

Fig. 4. Similar analysis of childhood ALL patients as shown in Fig. 3, but now only within the clinically good prednisolone (PRD) responders as shown in Fig. 2. The extent of in vitro prednisolone resistance (MTT assay) still has prognostic significance within this subgroup and adds clinically relevant information to that obtained by measuring the clinical response to a systemic monotherapy with PRD. (Reprinted from Kaspers et al.: Prednisolone resistance in childhood acute lymphoblastic leukemia: vitro-vivo correlations and cross-resistance to other drugs. Blood 1990, 92: 259–266. Copyright American Society of Hematology, used by permission)

independent prognostic factor (Hongo et al. 1999). Asselin et al. (1999) reported on samples from 40 (of a cohort of 251) American children with ALL, tested with a dye exclusion assay for cytotoxicity of l-asparaginase (randomization between 3 different preparations). After combination chemotherapy, 18 of 19 in vitro l-asparaginase-sensitive patients were in CCR, compared with only 9 of 21 in vitro resistant patients (P=0.0008), with a median follow-up of more than 4 years. The relation between in vitro resistance to l-asparaginase and long-term clinical outcome remained significant on multivariate analysis (with the model also including risk group, sex and methotrexate randomization).

AML

Our group in Amsterdam is currently involved in two studies on the relation between in vitro cellular drug resistance and long-term clinical outcome in childhood AML. This is being done in collaboration with the German BFM-AML group and with the Dutch Childhood Leukemia Study Group/United Kingdom MRC Childhood Leukaemia Working Party. Both studies are in progress. In 49 adults with AML, we have shown that non-responders to induction chemotherapy had AML cells that were more resistant to daunorubicin (Klumper et al. 1996). However, patients who had AML cells that were more in vitro resistant to cytarabine had a fourfold higher risk of relapse (in fact, all relapsed within 18 months from CR) than those with cytarabine sensitive AML cells (pCCR 0.61 at 34 months). In a recent review (Kaspers et al. 1999) we summarized six studies on the relation between in vitro drug resistance and clinical outcome in childhood AML. Clinical correlations have been reported in 212 childhood AML patients, with overall positive and negative predictive accuracies of 77% and 74%, respectively. However, none of the studies included a long-term clinical follow-up.

Cellular Drug Resistance in Relation to Minimal Residual Disease

The above-mentioned studies in ALL included multivariate analyses of the prognostic significance of in vitro cellular drug resistance. However, the models did not include minimal residual disease. Yet this factor recently emerged as a very strong prognostic factor (Van Dongen et al. 1998; Sievers et al. 2000). Recently, we completed two small retrospective studies in childhood ALL on the correlation between in vitro drug resistance and minimal residual disease during and after induction chemotherapy. In both studies a weak but positive correlation (Spearman Rho of about 0.40) was found between (increased) resistance to prednisolone and (increased) minimal residual disease. For the other drugs used in induction, no such correlation was observed (De Haas et al. 2001; Schmiegelow et al. 2001). A number of ongoing studies (NOPHO, DCLSG, COALL) will reveal more information.

Discussion

Considering the factors that determine the success or failure of chemotherapy, it seems highly rational to study cellular drug resistance. Both the actual measurement of the sensitivity or resistance of leukemic cells to different drugs and the study of mechanisms of resistance and the possibilities of circumventing or modifying resistance are important. This review summarizes the data on cellular drug resistance profiles of childhood leukemia samples which we obtained in our research laboratory of pediatric oncology at the VU University Medical Center in Amsterdam over the past 15 years. Studies on mechanisms of resistance have been reviewed elsewhere (Kaspers et al. 1997b; Pieters et al. 1997). Most of the drug resistance profile data were obtained by using the semi-automated 4-day colorimetric total cell kill MTT assay. Although this assay has several advantages, such as being rapid, objective and capable of testing more than 10 different drugs successfully in the majority of samples, it has disadvantages as well. The two most important disadvantages are that methotrexate (and possibly similar antifolates as well) does not induce dose-dependent cell kill in the non-growing (generally non-dividing) patient samples and that the assay can not discriminate between malignant and non-malignant cells. The latter can be addressed by determining the percentage of leukemic cells in the control wells after 4 days of culture. We have demonstrated that as long as this is at least 70%, the MTT assay results are representative for the leukemic cell population (Kaspers et al. 1994a). Moreover, we have reported on a method to remove contaminating non-malignant cells from leukemic samples (Kaspers et al. 1994a). The first problem could not be solved by us, and we therefore adapted the so-called TS inhibition assay for testing the effects of methotrexate and novel antifolates on leukemic samples. Although this assay determines the extent of inhibition of TS and not cell kill, this concerns a key enzyme in the activity of methotrexate and cell line studies showed a good correlation between the TS inhibition assay and MTT assay results (Mauritz et al. 1998). Another disadvantage of the MTT assay is that it requires relatively high cell numbers, which sometimes is a limiting factor.

The data that we and others have reported demonstrate the clinical relevance of in vitro cellular drug resistance testing in childhood leukemia. In general, leukemia subgroups as defined by different clinical and cell biological features have markedly different cellular drug resistance profiles. This is summarized in Table 2. In general, these differences are in agreement with clinical experience, such as the increased resistance to glucocorticoids and methotrexate of T-cell ALL samples and the increased sensitivity to anti-metabolites of DNA hyperdiploid common ALL samples. On the other hand, the profiles reveal many differences that were not known, such as the increased sensitivity of pro-B ALL samples to cytarabine, the increased sensitivity of DNA hyperdiploid common ALL samples to l-asparaginase and the increased resistance of T-cell ALL samples to l-asparaginase. Another interesting finding is the general pattern of cross-resistance among different types of drugs. Although the extent of cross-resistance was clearly stronger for structurally related drugs, there was significant cross-resistance between non-related drugs as well (Kaspers et al. 1994b; 1998; Klumper et al. 1995a, 1995c). This does suggest a common final pathway of drug-induced cell death. This also implicates novel treatment targets involved in this pathway, with the possibility of increasing drug sensitivity to a broad range of anticancer agents. Another general finding is the significant relation between increased cellular drug resistance and a worse response to induction and combination chemotherapy. This was found for both ALL and AML, although in the latter disease no studies have been reported with long-term clinical follow-up. Finally, larger studies on the correlation between minimal residual disease and cellular drug resistance are still lacking.

The above discussion does indicate the usefulness of data on cellular drug resistance for clinical studies. A large number of potential applications has been defined (Table 1). Cellular drug resistance assays are being used to screen thousands of promising novel agents for their cytotoxicity on large numbers of cell lines, for instance by the National Cancer Institute. Agents that are relatively potent and that lack significant cross-resistance with known agents are of potential interest for further studies. As an example, we recently tested the activity of aplidine, a novel murine cyclic depsipeptide. We found that it had significant cytotoxicity at relatively low (nanomolar) concentra-

Table 2. Summary of significant differences in cellular drug resistance profiles between subgroups with different clinical and cell biological features in childhood ALL

Feature	Subgroup	Resistant/sensitive to:
Age[a]: (compared to 1.5–10 years)	<1.5 years	Glucocorticoids, l-asparaginase and teniposide; sensitive to cytarabine
	≥10 years	Glucocorticoids, l-asparaginase, mercaptopurine, idarubicin
Sex[b]:	Male versus female	No differences
WBC[b]:	High versus low	No differences
FAB type[b]:	L1 versus L2	No differences
Immunophenotype[a,c]: (versus common/pre-B ALL)	Pro-B	Glucocorticoids, l-asparaginase, daunorubicin, doxorubicin, thiopurines, 4-HOO-ifosfamide; sensitive to cytarabine
	T-cell	Glucocorticoids, l-asparaginase, vincristine, anthracyclines, cytarabine, 4-HOO-ifosfamide and methotrexate
Myeloid antigen expression[d]	Yes versus no	No differences
DNA ploidy[e] (within common ALL, versus non-hyperdiploid)	DNA hyperdiploid	More sensitive to anti-metabolites, l-asparaginase and 4-HOO-ifosfamide
TEL/AML1 gene fusion[f] (versus negative cases)	Positive cases	More sensitive to l-asparaginase
deletions of p16 within T-ALL[g]	Yes versus no homozygously deleted p16	No differences
Constitutional trisomy 21 (Down syndrome)[h]	Yes versus no	No differences

[a]Pieters et al. 1998.
[b]Kaspers et al. 1995a.
[c]Rots et al. 1999a.
[d]Den Boer et al. 1999.
[e]Kaspers et al. 1995b.
[f]Ramakers-Van Woerden et al. 2000.
[g]Ramakers-Van Woerden et al. 2001b.
[h]Zwaan et al. 2002.

tions and that there was no cross-resistance with other well-known agents. Normal bone marrow and peripheral blood samples were more resistant to aplidine than both ALL and AML samples (Bresters et al. 2002a,b). An appealing idea, but not (yet?) being applied, is the non-random selection of patients for phase II studies, based on relative sensitivity in vitro for the drug of interest. This approach might help in the earlier and faster identification of valuable new anticancer agents. It might also diminish the possibility that valuable agents are discarded as useless because the wrong patients were selected to test the drug. Chemotherapy with curative intention nearly always means a combination of different drugs. Potential drug interactions may then occur.

Obviously, one would want to benefit from beneficial – synergistic or at least additive – interactions, whereas antagonistic combinations should ideally be identified and omitted from the beginning. Cellular drug resistance testing is valuable in this respect (Kaspers et al. 1995c). Studies on drug resistance modulation and circumvention have a similar background. Although not the subject of this review, we have done a number of studies on modulation of resistance. Meta-iodobenzylguanidine (MIBG) appeared to interact favorably with glucocorticoids in childhood ALL, especially in relatively glucocorticoid resistant samples (Haarman et al. 2001b). Another example is the favorable interaction between fludarabine and cytarabine in childhood AML (Kaspers et al. 2001a), and between aphidicolin and cytarabine in childhood acute leukemia (Sargent et al. 2001). Similarly, the finding that in vitro resistance to methotrexate of AML cells could be overcome by a continuous 21-h exposure (Rots et al. 2001) led to a recently completed phase II window study with methotrexate in childhood relapsed and refractory AML. Circumvention of drug resistance mainly addresses the issue of non-cross-resistance between otherwise related drugs. Especially with respect to antifolates, we have shown that seemingly small differences between drugs can be associated with significant differences in cytotoxicity and inhibition of the key enzyme TS (Mauritz et al. 1998, Rots et al. 1999b). We also found that although ALL cells were strongly cross-resistant to prednisolone and dexamethasone, the latter drug seemed more potent than what was assumed based on anti-inflammatory potencies (Kaspers et al. 1996). Several clinical studies have now shown that the use of dexamethasone gives superior results in terms of efficacy, although toxicity may also be increased (Jones et al. 1991; Veerman et al. 1990b, 1996; Gaynon et al. 2000; Hurwitz et al. 2000; Mattano et al. 2000). Rational improvements of current treatment protocols with subgroup-specific treatment modifications is an approach that is more and more being suggested by molecular biological and cellular drug resistance studies (Kaspers, 2001b). Each subgroup has its own characteristics, and it appears that most if not all subgroups have their own specific drug resistance profiles. Thus the finding that samples of infants with ALL are relatively more resistant to several drugs but more sensitive to cytarabine (Pieters et al. 1998), was one of the reasons for developing an international collaborative infant ALL study, in which large amounts of cytarabine are being used. The prognostic significance of cellular drug resistance data made the German COALL Group decide to include such information for risk-group stratification and subsequent risk-group adapted chemotherapy in their ongoing COALL 97 study. The initial conventional risk-group stratification is based on age, white blood cell count, immunophenotype, and a limited number of cytogenetic abnormalities. If possible (in about 80% of patients), a second stratification is done based on the cellular drug resistance profile. In the case of an intermediately sensitive profile, no treatment modifications are made. In the case of a sensitive profile, treatment is reduced, whereas a resistant profile leads to intensified treatment. Outcome data are not available yet, but it does appear to be feasible (Den Boer and Janka-Schaub, personal communication). Finally, an ultimate goal might be individualized treatment. We have done such a clinical study in poor-risk relapsed ALL. It appeared to be feasible to make individual treatment modifications based on individual cellular drug resistance profiles, but the overall outcome of the patients did not seem to have been improved at a historical comparison (Agthe et al. 1997). However, patients might have been selected that could not be cured with chemotherapy anyway. Hongo et al. (1993) reported some promising experiences with tailored therapy in childhood leukemia. In a recent review of 12 prospective studies including more than 1,000 patients, it was concluded that chemotherapy selected by drug sensitivity testing resulted in higher response rates than empiric chemotherapy (Cortazar et al. 1999). We and others have reported good experiences with assay-selected chemotherapy in individual patients outside clinical protocols (Parker et al. 1992; D'Haens et al. 1998).

In conclusion, cellular drug resistance testing provides clinically relevant information that can be available within 1 week and can be performed successfully in the vast majority of leukemia samples. The data are more and more being used and being considered for use in clinical trials in childhood leukemia. Together with the implementation of other developments, such as pharmacogenomics, minimal residual disease measurements and novel, more selective anti-cancer agents, an improved, individualized treatment of childhood leukemia is feasible.

Acknowledgements. We thank the past and present technicians of the research laboratory of pediatric oncology of the VU University Medical Center of Amsterdam, who contributed greatly to the work summarized here: A.J.F. Broekhuizen, P.A.J.M. de Laat, D.R. Huismans, K.M. Kazemier, A.H. Loonen, M.M.A. Rottier, S. Van Schaick, R. Wünsche, C.H. Van Zantwijk. In addition, several – now or at that time – PhD students/medical doctors have made a essential contribution as well: M.L. den Boer, I. Hubeek, E. Klumper, M.G. Rots, and Ch.M. Zwaan. We also thank A. Heus for her excellent secretarial support. Most of the presented work could only be accomplished because of collaboration with the Sophia Children's Hospital/University Hospital Rotterdam (K. Hählen, M.L. den Boer, R. Pieters), the Dutch Childhood Leukemia Study Group (especially A. Van Der Does-Van Den Berg and E.R. Van Wering), the Juliane Marie Centre/National University Hospital, Copenhagen, Denmark (K. Schmiegelow), the MRC Childhood Leukaemia Working Party (B. Gibson), the German COALL Study Group (G.E. Janka-Schaub), the German BFM-AML Group (U. Creutzig) and the German BFM-ALL-REZ Group (G. Henze).

References

Agthe AG, Dörffel W, Neuendank A, Hartmann R, Brühmüller S, Klumper E, Pieters R, Veerman AJP, Henze G (1997) Tailored therapy for relapsed or refractory childhood acute lymphoblastic leukemia. In: Pieters R, Kaspers GJL, Veerman AJP (eds) Drug resistance in leukemia and lymphoma II. Harwood Academic, Amsterdam, pp 51–57

Asselin BL, Kreissman S, Coppola DJ, Bernal SD, Leavitt PR, Gelber RD, Sallan SE, Cohen HJ (1999) Prognostic significance of early response to a single dose of asparaginase in childhood acute lymphoblastic leukemia. J Pediatr Hematol Oncol 21:6–12

Bresters D, Broekhuizen R, Jimeno J, Faircloth GT, Kaspers GJL (2002a) Different cytotoxic activity in vitro of aplidine in pediatric leukemic and normal bone marrow and blood samples. Proc Am Assoc Cancer Res 43:924 (#4579)

Bresters D, Broekhuizen R, Jimeno J, Faircloth GT, Kaspers GJL (2002b) Lack of in vitro cross-resistance between Aplidine and other drugs in childhood leukemia and normal bone marrow and blood samples. Proc Am Assoc Cancer Res 43:925 (#4583)

Cortazar P, Johnson BE (1999) Review of the efficacy of individualized chemotherapy selected by in vitro drug sensitivity testing for patients with cancer. J Clin Oncol 17:1625–1631

Creutzig U, Ritter J, Zimmermann M, Reinhardt D, Hermann J, Berthold F, Henze G, Jurgens H, Kabisch H, Havers W, Reiter A, Kluba U, Niggli F, Gadner H (2001) Improved treatment results in high-risk pediatric acute myeloid leukemia patients after intensification with high-dose cytarabine and mitoxantrone: results of Study Acute Myeloid Leukemia-Berlin-Frankfurt-Munster 93. J Clin Oncol 19:2705–2713

De Haas V, Kaspers GJL, Oosten L, Bresters D, Wijkhuijs AJM, Van Den Berg H, Van Der Schoot CE (2001) In vitro resistance to prednisolone is related to minimal residual disease (MRD) after induction therapy in childhood acute lymphoblastic leukemia (ALL). Leukemia 15:510 (abstract P62)

Den Boer ML, Kapaun P, Pieters R, Kazemier KM, Janka-Schaub GE, Veerman AJP (1999) Myeloid antigen co-expression in childhood acute lymphoblastic leukaemia: relationship with in vitro drug resistance. Br J Haematol 105:876–882

D'Haens EJ, Veerman AJP (1998) Complete remission in a boy with treatment refractory acute lymphoblastic leukemia based on in vitro drug resistance testing with the MTT assay (in Dutch, English abstract). Tijdschr Kindergeneeskd 66:129–132

Dübbers A, Würthwein G, Müller HJ, Schulze-Westhoff P, Winkelhorst M, Kurzknabe E, Lanvers C, Pieters R, Kaspers GJL, Creutzig U, Ritter J, Boos J (2000) Asparagine synthetase activity in pediatric acute leukaemias: AML-M5 subtype shows lowest activity. Br J Haematol 109:427–429

Evans WE, Relling MV, Rodman JH, Crom WR, Boyett JM, Pui CH (1998) Conventional compared with individualized chemotherapy for childhood acute lymphoblastic leukemia. N Engl J Med 338:499–505

Gaynon PS, Trigg ME, Heerema NA, Sensel MG, Sather HN, Hammond GD, Bleyer WA (2000) Children's Cancer Group trials in childhood acute lymphoblastic leukemia: 1983–1995. Leukemia 14:2223–2233

Haarman EG, Kaspers GJL, Pieters R, Rottier MMA, Veerman AJP (2001a) Cell death regulator expression versus glucocorticoid resistance in childhood acute lymphoblastic leukemia. Leukemia 15:495 (abstract no. O56)

Haarman EG, Kaspers GJL, Pieters R, Rottier MMA, Veerman AJP (2001b) Modulation of glucocorticoid resistance in childhood acute lymphoblastic leukemia; preliminary results. Haematol Blood Transf 40:236–243

Haarman EG, Kaspers GJL, Pieters R, Rottier MMA, Veerman AJP (2001c) A comparison of the antileukemic activity in vitro of cortivazol, prednisolone and dexamethasone in childhood leukemia. Ann Hematol 80 [Suppl II]:S31 (abstract)

Hongo T, Fujii Y, Yajima S (1993) In vitro chemosensitivity of childhood leukemic cells and the clinical value of assay directed chemotherapy. In: Kaspers GJL et al. (eds) Drug resistance in leukemia and lymphoma I. Chur, Harwood, pp 313–319

Hongo T, Yajima S, Sakurai M, Horikoshi Y, Hanada R (1997) In vitro drug sensitivity testing can predict induction failure and early relapse of childhood acute lymphoblastic leukemia. Blood 89:2959–2965

Hongo T, Yamada S, Yajima S, Watanabe C, Fujii Y, Kawasaki H, Yazaki M, Hanada R, Horokoshi Y (1999) Biological characteristics and prognostic value of in vitro three-drug resistance to prednisolone, l-asparaginase, and vincristine in childhood acute lymphoblastic leukemia. Int J Hematol 70:268–277

Hurwitz CA, Silverman LB, Schorin MA, Clavell LA, Dalton VK, Glick KM, Gelber RD, Sallan SE (2000) Substituting dexamethasone for prednisone complicates remission induction in children with acute lymphoblastic leukemia. Cancer 88:1964–1969

Ito C, Evans WE, McNinch L, Coustan-Smith E, Mahmoud H, Pui CH, Campana D (1996) Comparative cytotoxicity of dexamethasone and prednisolone in childhood acute lymphoblastic leukemia. J Clin Oncol 14:2370–2376

Jones B, Freeman AI, Shuster J, et al. (1991) Lower incidence of meningeal leukemia when prednisone is replaced by dexamethasone in the treatment of acute lymphoblastic leukemia. Med Pediatr Oncol 19:269–275
Kaspers GJL, Pieters R, Van Zantwijk CH, De Laat E, De Waal FC, Van Wering ER, Veerman AJP (1991) In vitro drug sensitivity of normal peripheral blood lymphocytes and childhood leukaemic cells from bone marrow and peripheral blood. Br J Cancer 64:469–474
Kaspers GJL, Veerman AJP, Pieters R, Broekema GJ, Huismans DR, Kazemier KM, Loonen AH, Rottier MMA, Van Zantwijk CH, Hählen K, Van Wering ER (1994a) Mononuclear cells contaminating leukemic samples tested for cellular drug resistance using the methyl-thiazol-tetrazolium assay. Br J Cancer 70:1047–1052
Kaspers GJL, Pieters R, Klumper E, Van Zantwijk CH, Hählen K, De Waal FC, Van Wering ER, Veerman AJP (1994b) In vitro cytotoxicity of mitoxantrone, daunorubicin, and doxorubicin in untreated childhood acute leukemia. Leukemia 8:24–29
Kaspers GJL, Kardos G, Pieters R, Van Zantwijk CH, Klumper E, Hählen K, De Waal FC, Van Wering ER, Veerman AJP (1994c) Different cellular drug resistance profiles in childhood lymphoblastic and non-lymphoblastic leukemia: a preliminary report. Leukemia 8:1224–1229
Kaspers GJL, Pieters R, Van Zantwijk CH, Van Wering ER, Veerman AJP (1995a) Clinical and cell biological features related to cellular drug resistance of childhood acute lymphoblastic leukemia cells. Leukemia Lymphoma 19:407–417
Kaspers GJL, Smets LA, Pieters R, Van Zantwijk CH, Van Wering ER, Veerman AJP (1995b) Favorable prognosis of hyperdiploid common acute lymphoblastic leukemia may be explained by sensitivity to antimetabolites and other drugs: Results of an in vitro study. Blood 85:751–756
Kaspers GJL, Pieters R, Van Zantwijk CH, Hählen K, Van Wering ER, Veerman AJP (1995c) Drug combination testing in acute lymphoblastic leukemia using the MTT assay. Leuk Res 19:175–181
Kaspers GJL, Veerman AJP, Popp-Snijders C, Lomecky M, Van Zantwijk CH, Swinkels LMJW, Van Wering ER, Pieters R (1996) Comparison of the antileukemic activity in vitro of dexamethasone and prednisolone in childhood acute lymphoblastic leukemia. Med Pediatr Oncol 27:114–121
Kaspers GJL, Veerman AJP, Pieters R, Van Zantwijk CH, Smets LA, Van Wering ER, Van Der Does-Van Den Berg A (1997a) In vitro cellular drug resistance and prognosis in childhood acute lymphoblastic leukemia. Blood 90:2723–2729
Kaspers GJL, Pieters R, Veerman AJP (1997b) Glucocorticoid resistance in childhood leukemia. Int J Pediatr Hematol Oncol 4:583–596
Kaspers GJL, Pieters R, Van Zantwijk CH, Van Wering ER, Van Der Does-Van Den Berg A, Veerman AJP (1998) Prednisolone resistance in childhood acute lymphoblastic leukemia: vitro-vivo correlations and cross-resistance to other drugs. Blood 92:259–266
Kaspers GJL, Zwaan ChM, Veerman AJP, Rots MG, Pieters R, Bucsky P, Domula M, Göbel U, Graf N, Havers W, Jorch N, Kabisch K, Spaar H-J, Ritter J, Creutzig U (1999) Cellular drug resistance in acute myeloid leukemia: literature review and preliminary analysis of an ongoing collaborative study. Klin Pädiatr 211:239–244
Kaspers GJL, Litvinova E, Hubeek I, Haarman EG, Huismans DR, Peters GJ, Veerman AJP (2001a) Increased in vitro cytotoxicity of cytarabine when combined with fludarabine towards childhood acute myeloid leukemia cells. Leukemia 15:497 (abstract P08)
Kaspers GJL (2001b) Pediatric leukemia in the new millennium (editorial). Expert Rev Anticancer Ther 1:1–2
Klumper E, Pieters R, Veerman AJP, Huismans DR, Loonen AH, Hählen K, Kaspers GJL, Van Wering ER, Hartmann R, Henze G (1995a) Cellular drug resistance in children with relapsed and refractory acute lymphoblastic leukemia. Blood 86:3861–3868
Klumper E, Pieters R, Kaspers GJL, Huismans DR, Loonen AH, Rottier MMA, Van Wering ER, Van Der Does-Van Den Berg A, Hählen K, Creutzig U, Veerman AJP (1995b) In vitro chemosensitivity testing assessed with the MTT assay in childhood acute non-lymphoblastic leukemia. Leukemia 9:1864–1869

Klumper E, Pieters R, Den Boer ML, Huismans DR, Loonen AH, Veerman AJP (1995c) In vitro anthracycline cross-resistance patterns in childhood acute lymphoblastic leukemia. Br J Cancer 71:1188–1193

Klumper E, Ossenkoppele G, Pieters R, Huismans DR, Loonen AH, Rottier A, Westra G, Veerman AJP (1996) In vitro resistance to cytosine arabinoside, not to daunorubicin, is associated with the risk of relapse in de novo acute myeloid leukaemia. Br J Haematol 93:903–910

Krance RA, Hurwitz CA, Head DR, Raimondi SC, Behm FG, Crews KR, Srivastava DK, Mahmoud H, Roberts WM, Tong X, Blakley RL, Ribeiro RC (2001) Experience with 2-chlorodeoxyadenosine in previously untreated children with newly diagnosed acute myeloid leukemia and myelodysplastic syndrome. J Clin Oncol 19:2804–2811

Mattano LA Jr, Sather HN, Trigg ME, Nachman JB (2000) Osteonecrosis as a complication of treating acute lymphoblastic leukemia n children: a report from the Children's Cancer group. J Clin Oncol 18:3262–3272

Mauritz R, Bekkenk MW, Rots MG, Pieters R, Mini E, Van Zantwijk CH, Veerman AJP, Peters GJ, Jansen G (1998) Ex vivo activity of methotrexate versus novel antifolate inhibitors of dihydrofolate reductase and thymidylate synthase against childhood leukemia cells. Clin Cancer Res 4:2399–2410

Parker AN, Hutchinson RM, Chapman CS, Bosanquet AG (1992) Effective treatment of relapsed acute myeloid leukaemia with drugs chosen by DiSC assay. Br J Haematol 81:455–456

Pieters R, Huismans DR, Leyva A, Verman AJP (1988) Adaptation of the rapid automated tetrazolium dye based MTT assay for chemosensitivity testing in childhood leukemia. Cancer Lett 41:323–332

Pieters R, Huismans DR, Leyva A, Veerman AJP (1989) Comparison of a rapid automated tetrazolium based (MTT) assay with a dye exclusion assay for chemosensitivity testing in childhood leukemia. Br J Cancer 59:217–220

Pieters R, Loonen AH, Huismans DR, Broekeka GJ, Dirven MWJ, Heyenbrok MW, Hählen K, Veerman AJP (1990) In vitro drug sensitivity of cells from children with leukemia using the MTT assay with improved culture conditions. Blood 76:2327–2336

Pieters R, Huismans DR, Loonen AH, Hahlen K, Van Der Does-Van Den Berg A, Van Wering ER, Veerman AJP (1991) Relation of cellular drug resistance to long-term clinical outcome in childhood acute lymphoblastic leukaemia. Lancet 338:399–403

Pieters R, Klumper E, Kaspers GJL, Veerman AJP (1997) Everything you always wanted to know about cellular drug resistance in childhood acute lymphoblastic leukemia. Crit Rev Hematol/Oncol 25:11–26

Pieters R, Den Boer ML, Durian M, Janka G, Schmiegelow K, Kaspers GJL, Van Wering ER, Veerman AJP (1998) Relation between age, immunophenotype and in vitro drug resistance in 395 children with acute lymphoblastic leukemia – implications for treatment of infants. Leukemia 12:1344–1348

Preisler HD, Gopal V (1994) Regrowth resistance in leukemia and lymphoma: the need for a new system to classify treatment failure and for new approaches to treatment. Leuk Res 18:149–160

Pui C-H, Evans WE (2000) Acute lymphoblastic leukemia in children. Curr Opin Oncol 12:3–12

Ramakers-Van Woerden NL, Pieters R, Loonen AH, Hubeek I, Van Drunen E, Beverloo HB, Slater RM, Harbott J, Seyfarth J, Van Wering ER, Hählen K, Schmiegelow K, Janka-Schaub GE, Veerman AJP (2000) TEL/AML1 gene fusion is related to in vitro drug sensitivity for l-asparaginase in childhood acute lymphoblastic leukemia. Blood 96:1094–1099

Ramakers-van Woerden NL, Pieters R, Rots MG, Kaspers GJL, Van Wering ER, Loonen AH, Slater RM, Harbott J, Schmiegelow K, Janka-Schaub GE, Veerman AJP (2001a) Ploidy status and drug resistance profiles in childhood acute lymphoblastic leukemia: an analysis of 425 cases. Leukemia 15:506 (abstract no. P45)

Ramakers-van Woerden NL, Pieters R, Slater RM, Loonen AH, Beverloo HB, Van Drunen E, Heyman M, Moreno TC, Rots MG, Van Wering ER, Kamps WA, Janka-Schaub GE, Veerman AJP (2001b) In vitro drug resistance and prognostic impact of p16INK4A/p15INK4B deletions in childhood T-cell acute lymphoblastic leukaemia. Br J Haematol 112:680–690

Rots MG, Pieters R, Kaspers GJL, Van Zantwijk CH, Noordhuis P, Mauritz R, Veerman AJP, Jansen G, Peters GJ (1999a) Differential methotrexate resistance in childhood T- versus common/pre-B acute lymphoblastic leukemia can be measured by an in situ thymidylate synthase inhibition assay, but not by the MTT assay. Blood 93:1067–1074

Rots MG, Pieters R, Peters GJ, Van Zantwijk CH, Mauritz R, Noordhuis P, Willey JC, Hählen K, Creutzig U, Janka-Schaub G, Kaspers GJL, Veerman AJP, Jansen G (1999b) Circumvention of methotrexate resistance in childhood leukemia subtypes by rationally designed antifolates. Blood 94:3121–3128

Rots MG, Pieters R, Kaspers GJL, Veerman AJP, Peters GJ, Jansen G (2000) Classification of ex vivo methotrexate resistance in acute lymphoblastic and myeloid leukaemia. Br J Haematol 110:791–800

Rots MG, Pieters R, Peters GJ, Kaspers GJL, Van Zantwijk CH, Noordhuis P, Voorn DA, Van Wering ER, Creutzig U, Veerman AJP, Jansen G (2001) A possible role for methotrexate in the treatment of childhood acute myeloid leukemia in general, and for acute monocytic leukemia in particular. Eur J Haematol 37:492–498

Sargent JM, Williamson CJ, Taylor CG, Pieters R, Peters GJ, Kaspers GJL (2001) Aphidicolin decreases in vitro resistance to ara-C in childhood acute leukaemia. Leukemia 15:497 (abstract P09)

Schmiegelow K, Nyvold C, Seyfarth J, Pieters R, Knabe N, Rottier N, Ryder LP, Madsen HO, Kaspers GJL (2001) Post-induction residual disease in childhood acute lymphoblastic leukemia quantified by PCR is related to in vitro prednisolone resistance. Leukemia 15:1066–1071

Sievers EL, Radich JP (2000) Detection of minimal residual disease in acute leukemia. Curr Opin Hematol 7:212–216

Stevens RF, Hann IM, Wheatley K, Gray RG (1998) Marked improvements in outcome with chemotherapy alone in paediatric acute myeloid leukaemia: results of the United Kingdom Medical Research Council's 10th AML trial. MRC Childhood Leukaemia Working Party. Br J Haematol 101:130–140

Van Dongen JJM, Seriu T, Panzer-Grumayer ER, et al. (1998) Prognostic value of minimal residual disease in acute lymphoblastic leukemia. Lancet 352:1731–1738

Veerman AJP, Pieters R (1990a) Drug sensitivity assays in leukaemia and lymphoma. Br J Haematol 74:381–384

Veerman AJP, Hählen K, Kamps WA, Van Leeuwen EF, De Vaan GAM, Van Wering ER, Van der Does-Van Den Berg A, Solbu G, Suciu S (1990b) Dutch Childhood Leukemia Study Group: Early results of study ALL-VI (1984–1988). Haematol Blood Transf 33:473–477

Veerman AJP, Hählen K, Kamps WA, Van Leeuwen EF, De Vaan GAM, Solbu G, Suciu S Van Wering ER, Van der Does-Van Den Berg A (1996) High cure rate with a moderately intensive treatment regimen in non-high-risk childhood acute lymphoblastic leukemia. Results of protocol ALL VI from the Dutch Childhood Leukemia Study Group. J Clin Oncol 14:911–918

Zwaan ChM, Kaspers GJL, Pieters R, Huismans DR, Van Wering ER, Janka-Schaub GE, Creutzig U, Henze G, Veerman AJP (2000a) Circumvention of cytarabine resistance by 2-chlorodeoxyadenosine in pediatric acute myeloid and acute lymphoblastic leukemia: an in vitro study. Blood 96 (11, part 1):307a (abstract)

Zwaan ChM, Kaspers GJL, Pieters R, Ramakers-Van Woerden NL, Den Boer ML, Wünsche R, Rottier MMA, Hählen K, Van Wering ER, Janka-Schaub GE, Creutzig U, Veerman AJP (2002b) Cellular drug resistance profiles in childhood acute myeloid leukemia: differences between FAB types and comparison with acute lymphoblastic leukemia. Blood 96:2879–2886

Zwaan ChM, Kaspers GJL, Pieters R, Hählen K, Janka-Schaub GE, Van Zantwijk CH, Huismans DR, De Vries E, Rots MG, Peters GJ, Jansen G, Creutzig U, Veerman AJP (2002a) Different drug sensitivity profiles of acute myeloid and lymphoblastic leukemia and normal peripheral blood mononuclear cells in children with and without Down syndrome. Blood 99:245–251

Zwaan ChM, Kaspers GJL, Pieters R, Hählen K, Huismans DR, Zimmermann M, Harbott J, Släter RM, Creutzig U, Veerman AJP (2002b) Cellular drug resistance is related to chromosomal abnormalities in childhood AML. Blood (in press)

ATP Chemosensitivity Testing in Ovarian and Breast Cancer: Early Clinical Trials

Christian M. Kurbacher, Ottilia M. Grecu, Ursula Stier, Tobias J. Gilster, Margit-M. Janát, Michael Untch, Gottfried Konecny, Howard W. Bruckner, Ian A. Cree

C.M. Kurbacher (✉)
Division of Clinical and Experimental Gynecologic Oncology,
Department of Gynecology and Obstetrics, University of Cologne
Medical Center, Kerpener Straße 34, 50931 Köln, Germany
e-mail: Christian.Kurbacher@medizin.uni-koeln.de

Abstract

After disappointing results achieved with older chemosensitivity tests such as the human tumor clonogenic assay (HTCA) during the 1980s, the last decade has seen a renaissance of the concept of individualized chemotherapy in oncology, markedly stimulated by the development of newer nonclonogenic assays. These methods appear to be able to overcome major technical limitations associated with older assays, now allowing for successful testing of most of the tumor specimens submitted. Currently, the ATP-based tumor chemosensitivity assay (ATP-TCA) can be regarded as the most sophisticated assay to investigate both solid samples and effusions derived from patients with various organ tumors.

During the last 5 years, the ATP-TCA has been used successfully to screen for novel drug combinations for further clinical use in both ovarian and breast cancer such as mitoxantrone plus paclitaxel (NT) and treosulfan plus gemcitabine (TG), respectively. Clinical trials that have been set up in heavily pretreated patients with recurrent ovarian or breast cancer have convincingly confirmed the high activity of these combinations previously demonstrated in preclinical investigations using the ATP-TCA. In a recent phase II trial performed in 59 patients with relapsed ovarian carcinoma, ATP-TCA-directed therapy was able to triple the response rate and to double the survival time, compared with published empirical chemotherapy regimes. Preliminary results with ATP-TCA-directed therapy in breast cancer also evidenced promising response rates. These results have been confirmed by additional prospective clinical trials using other types of modern nonclonogenic assays. A phase III trial that is now actively recruiting patients with platinum-refractory ovarian cancer to verify the promising phase II studies will prove the further value of the ATP-TCA as a predictor applicable in routine clinical oncology.

Introduction

Chemotherapy has become an integral component of various therapeutic scenarios in gynecologic oncology, particularly in patients suffering from breast (BC) or ovarian cancer (OC). Despite its well-documented efficacy reported in numerous controlled trials, the uncertainty of individual response to chemotherapy remains one of the unresolved problems for the majority of patients treated.

During the last three decades, considerable efforts have been made to develop a laboratory method that allows accurate prediction of an individual patient's response to chemotherapy [1–3]. The most popular of these assays is the human tumor clonogenic assay (HTCA) [4]. This test, as many others that have been introduced up to now, provided a satisfactory predictive accuracy with a positive predictive value (PPV) of around 65% and a negative predictive value (NPV) of 90% or more [2, 4]. These data are very close to those achieved with worldwide accepted predictive tests for hormonal responsiveness of breast cancer or antibiotic sensitivity of microbes.

However, the HTCA suffered from major technical limitations such as low evaluability rates, a long incubation period, and the large number of tumor cells required [1, 2, 5]. Nonetheless, a number of clinical trials have been set up during the last two decades to test the ability of the HTCA and other assays to direct chemotherapy for different human malignancies [6]. Except for lung cancer, OC has been the most intensively investigated tumor type in these trials, including two of three randomized studies published so far. Although mostly encouraging results have been reported, older studies failed to univocally demonstrate predictive assays to be able to improve survival [6, 7]. One of the major problems of these trials was the low assay success rate, which resulted in insufficient recruitment. Nonetheless, it is also very clear from these trials that the use of any predictive assay to direct individualized chemotherapy is extremely unlikely to harm patients [6].

More recently, a number of nonclonogenic assays have been developed that may well be able to overcome the major technical limitations of older methods. Among these, the ATP tumor chemosensitivity assay (ATP-TCA), one of the different types of ATP-based viability assays, has the best documented track record in solid tumors [2, 8]. The ATP-TCA is easy to handle and highly reproducible and utilizes a standardized methodology that provides success rates of more than 90% in both BC and OC when surgical specimens or malignant effusions are used. Retrospective analyses revealed that the NPV approximates 100% and the PPV is around 90%, resulting in a predictive accuracy of 90% or more [2, 8, 9]. In a recent publication, we were able to demonstrate that the ex vivo sensitivity found in the ATP-TCA is also a strong predictor of long-term survival in patients with advanced primary OC treated with platinum-based chemotherapy [10]. Therefore, we have initiated several trials using the ATP-TCA both to screen for innovative drug combinations for further clinical use and to select individualized chemotherapy in patients suffering from metastatic BC (MBC) or recurrent OC (ROC). The major findings of these trials are summarized in this review.

New Regimen Screening Guided by the ATP-TCA

Two major combinations in ROC or MBC that have recently been developed by using previous preclinical data achieved with the ATP-TCA are NT – mitoxantrone (MX) plus paclitaxel (PCT) – and TG – treosulfan (TREO) combined with gemcitabine (dFdC).

The first study was based on the preclinical evaluation of NT, which produced ex vivo chemosensitivity in 83% of native tumor samples derived from patients with platinum-refractory ROC. In a substantial number of samples showing resistance to both single agents, significant sensitivity to NT could be recorded. A typical example is shown in Fig. 1. These results prompted a subsequent pilot trial, in which NT was administered at two different schedules to 18 patients with heavily pretreated ROC, a classical 3-weekly protocol with 8 mg/m^2 MX and 180 mg/m^2 PCT, and a dose-dense protocol with 6 mg/m^2 MX given on day 1 and 100 mg/m^2 PCT given on days 1 and 8 repeated every second week. Lacking any differences between both NT variants, therapy resulted in a high clinical activity with five complete (CR) and nine partial remissions (PR) accounting for an objective response rate (ORR) of 78% and a median progression-free survival (PFS) of 11.1 months [11].

Because of these encouraging results, which were in perfect agreement with the preclinical data achieved previously, we decided to reopen the trial. Recently, we were able to report on mature results of this feasibility study after recruiting a total of 39 heavily pretreated ROC patients with all but 5 suffering from platinum-refractory disease [12]. The remainder had failed at least two prior chemotherapy regimens, underlining the poor prognosis of the entire

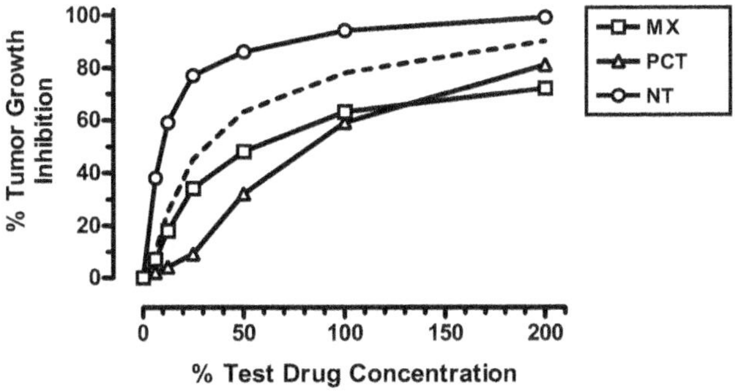

Fig. 1. Dose–response curves of mitoxantrone (MX), paclitaxel (PCT), and the combination (NT) tested with the ATP-TCA in a tumor specimen derived from a patient with platinum-refractory pretreated ovarian carcinoma. The tumor is resistant to both single agents but highly sensitive to the combination. The dotted line represents the theoretical dose-response curve of the combination assuming that both single agents act additively. The strong synergistic effect of both cytostatics should be noted

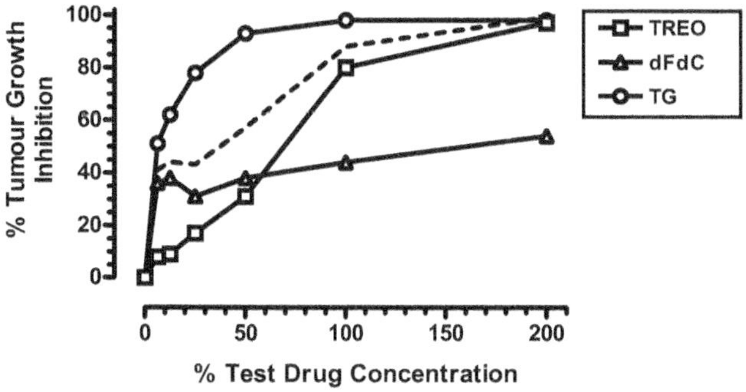

Fig. 2. Dose-response curves of treosulfan (TREO), gemcitabine (dFdC), and the combination (TG) tested with the ATP-TCA in a tumor specimen derived from a patient with platinum-refractory pretreated ovarian carcinoma. The tumor is resistant to both single agents but highly sensitive to the combination. The dotted line represents the theoretical dose-response curve of the combination assuming that both single agents act additively. The strong synergistic effect of both cytostatics should be noted

population treated. NT-associated myelosuppression was remarkable but did generally not compromise dose intensity. Except for alopecia, nonhematological side effects were infrequent. In particular, we did not observe any severe acute or prolonged neurotoxicity. A total of 14 CR and 12 PR were achieved, resulting in a 67% ORR. PFS was 9 months and median overall survival (OS) was 19.8 months. These encouraging results, which were able to prove the ATP-TCA to be a valuable tool to screen for active and clinically feasible drug combinations, were confirmed by additional studies of NT in prognostically comparable patients with platinum-refractory or at least heavily pretreated ROC showing response rates between 70% and 85% and a PFS of 8–15 months [13, 14].

In a second study, which was stimulated by preclinical work in OC and melanoma [15, 16], we investigated TG in patients with refractory ROC or heavily pretreated MBC [17, 18]. This combination was chosen in an attempt to overcome resistance against platinum and alkylating agents by dFdC-induced inhibition of DNA repair without sharing major platinum-associated organ toxicities. In an initial laboratory study, a total of 42 tumor specimens derived from patients with either platinum-refractory ROC or pretreated MBC were tested with the ATP-TCA against TREO, dFdC, and TG. Only 24% and 42% of tumors showed ex vivo sensitivity to TREO and dFdC, respectively. In contrast, 79% of tumors were responsive to TG, with the majority exhibiting high sensitivity ex vivo. A typical example is shown in Fig. 2.

Subsequently, a clinical pilot trial was set up recruiting 14 patients with platinum-refractory ROC and 12 MBC patients mostly pretreated with anthracyclines. Ten patients with ROC and another three with MBC had received prior taxanes. Patients had failed one to six prior chemotherapies with a median number of three. TG was given with TREO at 5 g/m^2 on day 1 and dFdC at 1,250 mg/m^2 on days 1 and 8 of a 3-week schedule. All but one patient were evaluable for response with 4 CR and 8 PR accounting for an ORR of 48%

(52% in evaluable patients). The median PFS was 21 weeks, and the median OS was 110+ weeks. Patients with MBC and ROC did not differ significantly in terms of ORR and survival. Nonhematological side effects of TG were infrequent and generally mild. In contrast, the hematological toxicity was substantial, with WHO grade 3–4 leukopenia observed in 30 of 93 cycles administered. However, no patient required hospitalization because of neutropenic complications. Severe thrombocytopenia and anemia were less frequent but sometimes of long duration. Although colony-stimulating factors were given liberally, dose reduction and/or interval prolongation was necessary in 13 of 25 patients treated. Thus the actuarial relative dose intensity (RDI) in this trial was 92% for TREO and 84% for dFdC. Generally, reduction of RDI did not adversely affect the chance to respond to TG. However, all but one patient progressing on therapy had TG treatment at a reduced RDI. Corresponding to the NT trial, this study confirms that the ATP-TCA is able to screen for new active chemotherapy regimes even in heavily pretreated patients. Nevertheless, the TG regimen used here clearly needs to be modified to allow the majority of patients to be treated with the full RDI, which has been found to be crucial to achieve long-term survival.

Using the ex vivo apoptotic (EVA) assay for the clinical development of the cisplatin/gemcitabine regimen (PG) in ROC and MBC, Nagourney and coworkers made very similar experiences [19, 20]. In accordance with our results with NT or TG, they were able to achieve a high preclinical activity in both breast and ovarian tumors, which subsequently translated into convincing clinical results within different phase II trials.

Individualized Chemotherapy Directed by the ATP-TCA

On the basis of the encouraging results of the aforementioned studies, we initiated a prospective clinical trial using chemotherapy individually selected by the ATP-TCA in patients with intensively pretreated ROC. Results achieved in the first 25 patients were retrospectively compared with 30 patients treated simultaneously on an empirical basis [21]. Both ORR (64% vs. 37%) and PFS (50 vs. 20 weeks) were significantly higher in the ATP-TCA group. Additionally, significantly more patients receiving assay-directed therapy achieved CR (32% vs. 7%). There was also a trend toward improved OS in the ATP-TCA group, but not significantly so (Fig. 3). In particular, patients with platinum-refractory appeared to benefit from assay-directed chemotherapy.

Mature results of this trial have recently been reported (22, 23). A total of 59 patients (31 with platinum-sensitive ROC, 28 with platinum-refractory ROC) who had failed one to five prior chemotherapies (median 2) were included, with 28 of each subgroup being evaluable for response. The ORR was 66% (70% in evaluable patients), with 20 CR and 19 PR seen. The false positive rate was very low with only six patients (10%) progressing on ATP-TCA-directed therapy. Median PFS was 45 weeks, and median OS was 90 weeks. As a unique finding regarding the published results on empirical salvage chemo-

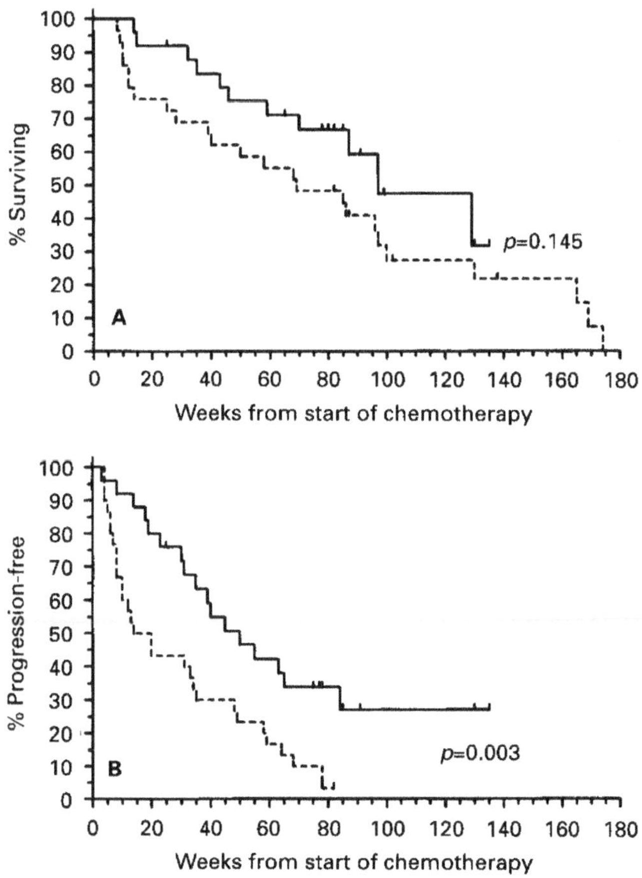

Fig. 3. Kaplan-Meier curves for (**A**) progression-free (PFS) and (**B**) overall survival (OS) achieved with ATP-TCA-directed chemotherapy in 25 patients with recurrent ovarian cancer versus 30 patients treated empirically in the same period. (From Kurbacher et al. 1998, reproduced with the permission of the publisher)

therapy for recurrent ovarian cancer, ORR and survival (PFS and OS) were identical in both platinum-refractory and -sensitive subsets of patients. Including additional clinicopathological parameters (age, type of chemotherapy, number of preceding treatments, residual tumor volume), response to therapy was the only significant determinant of long-term survival in both a univariate and a multivariate analysis.

Generally, the ATP-TCA favored the use of novel drug combinations instead of standard single agents. These new regimens (i.e., NT, doxorubicin plus PCT, platinum plus either cytarabine or dFdC) produced 31 of 39 remissions. It should be emphasized, however, that the frequent use of polychemotherapy did not result in a higher incidence of severe hematological or nonhematological side-effects. During 316 evaluable cycles of assay-directed chemotherapy,

WHO grade 3 leukopenia was seen in $\leq$13%, grade 3 anemia in $\leq$10%, and grade 3–4 thrombocytopenia in $\leq$12% of courses related to the particular regimen given. One patient (1.7%) died of thrombocytopenic cerebral hemorrhage while experiencing disease stabilization after five courses of carboplatin plus cytarabine. Organ toxicity was infrequent and did not exceed grade 2. These results provide evidence that the use of the ATP-TCA to direct individualized chemotherapy allows for optimized treatment in terms of both increased antineoplastic efficacy and reduction of severe or life-threatening adverse effects.

In accordance with this trial, Dottino and co-workers reported on a study of the EVA assay as a means to direct chemotherapy in 44 patients with ROC after failure of up to six preceding chemotherapies [24]. Among 37 evaluable patients in this trial, the ORR trial was 52% with 5% CR, a PFS of 8 months, and a OS of 15 months. Toxicity data are not yet reported. Results were slightly inferior to those from our study with the ATP-TCA, which may indicate the particular suitability of this method as a true sensitivity assay. However, differences may also be a result of the particular characteristics of the patient populations treated. In general, findings of both trials were very supportive, demonstrating that the use of modern nonclonogenic assays to direct individualized chemotherapy for intensively pretreated ROC patients leads to extraordinary results in terms of both response and survival.

Recent results with ATP-TCA directed chemotherapy in MBC are less conclusive. However, we were able to achieve an encouraging ORR of 88% (15/17) with 6 CR and 9 PR in a small pilot trial including 17 patients [25]. Only one patient progressed on therapy that was selected by the ATP-TCA. Using the methylthiotetrazolium salt (MTT) assay, Xu and co-workers performed a larger feasibility study in MBC [26]. Seventy-three patients who were treated based on the assay results showed an ORR of 77%. In contrast, 73 patients simultaneously receiving empirical treatment presented with an ORR of 44%. In general, response data achieved in these trials correspond well to our previously reported results of ATP-TCA-directed therapy in ROC. However, long-term results are still pending for both these studies. Major findings of all clinical trials of salvage chemotherapy for ROC or MBC selected by modern nonclonogenic assays are summarized in Table 1.

Conclusions

During the last decade, clinical progress has been made with modern nonclonogenic assays as a successful means to individualize chemotherapy of BC and OC. In particular, the ATP-TCA has been found to provide a robust and reproducible methodology to test nonhematological malignancies, leading to evaluability rates of more than 90% and a high predictive accuracy for clinical response and survival. The ATP-TCA was thus intensively investigated both to screen for new active regimens and to direct chemotherapy in individual patients with both ROC and MBC. Until now, various drug combinations have

Table 1. Summary of prospective clinical trials investigating individualized chemotherapy for recurrent ovarian carcinoma or metastatic breast cancer selected by modern nonclonogenic chemosensitivity assays

Author	Assay	Patients	Results
Kurbacher et al. 1998	ATP-TCA	25 ROC 30 Controls treated empirically	ORR: 64% vs. 37% PFS: 50 weeks vs. 20 weeks OS: 116 weeks vs. 67 weeks
Dottino et al. 2000	EVA	44 ROC	ORR: 50% PFS: 8 months OS: 15 months
Kurbacher et al. 2001	ATP-TCA	59 ROC (31 platinum-sensitive; 28 platinum-refractory)	ORR: 66% PFS:45 weeks OS: 90 weeks No difference between sensitive and refractory patients
Xu et al. 1999	MTT	73 MBC 73 Controls treated empirically	ORR: 77% vs. 44%
Kurbacher et al. 2000	ATP-TCA	17 MBC	ORR: 88%

been identified to display major antineoplastic effects in the ATP-TCA, including TG or NT. These regimens are now successfully used in intensively pretreated patients with ROC and MBC.

Individualized chemotherapy for patients with both ROC and MBC directly selected by pretherapeutic sensitivity testing with the ATP-TCA has resulted in exceptionally high response rates, with many patients achieving CR and a PFS and OS that are clearly superior to those seen with empirical chemotherapy regimens. Results of ATP-TCA-directed chemotherapy in platinum-refractory ROC were particularly promising in that both response rates and long-term results in these patients were comparable to those normally seen exclusively in patients with platinum-sensitive disease.

At present, the ATP-TCA can be regarded the best documented modern nonclonogenic chemosensitivity assay. Nonetheless, findings obtained with other new-generation test systems such as the EVA assay or the MTT assay are generally in good agreement with those that we were able to make with the ATP-TCA. Randomized trials that are currently active in patients with platinum-refractory ROC (see Fig. 4) are now warranted to verify the promising results achieved in the aforementioned studies.

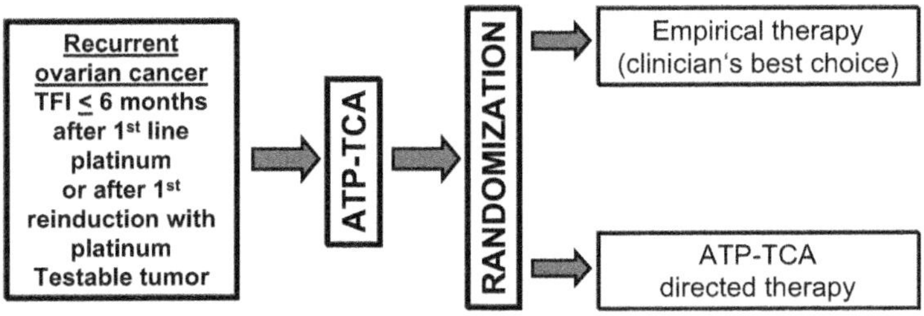

Fig. 4. Design of a currently active multinational phase III study comparing ATP-TCA-directed chemotherapy versus clinician's best choice in patients with platinum-refractory recurrent ovarian carcinoma

References

1. Bellamy WT (1992) Prediction of response to drug therapy of cancer. A review of in vitro assays. Drugs 44:690–708
2. Cree IA, Kurbacher CM (1997) Individualizing chemotherapy for solid tumors – is there any alternative? Anti-Cancer Drugs 8:541–548
3. DeVita VT (1997) Principles of cancer management: chemotherapy. In: DeVita VT, Hellman S, Rosenberg SA (eds) Cancer: principles and practice of oncology, 5th edn. Lippincott-Raven, Philadelphia, pp 333–347
4. Hamburger AW, Salmon SE (1977) Primary bioassay of human tumor stem cells. Science 197:161–163
5. Von Hoff DD (1990) He's not going to talk about in vitro predictive assays again, is he? J Natl Cancer Inst 82:97–101
6. Cortazar R, Johnson BE (1999) Review of the efficacy of individualized chemotherapy selected by in vitro drug sensitivity testing for patients with cancer. J Clin Oncol 17:1625–1631
7. Brown E, Markman M (1996) Tumor chemosensitivity and chemoresistance assays. Cancer 77:1020–1025
8. Andreotti PE, Cree IA, Kurbacher CM et al (1995) Chemosensitivity testing of human tumors using a microplate adenosine triphosphate luminescence assay: clinical correlation for cisplatin resistance of ovarian carcinoma. Cancer Res 55:5276–5282
9. Cree IA, Kurbacher CM, Untch M et al (1996) Correlation of the clinical response to chemotherapy in breast cancer with ex vivo chemosensitivity. Anti-Cancer Drugs 7:630–635
10. Konecny G, Cohns C, Pegram M et al (2000) Correlation of drug response with the ATP tumorchemosensitivity assay in primary FIGO stage III ovarian cancer. Gynecol Oncol 77:258–263
11. Kurbacher CM, Bruckner HW, Cree IA et al (1997) Mitoxantrone combined with paclitaxel as salvage therapy for platinum-refractory ovarian cancer: laboratory study and clinical pilot trial. Clin Cancer Res 3:1527–1533
12. Janát M, Kurbacher CM, Rein D et al (2000) Mitoxantrone plus paclitaxel: a highly active regimen for heavily pretreated ovarian cancer. Proc Am Soc Clin Oncol 19:384a
13. Flaskamp C, Köhler S, Kurbacher C et al (1998) Kombinationschemotherapie des rezidivierten Ovarialkarzinoms mit Mitoxantron und Paclitaxel. Arch Gynecol Obstet 261 (Suppl 1):S17
14. Salimichokami M (2001) Weekly paclitaxel and mitoxantrone: a highly active salvage regimen for recurrent ovarian cancer. Proc Am Soc Clin Oncol 20:214a
15. Neale MH, Myatt N, Cree IA et al (1999) Combination chemotherapy for choroidal melanoma: ex vivo sensitivity to treosulfan with gemcitabine or cytosine arabinoside. Br J Cancer 79:1487–1493
16. Cree IA, Neale MH, Myatt NE et al (1999) Heterogeneity of chemosensitivity of metastatic cutaneous melanoma. Anti-Cancer Drugs 10:437–444

17. Grecu OM, Kurbacher CM, Mallmann P et al (2001) Treosulfan and gemcitabine in heavily pretreated patients with breast and ovarian cancer: laboratory study and clinical pilot trial of the ISCO Clinical Study Group. Proc Am Soc Clin Oncol 20:187b
18. Grecu OM, Kurbacher CM, Stier U et al (2001) Salvage therapy of patients with heavily pretreated breast and ovarian carcinoma: a clinical pilot trial based on results of an ex vivo study. Anti-Cancer Drugs 12 (Suppl 4):A15
19. Nagourney RA, Su YZ, Link J et al (1998) Gemcitabine synergy with cisplatin. Clinical and laboratory correlates. Proc Am Assoc Cancer Res 39:310
20. Nagourney RA, Link JS, Blitzer JB et al (2000) Gemcitabine plus cisplatin repeating doublet therapy in previously treated, relapsed breast cancer patients. J Clin Oncol 18:2245–2249
21. Kurbacher CM, Cree IA, Bruckner HW et al (1998) Use of an ex vivo ATP luminescence assay to direct chemotherapy for recurrent ovarian cancer. Anti-Cancer Drugs 9:51–57
22. Kurbacher CM, Stier U, Janát M et al (2001) ATP-assay-directed chemotherapy for recurrent ovarian cancer: mature results of an ISCO Clinical Study Group Trial. Proc Am Soc Clin Oncol 20:184b
23. Kurbacher CM (2001) ATP chemosensitivity testing in ovarian cancer: early clinical trials. Anti-Cancer Drugs 12 (Suppl 4):A14
24. Dottino R, Evans SS, Segna R et al (2000) EVA-assay directed therapy of advanced ovarian cancer. Proc Amer Soc Clin Oncol 19:387a
25. Kurbacher CM, Janát MM, Brenne U et al. Chemosensitivitätstestung beim Mammakarzinom. In: Untch M, Konecny G, Sittek H, et al (eds) Diagnostik und Therapie des Mammakarzinoms – State of the Art 2000. Zuckschwerdt, Munich
26. Xu JM, Song ST, Zang ZM et al (1999) Predictive chemotherapy of advanced breast cancer directed by MTT assay in vitro. Breast Cancer Res Treat 53:77–85

Chemosensitivity Testing – Present and Future in Japan

Tetsuro Kubota, Yoshihide Otani, Toshiharu Furukawa,
Hirotoshi Hasegawa, Masahiko Watanabe, Masaki Kitajima

T. Kubota (✉)
Department of Surgery, School of Medicine, Keio University,
35 Shinanomachi, Shinjuku-ku, Tokyo 160-8582, Japan
e-mail: tkubota@sc.itc.keio.ac.jp

Abstract

Radical surgery with extended lymph node dissection is the first and only curative treatment of gastrointestinal cancer. Although the combined cancer chemotherapy has achieved 30%~50% response rates, a controversy still remains over the significance of the adjuvant cancer chemotherapy after surgery. To break through this limitation, we have introduced the chemosensitivity test to evaluate the appropriate adjuvant cancer chemotherapy for advanced gastrointestinal cancer. Our plural studies indicated that the chemosensitivity test would be useful in evaluating the appropriated adjuvant chemotherapy by increasing survival in the sensitive group. Recently, the molecular targets have been clarified for the conventionally available antitumor agents, e.g., thymidylate synthetase for 5-fluorouracil, ATP-binding cassette transporters for anthracyclines, glutathione-related detoxification for platins, and topoisomerase I for CPT-11, which will be applied for clinical use in evaluating the appropriate cancer chemotherapy. The chemosensitivity test is approved as "advanced clinical medicine" by the Japanese Ministry of Health, Welfare, and Labor in five institutes at present. Because complete dissection and chemosensitivity test-guided adjuvant chemotherapy will result in a survival benefit for patients with advanced gastrointestinal cancer, this test should be approved as "social insurance" for further wide clinical application.

Introduction

There is no doubt that gastrectomy with extended lymph node resection is the first and only curative treatment of choice for gastric cancer. However, because a portion of patients undergoing curative resection will relapse, adjuvant cancer chemotherapy has been actively studied in gastric cancer. Although many drugs have shown activity on recurrent and advanced gastric

Recent Results in Cancer Research, Vol. 161

Table 1. Efficacy rate of antitumor agents and their combination on advanced gastric carcinoma

	Efficacy rate	Evaluable patients
Mitomycin C	30%	211
Cisplatin	19%	139
5-FU	21%	392
Adriamycin	17%	141
FAM	29%	941
EAP	48%	509
FLEP	41%	318
FP	38%	261

A, adriamycin; E, epirubicin; F, 5-fluorouracil; L, leucovorin; P, cisplatin.

cancer, the efficacy of single-agent chemotherapy was limited, without increased survival benefit [1]. The response rates for single agents were reported to be less than 20% as shown in Table 1, except mitomycin C (MMC), which was tested as a single-agent therapy before the present response criteria were introduced. Cisplatin (DDP) was tested with the present criteria of response and 5-fluorouracil (5-FU) was tested on many patients with gastric cancer, and their response rates (21% and 19%, respectively) are considered to be a standard efficacy of single agents on gastric cancer. Because of the low efficacy of single agents, several combination regimens have been developed, including 5-FU plus adriamycin (ADM) plus MMC (FAM), etoposide plus ADM plus DDP (EAP), 5-FU plus leucovorin (LV) plus epirubicin (EPI) (FLEP), and 5-FU plus DDP (FP). These regimens have achieved 29%–48% response rates (Table 1), although the overall complete response (CR) rate was only 2% [2]. Because long-term survival of patients with disseminated malignancy is only achieved when treatments produce CR of disease, there has been no impact on patient survival in advanced gastric cancer treated with the combined regimen of cancer chemotherapy.

Cumulative Results of Chemosensitivity Tests for Antitumor Agents in Japan

The Japan Research Society for Appropriate Cancer Chemotherapy set out to summarize the present status of chemosensitivity testing for antitumor agents in Japan [3]. Two different questionnaires were sent to 122 and 94 institutes, respectively, and responses were received from 87 (71.3%) and 41 (43%) institutes, respectively. The results showed that chemosensitivity tests were performed in 42 institutes, where a total of 2 in vivo and 10 in vitro assays were performed. Actual cases of chemosensitivity detected by the tests varied from 1 to 368 cases/year/institute, with a median of 15 cases and mean±standard deviation of 48±65 cases. The total number of tested cases increased from 1,747 cases in 1993 to 1,934 cases in 1994 and to 2,147 cases in 1995, resulting in an average of 1,891 cases/year. Assays used included the adenosine triphos-

Table 2. Predictive values for chemosensitivity tests

No. of correlations attempted	S/S	S/R	R/S	R/R	Accuracy
1,101	215	246	45	595	74%

True positives: 47%; true negatives: 93%; sensitivity: 83%; specificity: 71%.

phate inhibition assay, collagen droplet embedded drug response assay, fluorescent dye assay, growth chamber assay, histoculture drug response assay, human tumor clonogenic assay, MTT assay (SDI test), nuclear damage assay, nude mouse model, subrenal capsule assay, and thymidine incorporation assay (scintillation assay). The correlation of in vitro and in vivo results revealed 215 true positive (S/S), 246 false positive (S/R), 45 false negative (R/S), and 595 true negative (R/R) cases, resulting in rates of 47% for true positives and 93% for true negatives and a 74% accuracy (Table 2). We conclude that chemosensitivity testing is widely applied in this country and has a high accurate predictive value for advanced carcinomas. As a result, chemosensitivity testing appears to have advantages for the clinician for several kinds of carcinomas. This requires further clarification with randomized prospective trials consisting of a "chemosensitivity test-guided arm" and an "empirical arm." However, as this trial would be a late phase II study, it should only be conducted after the confirmation of the usefulness of chemosensitivity testing in early phase II studies. For this reason, chemosensitivity testing should be widely used in our country, after approval by social insurance, based on the cumulative results obtained from the 15-year history of chemosensitivity testing.

Drug Sensitivity Test in Evaluating the Appropriate Adjuvant Cancer Chemotherapy

Hermans et al. have reviewed 14 randomized trials and analyzed data from 11 of these trials consisting of 2,096 patients [4]. When they calculated the odds ratios by comparing the adjuvant treatment arm with the observation-only arm, the results suggested that the adjuvant chemotherapy regimens do not improve survival, despite their effectiveness in phase II studies. On the other hand, Nakajima has reviewed single-drug therapy with MMC and combination therapy with 5-FU and methyl-CCNU, MFC, and reported that FAM seems to have potential survival benefit for patients with curative surgery [5]. These contradictory results for adjuvant cancer chemotherapy after gastric surgery might be due to the insufficient power of the conventionally available antitumor agents on gastric cancer. This hypothesis might be also supported by the results that the efficacy rates of these drugs remain at 20% for single-agent and 29%~48% for combined regimens [1, 2].

MTT Assay

To break through this limitation, we have introduced the chemosensitivity test to evaluate the appropriate adjuvant cancer chemotherapy for advanced gastric cancer. The initial study [6] was conducted using 148 patients with gastric cancer admitted to Keio University Hospital between July 1988 and October 1992, who underwent resection of the primary lesion as well as single-cell suspension assay of fresh surgical materials with 3-(4,5-dimethylthiazol-2-yl)-2,5-diphenyltetrazolium bromide (MTT assay), which was reported by Mosmann [7] with some modifications [8–10]. The method of the MTT assay is shown in Fig. 1. Fifty patients with histological stage III or IV gastric cancer were enrolled in this study, among whom 10 received no chemotherapy after surgery whereas 40 received chemotherapy at equivalent dose levels after surgery. The patients given chemotherapy were divided into two groups consisting of a sensitive group treated with at least one agent identified as effective by the assay and a resistant group treated with agents to which the cells were not sensitive in the assay to identify the optimal cut-off inhibition rate (IR) in the MTT assay for evaluation of the appropriate adjuvant cancer chemotherapy after surgery. A cut-off IR of 30% was optimal for differentiating the survival rates between the sensitive and resistant groups. Patients treated with drugs that showed more than 30% IR on their surgical specimens showed a better survival rate than patients treated with drugs that were ineffective in the assay. In addition, there were no statistically significant differences between the survival rates of the resistant group and the surgery-alone group who were treated only with surgery (Fig. 2).

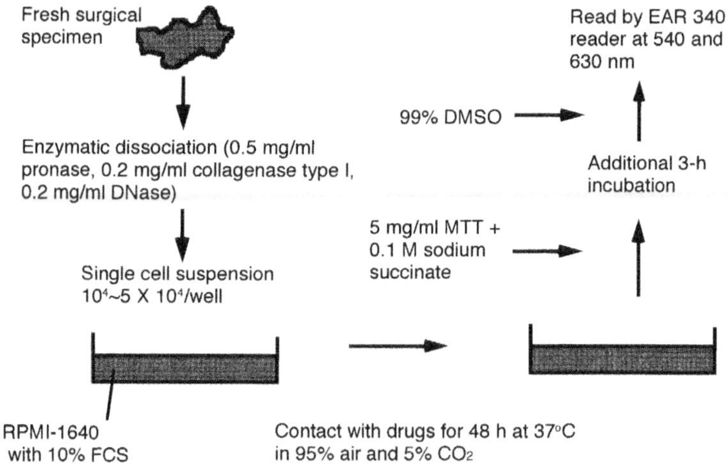

Fig. 1. Method of 3-(4,5-dimethylthiazol-2-yl)-2,5-diphenyltetrazolium bromide (MTT) assay. The MTT assay is a single-cell monolayer culture with MTT end point. For details, see [6–10]

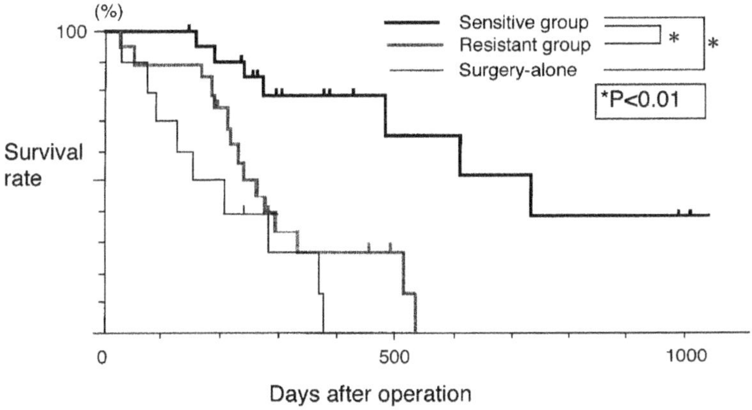

Fig. 2. Survival rates of patients with advanced gastric cancer detected by MTT assay. A sensitive group was treated with at least one drug shown to be effective by MTT assay, a resistant group was given chemotherapy with drugs resistant in the assay, and a surgery-alone group was treated with surgery alone. The sensitive group showed a better outcome than the resistant group and surgery-alone group with a statistically significant difference at P<0.01, whereas there was no significant difference between the resistant group and the surgery-alone group

Histoculture Drug Response Assay

After this retrospective study, we introduced the histoculture drug response assay (HDRA) [11–13] to evaluate the appropriate adjuvant cancer chemotherapy for advanced gastric cancer. The method of the HDRA is shown in Fig. 3. To investigate the potential of the HDRA to contribute to patient survival, 215 patients with gastric cancer from 45 medical centers were tested with the HDRA in a blinded study after resection of the primary lesion (Fig. 4) [14].

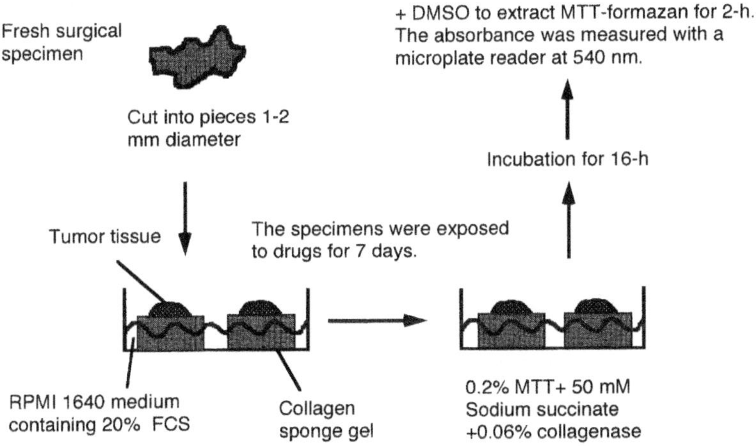

Fig. 3. Method of histoculture drug response assay (HDRA). The HDRA is a histoculture with MTT end point. For details, see [11–14]

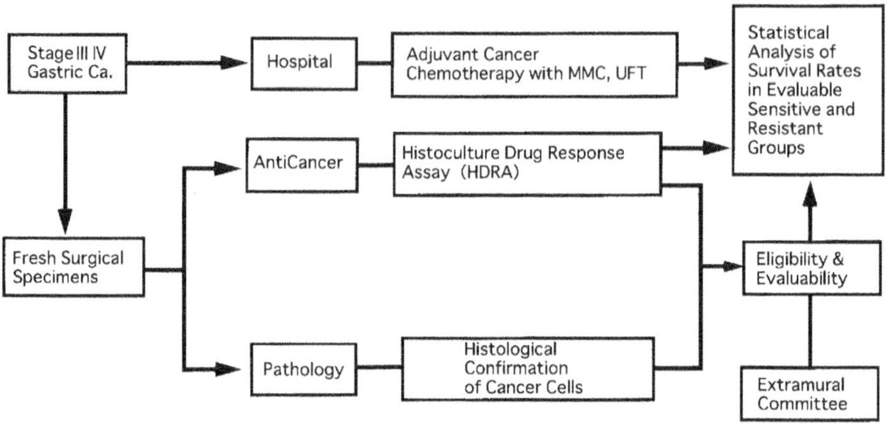

Fig. 4. Study design. To investigate the potential of HDRA to contribute to patient survival, 215 patients with gastric cancer from 45 medical centers were tested with the HDRA in a blinded study after resection of the primary lesion. All of the registered cases were treated with the same protocol without knowledge of the results of the HDRA. One hundred sixty-eight patients received at least 20 mg/m^2 of MMC and a minimum of 30 g UFT, thereby making them eligible for the study. Of these, 128 cases were evaluated by HDRA

All of the registered cases were treated with the same protocol without knowledge of the results of the HDRA. One hundred sixty-eight patients received at least 20 mg/m^2 of MMC and a minimum of 30 g UFT, thereby making them eligible for the study. Of these 128 cases were evaluated by HDRA. The evaluable patient tumors were tested by HDRA with the [^{3}H]thymidine incorporation end point measured by microautoradiography to be drug "sensitive" or "resistant." In the correlation of the overall survival rate of MMC- and UFT-treated stage III and IV gastric cancer patients and the HDRA to MMC, the sensitive group consisted of 25 patients whose tumors were sensitive to MMC in the HDRA. The resistant group consisted of 98 patients whose tumors were resistant to MMC in the HDRA. The overall survival rate of the sensitive group was better than that of the resistant group (P=0.014 by log-rank test and P=0.009 by generalized Wilcoxon test). This difference was also observed in the sensitivity to 5-FU. The sensitive group consisted of 20 patients whose tumors were sensitive to 5-FU in the HDRA. The resistant group consisted of 99 patients whose tumors were resistant to 5-FU. The overall survival rate of the sensitive group was better than that of the resistant group (P=0.031 by log-rank test and P=0.028 by generalized Wilcoxon test). When the sensitivity to MMC and/or 5-FU was assessed, the sensitive group consisted of 38 cases whose tumors were sensitive to MMC or 5-FU in the HDRA and the resistant group consisted of 89 patients whose tumors were resistant to MMC and 5-FU in the HDRA. The overall survival rate of the sensitive group was better than that of the resistant group (P=0.001 by log-rank test and P=0.0007 by generalized Wilcoxon test). Multivariate analysis was performed according to Cox's proportional hazard model. Risk ratios are shown for prolonged overall sur-

Table 3. Multivariate analysis of risk factors of gastric cancer patients for prolonged overall survival

Variable	Hazard ratio[a]	*P*
Sensitive or resistant to MMC in the HDRA		
Sensitive to MMC	0.180[b]	0.0218[c]
Pathological stage	2.801	0.0275[c]
T category	1.041	0.9247
N category	1.166	0.4550
Differentiation	3.118	0.0060[c]
Type of operation	0.715	0.3500
Curability of surgery	0.714	0.5023
Sensitive or resistant to 5-FU in the HDRA		
Sensitive to 5-FU	0.098	0.0266[c]
Pathological stage	2.822	0.0234[c]
T category	1.560	0.2369
N category	1.083	0.6962
Differentiation	1.901	0.1316
Type of operation	0.561	0.1121
Curability of surgery	0.571	0.2704
Sensitive to MMC or 5-FU or resistant to MMC and 5-FU		
Sensitive to MMC or 5-FU	0.137	0.0014[c]
Pathological stage	3.441	0.0078[c]
T category	1.133	0.7513
N category	1.152	0.4593
Differentiation	2.027	0.0843
Type of operation	0.754	0.4309
Curability of surgery	0.598	0.2903

[a]Risk ratios for overall survival rate.
[b]Risk ratios were calculated according to Cox's proportional hazard model using SAS Release 6.07 (Sun OS 4.1.1) software.
[c]$P<0.05$.

vival in Table 3 for each variable of the gastric cancer patients with tumors sensitive or resistant to MMC and/or 5-FU in the HDRA. The analysis demonstrated that the sensitivity to MMC and/or 5-FU in the HDRA is an independent risk factor for overall survival in each category. In this blinded study, the overall survival rates of the HDRA-sensitive group were found to be significantly higher than those of the HDRA-resistant group tested. The results demonstrated that the HDRA response correlates to patient survival, which suggests the potential of the HDRA to contribute to patient survival in gastric cancer.

Molecular Biological Chemosensitivity Test of 5-Fluorouracil

Patients and Methods

5-FU is widely used in the treatment of gastrointestinal carcinomas and is considered to be one of the most effective drugs against gastric cancer. Because the efficacy rate of 5-FU treatment alone for gastric cancer is only 10%–20% [15], one of the most frequently used protocols for gastric cancer is biomodulated 5-FU chemotherapy with folinic acid (leucovorin) and/or cisplatin [1]. However, the clinical effects of these regimens are still unsatisfactory with regard to long-term survival. One of the main modes of action of 5-FU is thought to be through its active metabolite, FdUMP. FdUMP suppresses thymidylate synthetase (TS; EC 2.1.1.45) by forming covalent ternary complexes with 5,10-methylenetetrahydrofolate, which subsequently inhibits DNA synthesis [16]. Several reports have indicated that tumoral TS expression is related to the response to 5-FU-based chemotherapy and patient survival in gastric and colorectal cancers [17, 18], although increased expression of TS is not always recognized as a determining factor for 5-FU resistance [19, 20]. We investigated the correlation between tumor sensitivity to 5-FU and enzymatic activities of TS and dihydropyrimidine dehydrogenase (DPD) in human gastric cancer specimens.

Forty-one patients with advanced gastric cancer were enrolled in this study at Keio University Hospital between May 1997 and July 1998 after giving their informed consent. Biopsy specimens of gastric cancer for the assay of TS mRNA and DPD mRNA by the RT-PCR method were obtained preoperatively through gastrofiberscopy. A total of five biopsy specimens of about 2–3 mm in size were collected and stored at -80°C with liquid nitrogen until use. After surgery, resected tumor tissues were divided into two pieces; one piece was brought to the laboratory as soon as possible for the MTT assay. The other piece of tumor tissue was immersed in liquid nitrogen and stored at -80°C until assayed for TS and DPD activities and mRNA levels. The TS binding activity to FdUMP was assessed according to the method of Spears et al. [21]. The DPD enzymatic assay was based on the method reported by Naguib et al. [22]. Semi-quantitative RT-PCR was performed using previously described methods [23]. The comparison of 5-FU sensitivity between groups of patients with high and low TS and DPD levels was performed with the Mann-Whitney test. The criterion of statistical significance was $P<0.05$.

Results and Discussion

A correlation between tumoral DPD activity in resected specimens and sensitivity to 5-FU was observed, with a correlation coefficient of 0.48, which was statistically significant ($P=0.0015$) (Fig. 5A). High DPD activity resulted in low sensitivity to 5-FU, whereas low DPD activity was associated with high sensitivity to 5-FU. This tendency was also observed between tumoral DPD

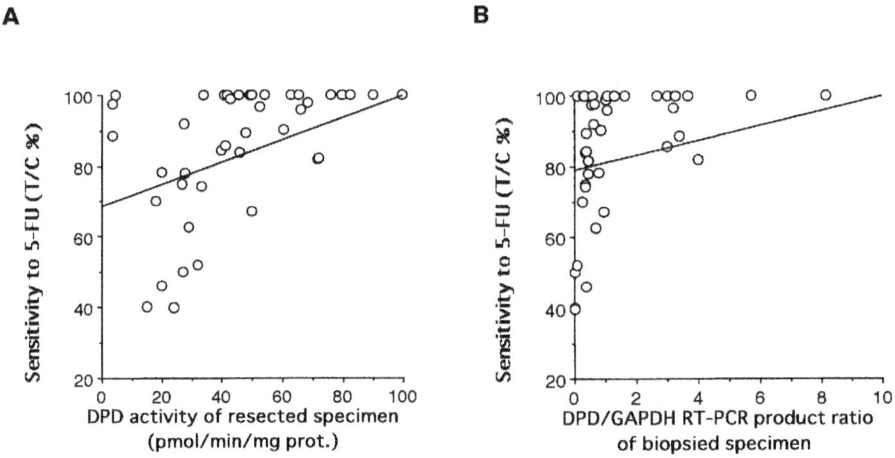

Fig. 5. Correlation between tumoral DPD levels and sensitivity to 5-fluorouracil. Plots show the correlation between DPD activity in resected specimens and sensitivity to 5-FU (**A**) and DPD:GAPDH RT-PCR product ratios in biopsied specimens and sensitivity to 5-FU (**B**) in gastric cancer patients. Sensitivity to 5-FU was measured by the MTT assay, and T/C values were calculated using the formula: A/B×100, where A and B represent the mean absorbance of the treated and control wells, respectively. **A** $y=0.37x+68.70$, $r=0.48$, $P=0.0015$. **B** $y=4.36x+79.00$, $r=0.41$, $P=0.0078$

mRNA levels in biopsy specimens and sensitivity to 5-FU, with a correlation coefficient of 0.41 ($P=0.0078$) (Fig. 5B). To estimate a possible cut-off point of DPD activity to determine resistance or sensitivity to 5-FU in gastric cancer patients, patients were categorized as having either high (≥50 pmol/min/mg protein) or low (<50 pmol/min/mg protein) DPD activity or high (≥2) or low (<2) DPD mRNA levels in biopsied specimens. The high-DPD activity group exhibited a significantly lower sensitivity to 5-FU than the low-DPD activity group (Fig. 6A). Likewise, low sensitivity to 5-FU was associated with the high-DPD mRNA group and high sensitivity to 5-FU with the low-DPD mRNA group (Fig. 6B).

The present study has shown a correlation of tumoral DPD activity and mRNA levels with 5-FU sensitivity in tumor specimens obtained from preoperative biopsy and surgical resection from 41 gastric cancer patients. High DPD activity and mRNA levels were associated with tumors with low 5-FU sensitivity, and low DPD activity was associated with high 5-FU sensitivity. This finding is consistent with our previous experimental study using seven human tumor xenografts in nude mice [23], in which both tumoral DPD activity and mRNA levels significantly correlated with 5-FU sensitivity. These findings suggested that in patients with high basal DPD levels in tumors, 5-FU is quickly catabolized to 2-fluoro-β-alanine, resulting in the suppression of the anabolic pathway of 5-FU phosphorylation and the reduction of 5-FU sensitivity. Because 5-FU-sensitive patients have a favorable outcome when treated with fluoropyrimidines as shown in our previous study [6, 14], tumoral DPD levels might influence the survival of patients treated with fluoropyrimidines.

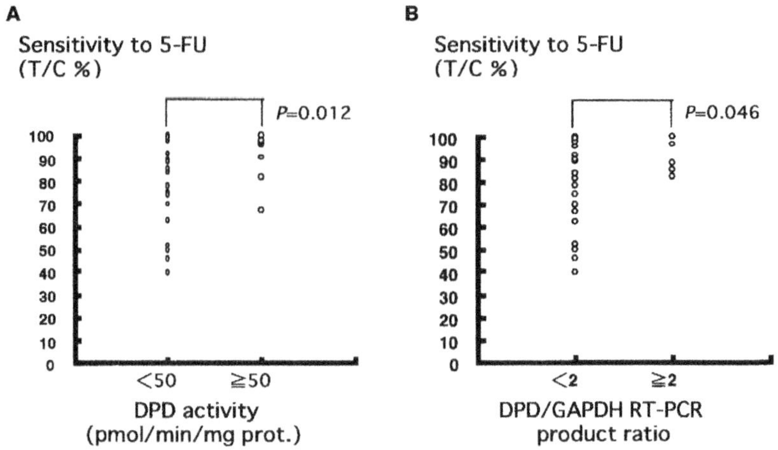

Fig. 6. Sensitivity to 5-fluorouracil according to DPD activity and DPD mRNA. Patients were categorized into a high-DPD activity group of resected specimens (≥50 pmol/min/mg protein) and a low-DPD activity group (<50 pmol/min/mg protein) (**A**) or a high-DPD mRNA group (≥2) and a low-DPD mRNA group (<2) in biopsied specimens (**B**). These cutoff levels successfully distinguished different sensitivities to 5-FU

Further investigation is required into the role of TS in 5-FU sensitivity and the prognosis of patients with advanced carcinoma.

Conclusion

The total kill assay originated from cellular biology is now being applied in clinical practice, and the approval as social insurance is coming up in Japan. The molecular biological technique may be useful in further investigating the chemosensitivity test using small samples by elucidating the known and unknown resistance-related genes.

References

1. Schipper DL, Wagener DJ (1996) Chemotherapy of gastric cancer. Anticancer Drugs 7:137–149
2. Macdonald JS, Gohmann JJ (1988) Chemotherapy of advanced gastric cancer: present status, future prospects. Semin Oncol 15:(Suppl 4) 42–49
3. Kondo T, Kubota T, Tanimura T, Yamaue H, Akiyama S, Maehara Y, Tanigawa T, Kitajima M, Takagi H, Japan Research Society for Appropriate Cancer Chemotherapy (2000) Cumulative results of chemosensitivity tests for antitumor agents in Japan. Anticancer Res 20:2389–2392
4. Hermans J, Bonenkamp JJ, Boon MC, Bunt AMG, Ohyama S, Sasako M, Van de Velde CJH (1993) Adjuvant therapy after curative resection for gastric cancer: meta-analysis of randomized trials. J Clin Oncol 11:1441–1447
5. Nakajima T (1995) Review of adjuvant chemotherapy for gastric cancer. World J Surg 19:570–574

6. Saikawa Y, Kubota T, Furukawa T, Suto A, Watanabe M, Kumai K, Ishibiki K, Kitajima M (1994) Single-cell suspension assay with an MTT end point is useful for evaluating the optimal adjuvant chemotherapy for advanced gastric cancer. Jpn J Cancer Res 85:762–765
7. Mosmann T (1983) Rapid colorimetric assay for cellular growth and survival: application to proliferation and cytotoxicity assays. J Immunol Methods 65:55–63
8. Shimoyama Y, Kubota T, Watanabe M, Ishibiki K, Abe O (1989) Predictability of in vivo chemosensitivity by in vitro MTT assay with reference to clonogenic assay. J Surg Oncol 41:12–18
9. Suto A, Kubota T, Shimoyama Y, Ishibiki K, Abe O (1989) MTT assay with reference to the clinical effect of chemotherapy. J Surg Oncol 42:28–32
10. Furukawa T, Kubota T, Suto A, Takahara T, Yamaguchi H, Takeuchi T, Kase S, Kodaira S, Ishibiki K, Kitajima M (1991) Clinical usefulness of chemosensitivity testing using the MTT assay. J Surg Oncol 48:188–193
11. Furukawa T, Kubota T, Watanabe M, Takahara T, Yamaguchi H, Takeuchi T, Kase S, Kodaira S, Ishibiki K, Kitajima M, Hoffman RM (1992) High in vitro-in vivo correlation of drug response using sponge-gel-supported three-dimensional histoculture and the MTT end point. Int J Cancer 51:489–498
12. Furukawa T, Kubota T, Watanabe M, Kase S, Takahara T, Yamaguchi H, Takeuchi T, Teramoto T, Ishibiki K, Kitajima M, Hoffman RM (1992) Chemosensitivity testing of clinical gastrointestinal cancers using histoculture and MTT endpoint. Anticancer Res 12:1377–1382
13. Furukawa T, Kubota T, Hoffman RM (1995) Clinical applications of the histoculture drug response assay. Clin Cancer Res 1:305–311
14. Kubota T, Sasano N, Abe O, Nakao I, Kawamura E, Saito T, Endo M, Kimura K, Demura H, Sasano H, Nagura H, Ogawa N, Hoffman RM, Chemosensitivity Group for HDRA (1995) Potential of the histoculture drug response assay to contribute to cancer patient survival. Clin Cancer Res 1:1537–1543
15. Macdonald JS, Gohmann JJ (1988) Chemotherapy of advanced gastric cancer: present status, future prospects. Semin Oncol 15 (Suppl. 4):42–49
16. Langenbach RJ, Danenberg PV and Heidelberger C (1972) Thymidylate synthetase: mechanism of inhibition by 5-fluoro-2'-deoxyuridylate. Biochem Biophys Res Commun 48:1565–1571
17. Peters GJ, van der Wilt CL, van Groeningen CJ, Smid K, Meijer S, Pinedo HM (1994) Thymidylate synthase inhibition after administration of fluorouracil with or without leucovorin in colon cancer patients: implications for treatment with fluorouracil. J Clin Oncol 12:2035–2042
18. Johnston PG, Fisher ER, Rockette H. Fisher B, Wolmark N, Drake JC, Chabner BA, Allegra CJ (1994) The role of thymidylate synthase expression in prognosis and outcome of adjuvant chemotherapy in patients with rectal cancer. J Clin Oncol 12:2640–2647
19. Peters GJ, Laurensse E, Leyva A, Lankelma J, Pinedo HM (1986) Sensitivity of human, murine, and rat cells to 5-fluorouracil and 5'-deoxy-5-fluorouridine in relation to drug-metabolizing enzymes. Cancer Res 46:20–28
20. Aschele C, Sobrero A, Faderan MA, Bertino JR (1992) Novel mechanism(s) of resistance to 5-fluorouracil in human colon cancer (HCT-8) sublines following exposure to two different clinically relevant dose schedule. Cancer Res 52:1855–1864
21. Spears CP, Shahinian AH, Moran RG, Heidelberger, Corbett TH (1982) In vivo kinetics of thymidylate synthetase inhibition in 5-fluorouracil-sensitive and -resistant murine colon adenocarcinomas. Cancer Res 42:450–456
22. Naguib FNM, el Kouni MH, Cha S (1985) Enzymes of uracil catabolism in normal and neoplastic human tissues. Cancer Res 45:5405–5412
23. Ishikawa Y, Kubota T, Otani Y, Watanabe M, Teramoto T, Kumai, K, Kitajima M, Takechi T, Okabe H, Fukushima M (1999) Dihydropyrimidine dehydrogenase activity and messenger RNA level may be related to the antitumor effect of 5-fluorouracil on human tumor xenografts in nude mice. Clin Cancer Res 5:883–889

Subject Index

GPSR Compliance

The European Union's (EU) General Product Safety Regulation (GPSR) is a set of rules that requires consumer products to be safe and our obligations to ensure this.

If you have any concerns about our products, you can contact us on ProductSafety@springernature.com

In case Publisher is established outside the EU, the EU authorized representative is:

Springer Nature Customer Service Center GmbH
Europaplatz 3
69115 Heidelberg, Germany

Batch number: 10755466

Printed by Printforce, the Netherlands